Development, Function
and Evolution of Teeth

edited by
A.H.Melcher
*Faculty of Dentistry, University of Toronto
Canada*

and W.H.Bowen
*Department of Dental Science, Royal College of
Surgeons of England, London, England*

Development, Function and Evolution of Teeth

Edited by

P. M. BUTLER
Department of Zoology,
Royal Holloway College

K. A. JOYSEY
University Museum of
Zoology, Cambridge

1978

ACADEMIC PRESS
LONDON . NEW YORK . SAN FRANCISCO

A Subsidiary of Harcourt Brace Jovanovich, Publishers

ACADEMIC PRESS INC. (LONDON) LTD.
24/28 Oval Road,
London NW1

United States Edition published by
ACADEMIC PRESS INC.
111 Fifth Avenue
New York, New York 10003

Library of Congress Catalog Card Number: 77 071811
ISBN: 0 12 148050 X

PRINTED IN GREAT BRITAIN BY
UNWIN BROTHERS LIMITED,
THE GRESHAM PRESS,
OLD WOKING SURREY

Contributors

A. C. BERRY, *Paediatric Research Unit, The Prince Philip Research Laboratories, Guy's Tower, London Bridge, London SE1 9RT.*

A. BOYDE, *Department of Anatomy and Embryology, University College London, Gower Street, London WC1E 6BT.*

P. M. BUTLER, *Department of Zoology, Royal Holloway College, Alderhurst, Bakeham Lane, Englefield Green, Surrey TW20 9TY.*

A. W. CROMPTON, *Museum of Comparative Zoology, Harvard University, Cambridge, Massachusetts 02138, U.S.A.*

A. A. DAHLBERG, *Department of Anthropology, University of Chicago, 1126 East 59th Street, Chicago, Illinois 60637, U.S.A.*

T. A. FINDLAY, *Department of Anatomy, University College, Cardiff, P.O. Box 78, Cardiff CF1 1XL.*

K. L. FLYNN-MILLER, *Department of Oral Biology, State University of New York at Buffalo, 4510 Main Street Buffalo, New York 14226, U.S.A.*

S. GLASSTONE HUGHES, *34, Porson Road, Cambridge CB2 2EU.*

K. HANIHARA, *Department of Anthropology, Faculty of Science, University of Tokyo, Hongo Bunkyo-ku, Tokyo, Japan.*

E. N. HEY, *Department of Child Health, The University, Newcastle upon Tyne NE1 7RU.*

K. HIIEMAE, *Department of Anatomy, Guy's Hospital Medical School, London Bridge, London SE1 9RT.*

R. F. KAY, *Department of Anatomy, Duke University Medical Center, Durham, North Carolina, U.S.A.*

Z. KIELAN-JAWOROWSKA, *Zaklad Paleobiologii, Polska Akademia Nauk, Al. Zwirki Wigury 93, 02–089 Warszawa, Poland.*

P. KIRVESKARI, *Institute of Dentistry, University of Turku, 20520 Turku, 52, Finland.*

E. J. KOLLAR, *Department of Oral Biology, Health Center, University of Connecticut, Farmington, Connecticut 06032, U.S.A.*

C. A. W. KORENHOF, *Tandheelkundig instituut, Rijksuniversiteit Utrecht, Sorbonnelaan 16, Utrecht 2506, The Netherlands.*

C. L. B. LAVELLE, *Department of Oral Biology, University of Manitoba, Faculty of Dentistry, 780 Bannatyne Avenue, Winnipeg, Manitoba, Canada, R3E 0W3.*

A. V. LOMBARDI, *2602,Wilmington Road, New Castle, Pennsylvania 16105, U.S.A.*

D. A. LUKE, *Department of Oral Anatomy, The Dental School, Northumberland Road, Newcastle upon Tyne NE1 8TA.*

D. A. LUNT, *Department of Oral Biology, Glasgow Dental Hospital and School, 378, Sauchiehall Street, Glasgow G2 3JZ.*

D. F. MAYHEW, *University Museum of Zoology, Downing Street, Cambridge CB2 3EJ.*

A. E. W. MILES, *Department of Anatomy, London Hospital Medical College, Turner Street, London E.1.*

W. A. MILLER, *Department of Oral Biology, State University of New York at Buffalo, 4510 Main Street Buffalo, New York 14226, U.S.A.*

J. R. E. MILLS, *Institute of Dental Surgery, Eastman Dental Hospital, Grays Inn Road, London WC1X 8LD.*

D. H. MORRIS, *Department of Anthropology, Arizona State University, Tempe, Arizona 85281, U.S.A.*

P. A. MORRIS, *Department of Zoology, Royal Holloway College, Alderhurst, Bakeham Lane, Englefield Green, Surrey TW20 9TY.*

M. L. MOSS, *Department of Anatomy, Columbia University, 630 West 168th Street, New York, N.Y. 10032, U.S.A.*

L. MOSS-SALENTIJN, *Department of Anatomy, Columbia University, 630 West 168th Street, New York N.Y. 10032, U.S.A.*

A. ORNOY, *The Hebrew University, Department of Anatomy, Hadassah Medical School, P.O. Box 1172, Jerusalem, Israel.*

J. W. OSBORN, *Department of Anatomy, Guy's Hospital Medical School, London Bridge, London SE1 9RT.*

J. M. RENSBERGER, *Department of Geological Sciences, University of Washington, Seattle, Washington 98195, U.S.A.*

D. SELIGSOHN, *Department of Anthropology, Hunter College, City University of New York, 695 Park Avenue, New York, N.Y. 10021, U.S.A.*

R. P. SHELLIS, *MRC Dental Unit, The Dental School, Lower Maudlin Street, Bristol BS1 2LY.*

P. SMITH, *The Hebrew University, Hadassah School of Dental Medicine, P.O. Box 1172, Jerusalem, Israel.*

J. A. SOFAER, *The School of Dental Surgery, Chambers Street, Ebinburgh, EH1 1JA.*

W. A. SOSKOLNE, *The Hebrew University, Department of Oral Pathology, Hadassah School of Dental Medicine, P.O. Box 1172, Jerusalem, Israel.*

M. V. STACK, *MRC Dental Unit, The Dental School, Lower Maudlin Street, Bristol, BS1 2LY.*

F. L. D. STEEL, *Department of Anatomy, University College Cardiff, P.O. Box 78, Cardiff CF1 1XL.*

F. S. SZALAY, *Department of Anthropology, Hunter College, City University of New York, 695 Park Avenue, New York, N.Y. 10021, U.S.A.*

W. D. TURNBULL, *Department of Geology, Field Museum of Natural History, Roosevelt Road at Lake Shore Drive, Chicago, Illinois 60605, U.S.A.*

G. H. R. VON KOENIGSWALD, *Forschunginstitut Senckenberg, 6 Frankfurt-M 1, Senckenberganlage 25.*

Preface

Teeth have long been intensively studied by comparative anatomists and palaeontologists. Because of the great variety of form that they display, especially among the mammals, they have great value in the identification of species and the investigation of phyletic relationships. Teeth are much used in anthropological studies of variability and microevolution. Their value is enhanced by the fact that, because of their durability and hardness, teeth provide the greater part of the fossil material on which the past history of the mammals, including man, has to be based.

At first primarily descriptive, interest in tooth form has increasingly become centred on its interpretation in terms of function and development. Palaeontologists are concerned to understand the adaptive aspects of evolutionary changes, while geneticists and embryologists are attempting to analyse dental forms in causal-developmental terms. Developmental and functional studies supplement each other, for evolution proceeds by the selection of gene systems that result in functionally viable dentitions.

The papers presented in this volume are based on contributions to an International Symposium on Dental Morphology held in Cambridge in September 1974. It was the fourth of a series of meetings, bringing together workers in a wide range of disciplines: dental anatomists, anthropologists, embryologists, geneticists, palaeontologists and zoologists. The proceedings of two previous symposia have been published, one as a supplement to the *Journal of Dental Research*, Vol. 46 (1967) and one as a book, *Dental Morphology and Evolution*, edited by A. A. Dahlberg, University of Chicago Press (1971).

In producing the present volume the contributions have been arranged in a sequence entirely different from the order of presentation at the Symposium itself. We are grateful to the authors for their patience during the necessary revision of their manuscripts and we are glad that they have been able to bring their contributions up to date while in press (1977). We hope that the rearrangement has woven the contributions together to form a coherent volume which reflects the present state of knowledge in this field.

Compared with many other organs, teeth are simple structures. Their shapes are basically surfaces of contact between the oral epidermis and mesenchyme that has migrated out of the neural crest. The two tissues form respectively the enamel organs and their associated papillae. Odontoblasts

vii

deposit dentine internally and ameloblasts deposit enamel externally to a surface which has previously folded to form the cusps, valleys and other features of crown topography. Much remains to be understood about epithelial–mesenchymal interactions during early stages of tooth development. Three problems can be distinguished. There is first the question of what determines the initiation of a tooth in a given position. This is discussed by J. W. Osborn, who believes that spacing is a crucial factor, the developing tooth germ inhibiting the formation of others in its immediate neighbourhood. He ascribes the order of appearance of tooth germs to growth of dentigerous mesenchyme, but there is at present only equivocal evidence that mesenchyme, rather than epithelium, is the primary initiator.

Then there is the problem of the folding of the epithelium–mesenchyme contact surface to form the cusp pattern. E. J. Kollar and co-workers have published experimental evidence that papillae, once formed, have the capacity to organize epithelium into enamel organs, and in his contribution to this volume he shows that collagen plays an essential part in the process. He also states that papilla cells retain their organizing power even after culture. W. A. Miller, in a study of the teeth of some mutants of the mouse, ascribes their departure from the normal patterns to a reduction in the quantity of mesenchyme taking part, perhaps due to its slower rate of migration from the neural crest.

A third aspect of tooth development is the histological differentiation of odontoblasts and ameloblasts. Here again, interactions between papilla and enamel organ are operative: odontoblasts develop only when in contact with ameloblasts, and enamel is formed only after the appearance of the adjacent dentine. L. Moss-Salentijn, in a discussion of the vestigial teeth that occur in a number of mammals, ascribes some of their characteristics to a breakdown of epithelial–mesenchymal interactions. In the teeth of teleost fish, described by R. P. Shellis, the inner dental epithelium in contact with the papilla resembles the mammalian ameloblast layer in many of its properties, although instead of producing enamel it takes part in the formation of enameloid internally to the basement membrane. It would be interesting to know more about tissue interactions during tooth formation in lower vertebrates. Among mammals, enamel structure is frequently complex, as is illustrated by A. Boyde's scanning electron microscope study of the incisor enamel of rodents, in which decussation of the prisms implies a relative movement of rows of ameloblasts during enamel secretion.

It is well known that human races differ in the frequency with which variations of tooth pattern occur, and P. Kirveskari compares the dentition of a Lapp population with those of Caucasoids and Mongoloids from this standpoint. D. H. Morris, S. Glasstone Hughes and A. A. Dahlberg describe an unusual premolar pattern which is confined to a limited number of Amerindian populations speaking related languages, and which they believe represents a mutation in the ancestral stock. The use of such details of tooth pattern in taxonomic and evolutionary studies is strongly indicative of a large genetic component in their determination, but direct evidence of this is limited. C. Berry shows that minor variants of human tooth patterns have a higher concordance among monozygous than among dizygous twins, though even among monozygous pairs 100% concordance is rare.

How genes influence individual teeth is still largely unsolved: we are confronted with the problem of the relation of genotype to phenotype, presented in a particularly intriguing way by the seemingly simple morphology of the tooth. The effects of mutant genes in the mouse, described by W. A. Miller and by K. L. Flynn–Miller and W. A. Miller, are widely dispersed through the dentition, and in the latter paper a humoral factor is postulated. Likewise the sex differences analysed in human teeth by K. Hanihara show the influence of regional factors affecting several teeth in both jaws. M. L. Moss, in a paper on sexual dimorphism in the human canine, argues that enamel thickness plays an important part in the dimensions of this tooth, and reviews the evidence for environmental influence on enamel development. A direct study of an environmental factor, rubella infection of the mother, is presented by P. Smith, W. A. Soskolne and A. Ornoy. Apart from direct local effects of the virus there is a reduction of growth rate due to inhibition of mitosis.

C. A. W. Korenhof reports on human lower molars from medieval Java, in which, owing to solution of the dentine subsequent to burial, it is possible to compare the outer and inner surfaces of the enamel. The inner surface shows a number of features that occur in lower primates, indicating that some of the characteristics of the human cusp pattern are due to enamel development.

Teeth are meristic organs, like vertebrae, arranged in series with regional differentiation. The genotype produces, not a single pattern but a sequence of patterns, each tooth differing from its neighbour. Again, we can only guess at the nature of the mechanisms at work. How does a given genetic constitution express itself differently in the histologically similar tooth germs that develop in different parts of the jaw? Speculation on this problem has been associated with the "Field Theory", which is critically discussed by J. W. Osborn. In its place he puts forward his Clone Theory. One of the consequences of this is a reassessment of the homologies of teeth in the neighbourhood of the canine in a number of mammals, a departure from orthodoxy with which palaeontologists may not agree. A different approach to regional organization is that of A. V. Lombardi, who by a multifactorial analysis of length and width measurements of the teeth from a Mexican population, shows that most factors are associated with regional tooth groups, but some, notably tooth width, are of more general application. His first two factors agree with those obtained by K. Hanihara. It is interesting that most factors apply to corresponding upper and lower teeth together. J. A. Sofaer's study of developmental stability in the vertebral column is of interest to students of the dentition, because its regions are longer and can be analysed in more detail. He finds that in general the vertebrae at the extremities of each region are the most stable, a result that conflicts with findings on the dentition, where the terminal teeth are the most variable.

The increasing use of tooth dimensions in statistical analysis was very apparent in the contributions to the symposium. C. L. Lavelle gives a timely critical review of the problems involved, in which he discusses not only the statistical techniques themselves, but also the difficulties involved in obtaining meaningful raw data.

Whatever the underlying genetic and ontogenetic processes may be, their result is the production of functional dentitions on which natural selection can operate. Mammalian teeth have a particular value for evolutionary studies because they carry on their surfaces direct evidence of their functioning, in the form of wear facets. These show not only how opposing teeth occlude but their relative movement during chewing. Structure can therefore be directly related to function even in fossils, and the adaptive significance of evolutionary changes can be realistically discussed. Thus A. W. Crompton and Z. Kielan-Jaworowska give a detailed description of the molar occlusal relations in Cretaceous mammals with tribosphenic molars, representative of a stage through which all later marsupials and placentals have passed.

That teeth are indeed adaptive is shown by D. Seligsohn and F. S. Szalay, who compare in detail the dentitions of two genera of lemurs with different diets. Further evidence for adaptation of the dentition is provided by R. F. Kay, who describes the molar function of Old World monkeys, and by a factorial analysis shows that there are dental differences between predominantly fruit-eating and predominantly leaf-eating species. However, though there are some allometric changes with size, the molars do not increase proportionately to food requirements, and other factors, such as the rate of feeding or the type of food eaten, must compensate for this. Another aspect of adaptation is described by J. R. E. Mills, who relates changes in human molar patterns to shortening of the jaws. He reminds us that teeth cannot be considered in isolation, for they are parts of a functional system that includes the jaws and their muscles.

The evolution of the human dentition may prove to be a more complex process than has sometimes been supposed. G. H. R. von Koenigswald briefly describes a palate from Java, dating $1 \cdot 9 \pm 0 \cdot 4$ million years, which possesses some very primitive (anthropoid) features that seemingly preclude its derivation from the African australopithecines.

K. M. Hiiemae provides a review of current knowledge, based on the observation of living mammals, of the masticatory movements and the muscle contractions that they involve. A common pattern is becoming discernible in a wide variety of mammals, one which must have been established early in the evolution of the class. The interaction between evolutionary modifications of this pattern and changes in the form of the teeth opens up a fascinating field for further study.

W. D. Turnbull, in a discussion of the marsupial sabre-tooth, *Thylacosmilus*, provides evidence that the posterior edge of the large upper canine was kept sharp by honing against the lower canine. This process of tooth-sharpening, or thegosis, has been held to account for a number of the molar facets. However, J. M. Rensberger, in a scanning electron microscope study of wear facets on rodent molars, failed to find evidence for thegosis there. He notes that supposed thegosis facets are usually scored by striations, which must be due to something harder than enamel, presumably grit in the food. In *Thylacosmilus*, exposed dentine on the upper canine is worn against enamel on the lower canine, but one wonders whether in some cases differences of enamel hardness might be used in a honing process. Rensberger finds considerable differences in the mode of wear in different rodents and even in different facets of a single tooth, and it would be interesting to know whether there are corresponding differences of enamel structure. What, for example, is the functional significance of the features of incisor enamel described by Boyde?

Although the great majority of those who describe molar teeth use the Osbornian names for the principal cusps, there is unfortunately no universally accepted nomenclature for many of the details of the crown. Even directional terms are not agreed: among the papers presented here, buccal–lingual, lateral–medial and external–internal are all used by different authors for the transverse axis, and the wear facets are numbered differently by Crompton and Kielan-Jaworowska on the one hand and by Mills on the other. P. M. Butler, while supporting the use of the Osbornian system of cusp nomenclature against that proposed by Vandebroek, makes a plea for parsimony in the introduction of additional technical terms.

One session of the symposium was devoted to the use of teeth for the estimation of individual age, and the papers are published in the final section of this book. A. E. W. Miles reviews the subject as it concerns man. After about 20 years of age, when development of the dentition is completed, age estimates have to be based on molar wear or on such features as the translucency of root dentine. Molar wear depends on the abrasiveness of food, and the gradient of wear from the first molar to the third varies from one population to another. D. A. Lunt discusses this problem in connection with her study of medieval Danish skulls. P. Morris reviews age estimation by teeth in wild mammals. Here, besides eruption and wear, use is made of incremental lines in the dentine and cementum. Although a high level of accuracy is often unattainable, the results may provide a useful insight into the age-structure of wild populations, and even, in favourable cases, of fossil populations. An example of the latter is D. F. Mayhew's study of a 3000–year–old population of beavers from the Cambridgeshire fen region, in which incremental layers in the cementum were used to age individuals. A short contribution by F. L. D. Steel and J. A. Findlay, on an aspect of the use of tetracyclines as a fluorescent marker, reminds us that growth of the jaw is another aspect of ageing.

Finally, the problem of ageing human foetuses on the basis of their tooth germs is discussed by D. A. Luke, M. V. Stack and E. N. Hey. They compare two methods, one based on the stages of cusp development of the deciduous molars, and the other on weights of calcified deciduous incisor crowns.

There are perhaps no organs that can be studied in so many different aspects as the teeth. Besides embryology, genetics and studies of variation in living populations, there is a rich palaeontological record. Function can be investigated in fossils by the direct evidence of wear, interpreted by the observation of living animals. By such studies the relations of genotype to phenotype, of form to function, are brought vividly into focus. The future of teeth as research media for the investigation of developmental and evolutionary problems seems bright.

In conclusion, on behalf of those who were privileged to attend the Symposium in Cambridge, we wish to thank the Royal Society and the British Council for their generous financial support which made the meeting possible. We would also like to thank the staff of Academic Press for their tremendous help during the process of publication. We are glad that the publication of this volume has now enabled us to make the results of an important meeting available to a wider audience.

September, 1977   P. M. BUTLER
                                                        K. A. JOYSEY

Contents

CONTENTS

CONTENTS

This volume is dedicated to Dr. Albert A. Dahlberg,
whose initiative has been responsible for the
International Symposia on Dental Morphology.

1. The Role of Collagen during Tooth Morphogenesis: Some Genetic Implications

EDWARD J. KOLLAR

Department of Oral Biology,
The University of Connecticut Health Center, U.S.A.

A number of papers in this symposium volume discuss functional aspects of tooth morphology from a variety of viewpoints using both fossil material and the morphology of extant species. But it was Dr. Butler's comments during a discussion at the symposium itself which provided me with my point of departure. That is, that adult tooth morphology is the product of genetic information translated during embryogenesis into complex, indeed elegant, form. The variation and plasticity of the genome provide the raw materials on which selection pressures will act ultimately to change the population phenotype. Understandably, the manifold genetic expressions related to the initiation and maintenance of adult tooth morphology are of interest to a variety of workers from the cell biologist to the population geneticist.

I will limit my discussion here, however, to some new developments in the study of the inductive tissue interactions that occur during the early stages of tooth morphogenesis. In an earlier series of papers, I demonstrated that the oral epithelium is responsive to the influence of the dental papilla and that the initiation of tooth morphogenesis is a function of the dental papilla. The lip furrow epithelium surfacing the oral epithelium which will line the lip sulcus, responds to the experimental addition of dental papillae cells and develops perfectly formed teeth with normal deposition of enamel and dentine matrices (Kollar and Baird, 1970a). In fact, the dental papilla can elicit tooth development from responsive embryonic integumental epithelium of non-oral origin (Kollar and Baird, 1970b).

Tooth morphology can be predicted very early in development when the basement membrane between the enamel organ epithelium and the dental papillae can be identified as the presumptive dentino–enamel junction. Indeed, this interface between the interacting tissue will eventually be exaggerated and replaced by hard tissue. Previous studies (Grobstein and Cohen, 1965; Kollar and Baird, 1970b; Koch, 1968; Kollar, 1972a) acknowledged that one of the easily identified protein components of the dentino–enamel interface, collagen, was likely to play an important role in the developmental process.

If collagenase (Koch, 1968) or the lathyrogenic agent β-aminopropionitrile (Kollar, 1972b) were administered to cultures of embryonic tooth germs, morphogenesis was disturbed. The enamel organ, in the presence of the lathyrogen, began to regress and after a relatively few days in culture the epithelium could no longer be identified as an enamel organ. If the agent continued to be present, the epithelium was eventually lost. However, the effect of the lathyrogen was reversible. If the tissues were removed to control medium, morphogenesis resumed and perfectly formed tooth buds once again appeared and proceeded to develop normally.

In addition, I observed earlier that when the dental epithelium was experimentally combined with non-dental connective tissue, the susceptibility of the epithelium to invasion was uncontrolled and tissue patterns resembling an enamel organ were not supported by the foreign connective tissue. I concluded that the connective tissue possibly acted via the collagenous framework by organizing, modelling and maintaining the epithelium into recognizable structures.

In one sense these findings were encouraging. The notion that a substance as ubiquitous throughout the organism and the animal kingdom could be involved in inductive tissue interactions suggested that collagen might provide the molecular basis of a general mechanism for biological induction. But the notion that so seemingly uninteresting a molecule could be responsible for the induction of such a variety of structures was problematical. How could one relatively simple, albeit universally distributed, molecule be involved in the manifold inductions of many unique structures found in the organism?

Recent advances in collagen biochemistry, however, have provided some intriguing possible solutions to the dilemma. Apparently the notion that the structure of collagen molecules was uniform and universal was an oversimplification. Collagen is not simply one molecular species; not all collagen is alike. An active area of research is rapidly defining the subtle complexities of the collagen molecule isolated from various tissue sources. The details of this work have been reviewed several times recently (Miller and Matukas, 1974; Bornstein, 1974; Trelstad, 1974; Stenzl et al., 1974). I wish only to mention a few general features of collagen biosynthesis and structure since it is the basis for our recent work on the factors that influence and control tooth morphogenesis.

The soluble precursor molecule that is secreted by the cell and which forms the mature cross-striated collagen fibre is a triple-stranded protein structure about 3000 Å long and 15 Å in diameter. The three polypeptide chains are called α-chains and contain more than 1000 amino acids. The structure and sequence of the amino acids in the α-chains have been determined because cyanogen bromide cleaves the α-chain into shorter peptides that can be separated on ion exchange columns. The partial characterization of the amino acid sequences indicated that not all α-chains showed the same amino acid sequences. Thus the biochemists have designated α1 and α2 chains, each with a unique amino acid composition and sequence. Further examination of the α-chains from collagens isolated from various sources have demonstrated even greater variety in molecular structure. Thus, four subclasses of α1 chains (I, II, III and IV) have been identified on the basis of amino acid composition. The molecular heterogeneity provided by the four classes of α1 chains and the α2 chain is a hint at the potential versatility of the collagen molecule. Since the triple-stranded molecule can be composed of combinations of these individual α-chains, it is clear that not all collagen is alike. Indeed, the composition of collagen isolated from dentine (as well as bone, tendon and dermis) is composed of two α1 (I) and one α2 chains combining in the triple-stranded collagen fibre precursor. Cartilage collagen, on the other hand, is composed of three α1 (II) chains. It is not necessary to review the controversies and advances in this research area. It is sufficient to emphasize the notion that the structural diversity displayed by the various collagen molecules suggests that this ubiquitous protein may function in ways not yet apparent from the traditional role of collagen as a structural fibrous protein.

The advances in understanding the molecular structure of collagen have been complemented by equally significant insights into the biosynthetic sequence which produces the α-chains. The identification of at least four distinct polypeptides suggests that there are correspondingly four distinct genetic loci for the transcription of distinct messenger RNAs necessary for protein synthesis. In the cytoplasmic milieu the mRNA message is translated into α chains. The proline in the chain is hydroxylated and then three chains are combined into a left-handed triple helix. This is the intracellular soluble form of the collagen precursor subunit called procollagen. The solubility of this collagen precursor is maintained by addition of amino acid sequences attached to the amino terminal end of the α-chains. When the completed procollagen molecule is secreted into the extracellular space, this amino terminal sequence is removed by a peptidase and the individual triple-stranded molecules may cross-link into the familiar cross-banded fibre known as collagen.

This cursory and superficial account of some of the critical steps involved in the biosynthesis of the various varieties of collagen is described here because the recent biochemical advances suggest several experimental approaches to the study of tooth morphogenesis and the role of collagen in initiating, controlling and maintaining tooth form.

Clearly, the experimental attack can be directed to the extracellular disruption of the collagen molecule, or alternatively, advantage may be taken of recently described intracellular events that I mentioned above. Both approaches have been used and it is the purpose of this paper to report the effects of disruption of collagen synthesis at several levels during the morphogenesis of embryonic tooth germs cultured *in vitro*.

The first indication that collagen might exert an important function during morphogenesis came from the studies of Grobstein and Cohen (1965) on salivary gland morphogenesis and, later, from a study by Koch (1968) on tooth germs. In both studies, collagenase was used to disrupt the mature collagen that was deposited during the morphogenesis of these two structures. When the collagen was disrupted, morphogenesis was stopped, the epithelium no longer responded in predictable ways and the complex structure of the salivary gland or tooth germ was lost. If the tissue was returned to control medium and collagen permitted to form, morphogenesis resumed.

An alternative procedure for this disruption of collagen in the extracellular space utilizes lathyrogens such as β-aminopropionitrile (BAPN). These agents do not alter procollagen synthesis or secretion, but the cross-linkage of the subunits into a collagen fibre is prevented. The action of β-aminopropionitrile (BAPN) prevents the action of lysyl oxidase, the enzyme necessary for the cross-linkage of the individual collagen subunits. Thus while intracellular collagen synthesis proceeds, the extracellular events do not occur normally. In earlier reports (Kollar and Baird, 1970c; Kollar, 1972b) it was demonstrated that when tooth buds are explanted at the early bell stage morphogenesis proceeds and differentiation of ameloblasts and odontoblasts occurs. If BAPN is added to the medium, the enamel organ regresses and is lost, Furthermore, the tissue remains healthy and mitotic figures are apparent in both the epithelium and mesoderm. But tooth morphogenesis is prevented by suppressing the final step in the maturation of the stable collagen fibre. Thus, suppression does not inflict irreversible loss of the capacity to form recognizable tooth germs and recovery is possible.

These data confirm the action of an anti-collagen agent on the morpho-differentiation of tooth germs at a biochemical locus just prior to the actual production of the stable collagen fibre. While the intracellular biosynthesis of the procollagen is not disturbed, the extracellular block to fibre formation is sufficient to inhibit morphogenesis. However, it is possible to use the new advances in the biochemistry of biosynthesis of collagen to make more direct attacks on the intracellular production of procollagen. The effects of agents that interrupt collagen synthesis or secretion into the extracellular space can now be examined. There are a number of agents with widespread debilitating effects on cellular function that suppress protein synthesis or prevent protein secretion into the extracellular space. For example, Schwartz and Kirsten (1974), have reported the suppressive but irreversible effects of a nucleic acid analogue bromodeoxyuridine (BUDR) on collagen synthesis in tooth buds *in vitro*. Presumably this agent acts at the genetic level; it certainly does not act specifically on collagen biosynthesis. In addition, since the tissue is irreversibly damaged such an agent is of limited usefulness. Rather, specific agents that can be shown to suppress collagen synthesis in the intracellular compartment at some identifiable point offer greater experimental advantage, especially if the tissue is not irreversibly damaged and can resume morphogenesis of identifiable structure.

Two such agents have been examined in my laboratory. They are L-azetidine-2-carboxylic acid, a proline analogue, that replaces proline and stops collagen synthesis at the ribosomal or immediate post-ribosomal level (Ruch *et al.*, 1973, 1974; Koch, 1974; Galbraith and Kollar, 1974) and α,α'-dipyridyl (Kollar, 1973) that chelates ionic iron and thus can prevent the hydroxylation of proline to hydroxyproline. Collagen secretion by the cell ceases in the presence of L-azetidine and α,α'-dipyridyl.

Figure 1 illustrates the degree of differentiation achieved by a 14-day embryonic mouse incisor cultured *in vitro* for 8 days. This germ has progressed from the late cap stage typical of the foetal mouse incisor of 14 days gestation to a well developed germ displaying odontoblasts and ameloblasts in the early stages of differentiation.

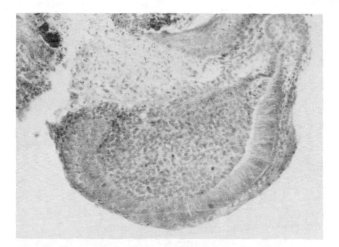

FIG. 1. A section of an incisor tooth germ explanted at the early bud stage (14 days gestation). Note the ameloblast differentiation, mitotic figures, and advanced histodifferentiation of this explant after 8 days of culture. × 189.

When L-azetidine is added to the cultures (Fig. 2), however, the epithelium regresses towards the surface and the mesenchymal cells of the papilla fail to differentiate as odontoblasts. Despite this reversal of the developmental process in these cultures, mitotic figures are present in the inhibited tooth germs indicating that some cell functions are unaffected by the action of L-azetidine.

Similar results are observed when cultures are treated with the iron chelating agent α,α'-dipyridyl (Fig. 3). The enamel organ begins to regress soon after the agent is added to the cultures and as the time of exposure is lengthened the enamel organ and any surface epithelium present at the time

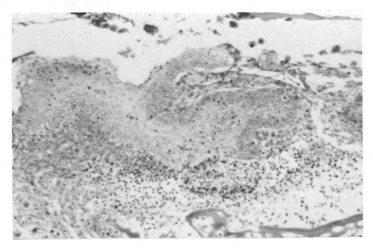

FIG. 2. The effect of L-azetidine (50 μg ml⁻¹) on the differentiation of a 15-day embryonic tooth germ. This section indicates the loss of the enamel organ, a general regression of the epithelium towards the surface and the presence of mitotic figures after 4 days of treatment *in vitro*. × 189.

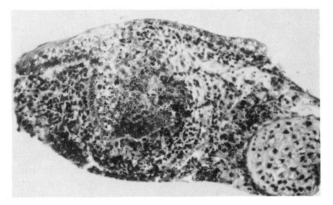

FIG. 3. The severe effects of α,α'-dipyridyl (0·1 mM) on a fifteen day molar tooth germ *in vitro* after 2 days *in vitro* are illustrated by the degenerative changes in the surface epithelium, the regression of the enamel organ and some cellular damage scattered throughout the explant. Mitotic figures are present in the dental papilla. × 189.

of explantation is sloughed from the mesenchymal bed. The action of the α,α'-dipyridyl is more severely disruptive of cell function since areas of cellular damage are obvious in many sections. Despite this impairment of cell function during the early stages of inhibition mitotic figures are present in the dental papilla.

The effect of these agents on the extracellular deposition of collagen has been confirmed by electron microscopy. L-azetidine (Ruch *et al.*, 1974) and α,α′-dipyridyl (Hetem *et al.*, 1975) both prevent the deposition of collagen into the extracellular space.

Interference with collagen synthesis at the ribosomal or post-ribosomal level clearly disrupts tooth morphogenesis in a manner reminiscent of our earlier studies with BAPN. The effect of BAPN seemed less intense and indeed the reversibility of the effect of BAPN indicated that the mechanisms of morphogenesis were not permanently disrupted. The recovery from BAPN inhibition prompted experiments to test the possible recovery from the more severe intracellular supression seen with L-azetidine and α,α′-dipyridyl.

Figure 4 illustrates an incisor tooth germ which has recovered from an α,α′-dipyridyl treated culture. The 15-day embryonic tooth germ was treated for 2 days and displayed obvious regressive changes when observed intact in the culture dish. After 2 days the regressing explant was moved to control medium and allowed to incubate for 4 additional days. The restoration of

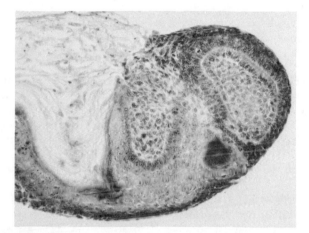

Fig. 4. Recovery of treated explants occurs *in vitro*. This is a well developed tooth growing in an explant that had been severely inhibited for two days with α,α′-dipyridyl (0·1 mM) and then moved to control medium free of the iron chelator for an additional 5 days. The differentiation of ameloblasts and odontoblasts as well as a stratified surface epithelium are apparent. ×189.

the enamel organ and surface epithelium is obvious; the recognizable histological configuration is remarkable. The resiliency of these treated tooth germs is exceptional and these studies bring to mind the dramatic demonstration by Dr. Glasstone (1952) of the recuperative and regulative abilities of halved tooth germs.

While these data have intrinsic interest because they further probe the relationship between collagen and morphogenesis, they suggest, in addition, that the tooth germ is capable of expressing its morphogenetic information even after severe and prolonged inhibition. But the exciting aspect of these data is in the potential use of inhibited explants as the basis for a more definitive analysis of the role of collagen in tooth development.

Certainly, the question raised at the beginning of this chapter can now be extended. If there are a variety of collagen precursor molecules that might be combined into a number of distinct types, and if these various collagens are involved in the induction and maintenance of specialized structures, then there should be some degree of biological specificity in terms of the function of these collagen molecules. That is to say, cartilage collagen should be less likely to support skin morphogenesis than collagen derived from dermis. Thus, if soluble procollagen could be obtained and added exogenously to intracellularly inhibited but responsive cultures, a test for the biological activity of the various collagen molecules and, therefore, a demonstration of the importance of collagen during tooth morphogenesis, would be available. As one might anticipate, my laboratory has begun to extend our analysis by utilizing just such an experimental device.

We have been aware for some time (Kollar, 1972a) that the dental papilla could be isolated and further dissociated into cell suspensions. The growth pattern of the isolated dental papilla cells after about one week of growth on plastic is typically fibroblastic and monolayer. In addition, it is clear that the dental papilla cells can be maintained by standard cell culture procedures. It is from such cells of primary cultures of other tissue sources and from established cell lines that the biochemists routinely have been able to isolate soluble procollagen for analysis. But it seemed important to show that by culturing the papilla cells we did not change the cells so that they were no longer able to function inductively as dental papillae cells.

Fortunately, we had already demonstrated in a previous study (Kollar, 1972a) that long-term culture of dental papillae does not destroy the ability to induce teeth, i.e. that cultured dental papillae cells retain their morphogenetic capabilities. If the monolayer of cultured cells is lifted from the plastic and recombined with epithelium, the epithelium participates with the dental papillae cells and a tooth is formed. Data such as these and the earlier report by Main (1966) that rat incisors can form after long-term growth in fibrin sponges suggest that the isolated cells retain their capability to act as papillae cells. Mr. D. Rohrbach in my laboratory is isolating the soluble procollagen secreted by monolayer cultures of cells extracted from the dental papilla and other cranial mesenchymal tissues. We are able to obtain sufficient quantities to permit testing these collagens on inhibited tooth germ cultures.

In the meantime, however, we have been fortunate to have a source of soluble procollagen samples from other tissue sources. One of the most interesting varieties of procollagen has been isolated from cultures of dermal cells obtained by Drs R. Church and M. Tanzer from Professor C. M. Lapière of Belgium. These cells are obtained from calves suffering from dermatosparaxis. Dermatosparaxis is a genetic disease in which the peptidase that converts procollagen to collagen by removing the amino terminal segment is defective or missing. Consequently, most of the collagen made remains in the soluble state resulting in very fragile skin—from whence the name of the disease is derived.

Lapière and his group (Lapière and Pierard, 1974) have shown that the peptidase acts in the extracellular space. Thus, in our cultures of normal mouse tooth germs, the peptidase activity should not be impaired, exogenously added procollagen should be converted to the cross-linked stable form and the effects of collagen inhibition should be circumvented. Figure 5

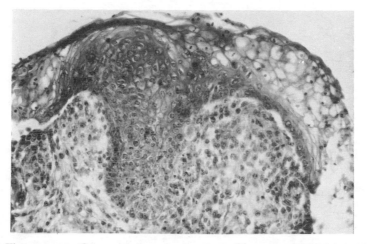

FIG. 5. The remnants of the epithelium can be seen in this explant of a 14-day-old molar tooth germ cultured for 5 days in the presence of α,α'-dipyridyl (0·05 mM). The surface epithelium is degenerating, the attachment to the connective tissue is lost and the tooth germ is absent. ×250.

illustrates a section of a tooth germ grown with a debilitating dosage of α,α'-dipyridyl for 4 days. It displays a typically regressing epithelium. Note that the keratinization and stratification pattern of the epithelium is defective and that the enamel organ has regressed, completing the inhibition of morphogenesis.

In contrast to this picture of severe inhibition, when some of the procollagen from the cultures of the dermatosparactic dermal cells is added exogenously to the cultures grown on medium containing the same dosage of α,α'-dipyridyl as in Fig. 5, it is shown in Fig. 6 that indeed the inhibition is circumvented and the cultures present a more normal appearance. Note that the keratinization and stratification of the surface epithelium are normal. A tooth germ is present and mitotic activity is apparent. Thus, the ability of inhibited cultures to respond to the addition of soluble procollagen suggests a promising approach to further testing of the morphogenetic role of collagen.

Clearly, the development of the tooth germ attained in Fig. 6 is not equivalent to the controls or to the recovering cultures described previously. But it should be noted that only one molecular species had been added, and

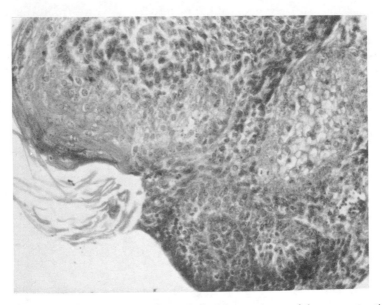

FIG. 6. In contrast to Fig. 5, if procollagen derived from cultures of dermatosparactic calf fibroblasts is added to inhibited tooth germ explants, the debilitating effects of the α,α'-dipyridyl are circumvented. The surface epithelium is normal and a rudimentary tooth germ is present. ×275.

with that the explant had begun to return to normal. It is obvious that a single collagen type derived from the mesenchymal component is not the complete and definitive composition of the extracellular milieu. Recent data from Trelstad and Slavkin (1974), for example, indicate that isolated enamel organ epithelium makes collagen and this collagen differs from the collagen derived from the dental papilla. Thus, several species of collagen may interact in any given epithelio–mesenchymal interacting system. In addition, there is increasing evidence of the importance of the acid mucopolysaccharides (the new terminology would demand the term proteoglycans) of the ground substance of the extracellular compartment which interact with the collagens and modify morphogenesis. Nonetheless, it seems that the ability of severely inhibited tooth germs to respond to the addition of molecules with suspected morphogenetic roles is a new and promising beginning in the studies of tooth morphogenesis.

The most exciting prospect, however, is that for the first time a molecule implicated in the origin and maintenance of histological structure can now be probed from the gross histological level all the way to the genome. Although many taxing problems are still unanswered, a well characterized biochemical sequence is known and genetic studies are underway. Perhaps now there is cause to be optimistic about understanding the relationship and pathway between genes and the expression of dental morphology.

REFERENCES

BORNSTEIN P. (1974). The biosynthesis of collagen. *A. Rev. Biochem.* **43**, 567–603.
GALBRAITH, D. B. and KOLLAR, E. J. (1974). Effects of L-azetidine-2-carboxylic acid, a proline analogue, on the *in vitro* development of mouse tooth germs. *Archs oral Biol.* **19**, 1171–1176.
GLASSTONE, S. (1952). The development of halved tooth germs in tissue culture. *J. Anat.* **86**, 12–15.
GROBSTEIN, C. and COHEN, J. (1965). Collagenase: Effect on the morphogenesis of embryonic salivary epithelium *in vitro*. *Science, N.Y.* **150**, 626–628.
HETEM, S., KOLLAR, E. J., CUTLER, L. S. and YAEGER, J. (1975). The effect of α,α'-dipyridyl on the basement membrane of tooth germs *in vitro*. *J. dent. Res.* **54**, 783–787.
KOCH, W. E. (1968). The effect of collagenase on embryonic mouse incisors growing *in vitro*. *Anat. Rec.* **160**, 377–378.
KOCH, W. E. (1974). The effects of azetidine-2-carboxylic acid on cultured incisors of embryonic mice. *Anat. Rec.* **178**, 393–394.
KOLLAR, E. J. (1972a). Histogenetic aspects of dermal-epidermal interactions. *In* "Developmental Aspects of Oral Biology" (Slavkin, H. C. and Bavetta, L., eds), Ch. 7, pp. 125–149. Academic Press, New York and London.
KOLLAR, E. J. (1972b). The development of the integument: spatial, temporal and phylogenetic factors. *Am. Zool.* **12**, 125 133.
KOLLAR, E. J. (1973). Effects of α,α'-dipyridyl on organ cultures of embryonic mouse tooth germs. *J. dent. Res.* **52**, 145.
KOLLAR, E. J. and BAIRD, G. R. (1970a). Tissue interactions in developing mouse tooth germs: I. Reorganization of the dental epithelium during tooth germ reconstruction. *J. Embryol. exp. Morph.* **24**, 159–171.
KOLLAR, E. J. and BAIRD, G. R. (1970b). Tissue interactions in developing mouse tooth germs: II. The inductive role of the dental papillae. *J. Embryol. exp. Morph.* **24**, 173–186.
KOLLAR, E. J. and BAIRD, G. R. (1970c). Inhibition of tooth germ development by beta-aminoproprionitrile. *Anat. Rec.* **166**, 333.
LAPIÈRE, C. M. and PIÉRARD, G. (1974). Skin procollagen peptidase in normal and pathological conditions. *J. invest. Derm.* **62**, 582–586.
MAIN, J. H. P. (1966). Retention of potential to differentiate in long-term cultures of tooth germs. *Science, N.Y.* **152**, 778–780.
MILLER, E. J. and MATUKAS, V. J. (1974). Biosynthesis of collagen. The biochemist's view. *Fedn Proc.* **33**, 1197–1204.
RUCH, J. V., KARCHER-DJURICIC, V., WOEHRLING, D. and HASSELMANN, M. (1973). Action de l'acide L-azetidine-2-carboxyl que sur la differentiation dentaire *in vitro*. Premiers resultats. *C. r. Séance. Soc. Biol.* **167**, 368.
RUCH, J. V., FABRE, M., KARCHER-DJURICIC, V. and STAUBLI, A. (1974). The effect of L-azetidine-2-carboxylic acid (analogue of proline) on dental cytodifferentiations *in vitro*. *Differentiation* **2**, 211–220.
SCHWARTZ, S. A. and KIRSTEN, W. H. (1974). Tissue-specific suppression of differentiation by 5-bromodeoxyuridine *in vitro*. *J. dent. Res.* **53**, 509–515.
STENZEL, K. H., MIYATA, T. and RUBIN, A. L. (1974). Collagen as a biomaterial. *A. Rev. Biophys. Bioeng.* **3**, 231–253.
TRELSTAD, R. L. (1974). Vertebrate collagen heterogeneity: a brief summary. *Devl. Biol.* **38**, f13–f16.

TRELSTAD, R. and SLAVKIN, H. C. (1974). Collagen synthesis by the epithelial enamel organ of the embryonic rabbit tooth. *Biochem. biophys. Res. Commun.* **59**, 443–449.

2. Vestigial Teeth in the Rabbit, Rat and Mouse; their Relationship to the Problem of Lacteal Dentitions

LETTY MOSS-SALENTIJN

Department of Anatomy, Columbia University, New York, U.S.A.

INTRODUCTION

In the past century sporadic reports have appeared on the occurrence of a small, transient, non-functional (vestigial) tooth in the incisor area of the foetal rabbit (Freund, 1892; Hirschfeld *et al.*, 1973; Peters and Strassburg, 1967, 1969; Woodward, 1894). A similar, though even smaller, structure has been noted in the foetal mouse (Fitzgerald, 1973; Peters and Strassburg, 1969; Strassburg *et al.*, 1971; Woodward, 1894), Vestigial incisor teeth had not been described earlier in rats. Recently, however, such a tooth was found in at least one rat species commonly used in the laboratory (Moss-Salentijn, 1975). The vestigial teeth in these three common laboratory animals are generally considered to be reduced members of the lacteal dentition. However, varied interpretations have been given on the nature of the neighbouring functional incisor teeth (Freund, 1892; Mayer, 1969, Moss-Salentijn, 1975). In this chapter the ontogenetic development and subsequent loss of the vestigial teeth in the rabbit are presented, as well as a summary on the ontogeny of such teeth in the rat and mouse. The data will serve as a point of departure for a reappraisal of the nature of the incisor teeth in these representative lagomorphs and rodents.

MATERIALS AND METHODS

Rabbits

Foetal specimens of New Zealand white rabbits were collected at 20, 21, 23, 25, 28 and 31 days post-conception (p.c.). Whole heads were freshly fixed in formalin, routinely embedded in paraffin, serially sectioned at 6 μm in coronal, sagittal and horizontal planes and stained either with haematoxylin and eosin or with Masson's trichrome. When necessary, certain structures were traced serially on acetate paper off an overhead viewer which was mounted on the microscope. Overlays of these tracings were used for a three-dimensional appraisal of the traced structures.

From selected specimens the teeth were dissected free, cleared and stained with Alizarin Red S.

Rats and Mice

Rats were studied from 17·5 days p.c. until 5 days after birth on serial coronal and sagittal sections, stained with haematoxylin and eosin (Moss-Salentijn, 1975). Mice were studied from 12·5 days p.c. until 15 days after birth on serial sections stained with several different stains (Fitzgerald, 1973).

OBSERVATIONS

Rabbits

Vestigial teeth were present in this material at 20, 21, 23 and 25 days p.c. At 20 days p.c. dentine was seen only in these vestigial teeth. Between 21 and 25 days p.c. dentine deposition was initiated in two functional incisors and three deciduous molars in the upper jaw, and in one functional incisor, two deciduous molars and one permanent molar in the lower jaw (Fig. 1).

There was one vestigial tooth in each quadrant. This tooth was located labially to the neighbouring incisor, its long axis nearly perpendicular to the long axis of that incisor (Fig. 2). The dental organs of the vestigial teeth consisted of a few layers of epithelial cells. No stellate reticulum was seen in any of the stages studied presently. The inner epithelial cell layer had locally differentiated into columnar cells, but no distinct enamel layer was formed. However, at 21 and 23 days p.c. a thin, refractive "cuticle" was found occasionally on the external dentine surface. A fully formed vestigial tooth consisted of a dentine shell surrounding a small core of pulpal cells. The dentine was atubular in nature; centrally, pulpal cells had become embedded within the calcified dentine tissue. A capillary loop was the vascular supply of the pulp (Fig. 3).

Towards the end of the tooth's development the enamel epithelium at the base of the tooth detached from the peripheral dentine, mesenchymal cells invaded the area between the dentine and the epithelium and formed a calcified, mostly acellular, cementum tissue. At 21 days p.c. the fully formed maxillary vestigial tooth was a cup-like shell measuring 90 μm in length and 80 μm in diameter at its widest point. At 23 days p.c. the fully mandibular vestigial tooth was projectile-shaped with a broad cementum base. It measured 175 μm in length and 160 μm in diameter at its widest point. An interesting finding was an "apical tail" of epithelium which could be seen in any longitudinal section as a triangular epithelial strand at the base of the developing vestigial tooth (Fig. 3A).

Careful observations were made especially on the relationship between

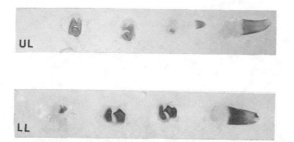

FIG. 1. Dissected, alizarinated developing teeth from a 23-day p.c. rabbit foetus. UL: upper left jaw; LL: lower left jaw. The molars are seen in occlusal view; the incisors in lingual view. In the upper jaw two functional incisors and three deciduous molars are in the stage of dentine deposition, while in the lower jaw the functional incisor, two deciduous molars and one permanent molar are in the stage of dentine deposition. The vestigial teeth, which are found anterior to the functional incisors, are not shown in this photograph. × 4.5.

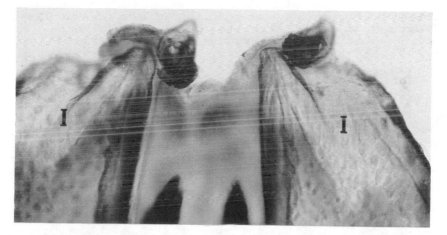

FIG. 2. Lower incisor teeth of a 23-day p.c. foetal rabbit. Dissected, alizarinated specimen, lingual view. The two vestigial teeth are found anteriorly near the tips of the functional incisors (I). The vestigial tooth on the right is in its correct position. The left vestigial tooth is dislodged medially. Note the morphology of this tooth with its relatively smooth dentine "crown" and the irregular cementum collar at its base. × 62.5.

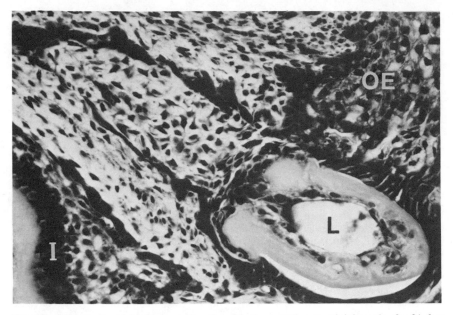

FIG. 3A. Longitudinal histologic section through the maxillary vestigial tooth of a 21-day p.c. foetal rabbit. A reduced enamel organ surrounds the crown part of the tooth; some epithelial cells are columnar. Cells are included in the dentine. Near the base of the tooth, mesenchymal cells are producing a cementum collar. Notice the wide lumen (L) of a capillary in the papilla on the triangular epithelial strand extending from the base of the tooth. OE: oral epithelium; I: enamel organ of the first functional incisor. × 335.

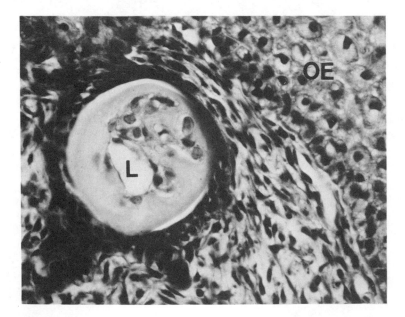

the enamel organs of the vestigial teeth and those of the neighbouring incisors. It could be shown repeatedly in serial sections of both upper and lower jaws that the vestigial teeth and each family of functional incisors all had separate attachments to the oral epithelium (Fig. 4A–C).

In the lower jaw one pair of functional incisors was developing. On the lingual surfaces of their enamel organs cap-shaped "enamel organs" appeared at 21 days p.c. At 23 days p.c. these structures were absent (Fig. 5). Similar abortive cap-shaped "enamel organs" were found at 21 days p.c. on the lingual surfaces of the enamel organs belonging to the first pair of functional incisors in the upper jaw.

The second pair of functional incisors located posterior to the first pair in the upper jaw was deciduous, to be replaced 35 days after birth by a permanent pair of incisors (Horowitz et al., 1973). In the foetal stages presently studied, the successional laminae of these replacing incisors developed from the lingual sides of their predecessors' enamel organs at 25 days p.c. and reached the bell stage at 31 days p.c.

By 23 days p.c. a massive resorption of the maxillary vestigial tooth was underway by multi-nucleated "dentinoclasts." At 25 days p.c. a small dentine fragment anterior to the erupting functional incisor was all that remained of this tooth. The mandibular vestigial tooth showed some dentino-clasia at its base by 23 days p.c. The "crown" of this tooth was lodged partially inside the oral epithelium. At 25 days p.c. the functional incisor was erupting. In one specimen of that age the mandibular vestigial tooth was still present; in others it was not seen and presumed shed.

Rats and Mice

Since more extensive descriptions have appeared elsewhere, only summaries of those findings are given here.

In rats the vestigial teeth were best seen shortly before birth at 20·5 days p.c. They were not present in all foetal specimens and they were never seen postnatally. One vestigial tooth was present in each quadrant, located anterior to the developing functional incisor. Its ill-defined enamel organ was immediately subjacent to the oral epithelium and was not attached to the dental lamina of the functional incisor. Dentine was present in both maxillary and mandibular teeth, the former being twice the size of the latter. No determination of the fate of these teeth could be made.

In mice, vestigial teeth were maximally developed at 15·5 days p.c. These teeth were found usually in the maxilla but only occasionally in the mandible. No distinct enamel organ was formed. These teeth developed as a "fold of mesenchyme" into the epithelium at the antero–lateral border of the enamel organ belonging to the functional incisor. Odontoblasts differentiated and

FIG. 3B. Transverse histologic section through the maxillary vestigial tooth of a 21-day p.c. foetal rabbit. Notice the reduced enamel organ surrounding the tooth, the cellular inclusions in the dentine, the wide lumen (L) of the capillary in the papilla. × 423.

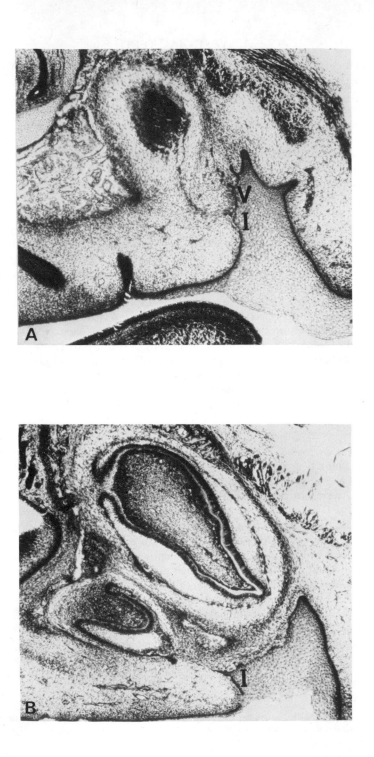

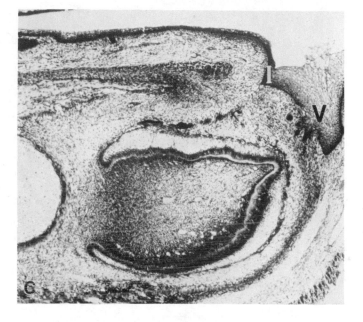

FIG. 4. Parasagittal histologic sections through the maxillary (A and B) and mandibular (C) incisor regions in a 21-day p.c. foetal rabbit. The points of attachment to the oral epithelium of the laminae of the vestigial tooth (V) and of the first functional incisor (I) are shown in A. In B, the point of attachment of the lamina of the second functional incisor (I) to the oral epithelium is shown. This section was 60 μm removed laterally from the section shown in A. The points of attachment of the laminae of the mandibular vestigial tooth (V) and of the functional incisor (I) to the oral epithelium are shown in C. × 215.

some irregular masses of dentine were formed between these cells. Around the time of birth the odontoblasts degenerated and the dentine disappeared, presumably by resorption.

DISCUSSION

The term "vestigial tooth" is reserved for those small teeth or tooth-like structures which do not actively erupt and become functional. Vestigial teeth develop in many mammalian species; they have a similarity in shape and structure, although the strength of actual morphologic expression may vary (compare the vestigial teeth of upper and lower jaw in the rabbit, or of rabbit and mouse!).

Vestigial teeth, occurring singly or in small groups, have been reported in a number of marsupials (Berkovitz, 1968a, b, 1972; Fosse and Risnes, 1972a, b; Wilson and Hill, 1896; Woodward, 1894), as well as in the hedgehog (Kindahl, 1959), the nine-banded armadillo (Röse, 1892a), the guinea pig (Santoné,

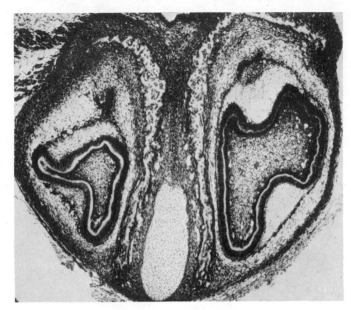

A

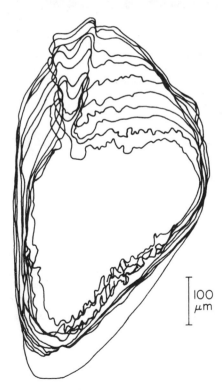

B

$\left[\begin{array}{c} 100 \\ \mu m \end{array}\right.$

1935) and shrews (Ziegler, 1971); these are in addition to the reports on such teeth in the rabbit, mouse and rat, referred to in the introduction.

An entire dentition may be vestigial. This has been reported for the deciduous dentition of the walrus (Cobb, 1933), the first tooth series in *Hatteria punctata* (Harrison, 1901) and the entire dentition (160–240 teeth) of the whalebone whale (Karlsen, 1962). Kubota (1963) described how an entire deciduous dentition in the fur seal developed, erupted and was shed before birth. These teeth, while reduced in size, were distinct incisors, canines and premolars with fully formed roots, which had to be resorbed before the teeth were shed. Strictly speaking, they were not vestigial teeth but, being quite non-functional in nature, they should be mentioned here.

On the other side of the spectrum are reports of isolated transient enamel organs, not developing beyond the cap stage. This has been seen in some marsupials (Röse, 1892c, d; Wilson and Hill, 1896), in the maxillary incisor and canine region of sheep (Hatt, 1967) and in the fur seal (Kubota and Togawa, 1970). Finally, claims have been made that a dental lamina is present (without any further future differentiation) in manis (Röse, 1892b), birds (Romanoff, 1960; Röse, 1892e) and turtles (Röse, 1892e). The regular development of vestigial teeth or transient enamel organs in a large number of species (without doubt many more may be added to this list) and in specific locations rules out the possibility that these teeth are supernumerary elements.

In all histologic descriptions of the enamel organs of vestigial teeth the absence of a stellate reticulum is uniformly noted. This and the absence of true secretory ameloblasts, producing a recognizable layer of enamel, other than a trace of it (Fosse and Risnes, 1972a; Hirschfeld *et al.*, 1973; Röse, 1892a) seem to be inseparable phenomena.

Dentine produced in a vestigial tooth is irregular, atubular and often cellular, especially towards the centre of the tooth, where odontoblastic cells may be trapped inside the dentine. At the base of a tooth a cementum-like tissue is formed jointly by odontoblasts in the papilla and cementoblasts from the dental sac. A similar tissue is formed near the apical foramina of dog teeth (Owens, 1974) and of rat molars (Lester, 1969) and is probably typical for the final stages of normal root formation.

The observation of a triangular epithelial strand near the bases of rabbit vestigial teeth is not clearly understood. Possible explanations are that the strand represents:

FIG. 5A. Coronal histologic section through the lower jaw of a 21-day p.c. foetal rabbit. Cap-shaped outgrowths are seen on the lingual surfaces of the enamel organs belonging to the functional mandibular incisors. The cap-shaped organ on the right is sectioned more posteriorly than the one on the left. ×55.

FIG. 5B. An overlay on serial tracings made on coronal histologic sections through the enamel organ of the mandibular functional incisor depicted above in Fig. 5A. The cap-shaped enamel organ on its lingual surface is present in all 30 sections represented in this overlay.

(a) an "epithelial tail" (Berkovitz, 1968a),
(b) a residual (and perhaps successional) dental lamina, and
(c) a vestigial root sheath (Hertwig).

Berkovitz (1968a) described solid epithelial tails extending from vestigial teeth in Macropodidae. No clear explanation was provided for this structure. However, it is to be distinguished from the residual dental lamina, lingual to vestigial teeth, which was described by Röse (1892a) and also by Berkovitz (op. cit. 1968a). A root sheath was noted by Karlsen (1962) adjacent to a number of vestigial teeth in the whalebone whale. But the interpretation of the present structure as a root sheath is unlikely. Owens (1974) demonstrated that during root formation Hertwig's root sheath progressively shortens, becoming inconspicuous near the apical foramen. If the processes of cementum and dentine formation in the base of a vestigial tooth are comparable to those near the apical foramen of an almost fully developed functional tooth, the long epithelial strand seen near the vestigial tooth here is an unlikely candidate for a root sheath. A final determination on the nature of this structure cannot be made presently.

Cobb (1933) listed three different fates for the vestigial teeth of the walrus:

(a) shedding soon after birth,
(b) resorption *in situ* before or soon after birth and
(c) persistence during the life of the animal (only in those teeth located away from the greatest functional activity).

Other authors claim the fate of vestigial teeth to be either shedding (Harrison, 1901; Hirschfeld *et al.*, 1973) or resorption (Fitzgerald, 1973; Freund, 1892; Karlsen, 1962; Kindahl, 1959).

The present observations in the rabbit would suggest that resorption will generally occur first and may lead to complete destruction of the vestigial tooth. Eruptive pressures of neighbouring teeth may force the partially resorbed tooth out of the jaw. The vestigial teeth of rabbits, rats and mice are found in an area of great functional activity. It is possible that in a different location no resorption or shedding would occur. The three different fates for the vestigial teeth of the walrus listed by Cobb (1933) may have applications for all vestigial teeth.

The Homology of Vestigial Teeth

Ever since the first descriptions on vestigial teeth in the rabbit by Huxley (1880) and Pouchet and Chabry (1884) and in the mouse by Woodward (1894), attempts have been made to establish the homology of these teeth. It may be generally stated that mammalian dentitions have a limited number of dental generations and in the broadest sense demonstrate one or two sets of teeth. Eutherian dentitions have undoubtedly evolved from the unreduced formula 3/3–1/1–4/4–3/3, some having developed by substantial reductions in the number of teeth. Most investigators describing vestigial teeth consider them as manifestations of an advanced stage in the reduction of a given tooth position; a relic of an earlier, more complete dentition. But to which dentition do they belong: the primary (deciduous) or secondary (permanent) dentition? And to which dentition do neighbouring functional teeth belong?

There seems to be a general agreement that the vestigial teeth in the rabbit and in the mouse belong to the deciduous dentition (Fitzgerald, 1973; Freund, 1892; Hirschfeld et al., 1973; Woodward, 1894). A similar conclusion was reached for the rat (Moss-Salentijn, 1975). However, the homology of the functional incisors and their relationship to the vestigial incisor remains debatable. Of the three species discussed here, the rabbit possesses in its upper jaw the most complete set of teeth, which may facilitate the answer to the above questions. In the upper jaw of a rabbit foetus the vestigial tooth is found anteriorly. Posterior to it the first functional incisor is present (which persists during the life of the animal). Posterior to this incisor a second functional incisor (characteristic for lagomorphs) is found. The latter is replaced postnatally by a permanent incisor. The following possibilities have been advanced (Mayer, 1969):

(a) The vestigial incisor is the deciduous predecessor to the first functional incisor (I^1). I^2 has been lost during evolution and the second functional incisor is really I^3.
(b) The vestigial incisor is the deciduous predecessor to the first functional incisor I^1. The second functional incisor is I^2, I^3 having been lost during evolution.
(c) The vestigial incisor is the deciduous predecessor to I^1, which has been lost during evolution. The first functional incisor is the deciduous predecessor to I^2, which has been lost during evolution. The second functional incisor is I^3.

Freund (1892) considered some of these possibilities seriously, but he did not arrive at a conclusion satisfactory to himself. Other authors simply stated that the vestigial teeth in the mouse and rabbit are the deciduous predecessors to the neighbouring functional incisors. Only Fitzgerald (1973) justified this statement by pointing out the appropriate topographic relationship between the vestigial tooth and the dental lamina of the functional incisor.

Establishing criteria for the determination of the deciduous or permanent nature of certain teeth has presented problems over the years. Wilson and Hill exclaimed in 1896:

There is too much unavoidable uncertainty about any question of this kind to encourage a genuinely dogmatic attitude in regard to it.

These authors cited (1896) some criteria (mostly negative) advanced by Leche, but they chose to retain only one: the criterion of "contemporaneousness of origin" of toothbuds to determine whether different teeth belong to the same dentition. More recently Berkovitz (1968a) provided some admittedly empirical criteria:

(a) The deciduous tooth develops buccal to the corresponding permanent one.

(b) The deciduous tooth develops and calcifies earlier than the corresponding permanent one.

(c) The deciduous tooth is replaced by the corresponding permanent one.

The same author immediately made an exception to one of these rules and other exceptions may be found (Berkovitz, 1973; Moss-Salentijn, 1975).

Many authors have considered the residual "free" dental lamina, lingual to an enamel organ, as an indication that a secondary dentition once formed from this lamina and therefore that the enamel organ belonged to a deciduous tooth (Gaunt, 1966; Kükenthal, 1891), but this was already disproved by Wilson and Hill (1896). Peters and Strassburg (1969) felt that two teeth belong to the same tooth family if they were seen in the same (frontal) plane of section. Kubota and Togawa (1970) studied the relation between an enamel organ and a known permanent lamina in the same jaw to establish whether the enamel organ belonged to a deciduous or a permanent tooth. The most useful criterion, which was used in this study, was presented by Ooë (1965). This author has restated an older observation that the successional lamina giving rise to a permanent tooth proliferates from the enamel organ of the corresponding deciduous tooth.

The rabbit is diphyodont. Its dental formula is 2/1–0/0–3/2–3/3. The formula for the deciduous dentition is usually given as 2/1–0/0–3/2 (which includes the two vestigial teeth). However, an evaluation of the present rabbit material, based on the origin of successional laminae, leads to the conclusion that in both upper and lower jaw the vestigial teeth and the functional incisors belong to different tooth families. Separate points of attachment were seen between the oral epithelium and the laminae of vestigial and functional teeth. This finding agrees with observations by Peters and Strassburg (1967) who described the development of three epithelial thickenings in the incisor area of each jaw quadrant in rabbit foetuses. The thickening near the midline in each jaw quadrant developed into the vestigial tooth (Hirschfeld et al., 1973; Peters and Strassburg, 1967). The first functional maxillary incisor was seen here in the second position. The development of a transient cap stage from the lingual surface of its enamel organ strongly suggested that the functional incisor was a deciduous tooth whose permanent successor did not develop beyond the cap stage. The second functional maxillary incisor was seen in third position. Both a deciduous and a permanent "third incisor" developed.

Palaeontologic data to support the embryological findings are not available at present. The earliest known lagomorph is *Palaeolagus* (Wood, 1940). It possesses an incisor formula similar to that of recent lagomorphs. In fact, all known lagomorphs, both ancient and recent, have similar incisor formulae (Sych, 1971). With regard to tooth reduction, Wood (1940) suggested out of functional anatomical considerations that if the maxillary I^3 had been lost during evolution, the one remaining mandibular incisor probably was an

I_2. On the other hand, if the maxillary I^1 had been lost (which appears to be the case), the one remaining mandibular incisor would be an I_3. It is with these considerations in mind that the incisors in the rabbit are presented here as follows (see Fig. 6):

$$\text{Deciduous dentition:} \quad \frac{i^1\ i^2\ i^3}{i_1\quad i_3}$$

$$\text{Functional dentition:} \quad \frac{i^2\ I^3}{i_3}$$

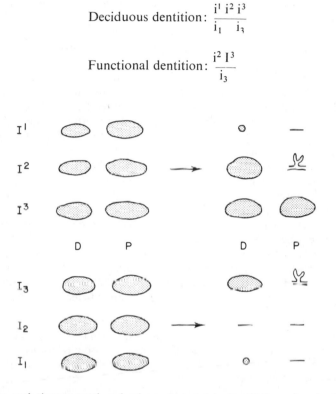

FIG. 6. The evolutionary tooth reductions suggested to have taken place in the rabbit incisor region. Top diagram represents the left upper jaw; bottom diagram represents the left lower jaw. The diagrams on the left portray the unreduced therian incisor formula (three incisors in each jaw quadrant, both in the deciduous (D) and in the permanent (P) dentition). To the right the present incisor formula is graphically represented in what are believed to be the homologously correct positions.

In the rabbit a determination of the individual incisors can be made with more assurance than in the rat or the mouse. These rodents are generally considered monophyodont with a dental formula 1/1-0/0-3/3. Rodents first appear in the late Paleocene; earlier transitional forms are not known at present (Romer, 1966; Wilson, 1949). It is reasonable to assume that all subsequent rodents are descended from the family of Paramyidae, whose dental formula was 1/1-0/0-2/1-3/3 and whose persistent incisors were constantly erupting (Wood, 1962). The palaeontologic record is of little assistance in determining homologies in the rodent incisor region.

In the mouse, as in the rabbit, Strassburg *et al.* (1971) described the occurrence of three epithelial thickenings in the incisor region of each jaw quadrant. These thickenings were considered by them as the sites of the three incisor teeth predicted in the ancient therian incisor forumula. The first and the third regressed rapidly and the second remained as the functioning incisor. If a similar event takes place in the rat, the vestigial tooth in this species, located slightly medially in relation to the functioning incisor and with a separate dental lamina, might be interpreted as a strongly reduced first incisor.

The description by Fitzgerald (1973) of the mouse vestigial tooth developing anteriorly in the dental lamina of the functioning incisor, appears at first sight to be different from the situation described for the rat. However, Gaunt (1966) makes the interesting observation that the mouse enamel organs arise directly from the oral epithelium without the presence of a definitive dental lamina. A dental lamina grows out later when the enamel organ has already developed. The mouse vestigial tooth may well have developed separately from the enamel organ of the functional incisor only to be drawn into its dental lamina later.

The ancestral method of evolutionary tooth loss in mammals consisted of a progressive retardation in the onset of ontogenetic development and tooth eruption (de Beer, 1958; Ziegler, 1971a). In evolutionary tooth loss the successor tooth at a particular tooth position generally disappears first (Ziegler, 1971a). It is, therefore, likely that all teeth of the dentition in rats and mice, including the vestigial incisors, belong to the same (deciduous) dental generation. With regard to the reduction of deciduous teeth Ziegler (1971b) states:

> well developed milk teeth quite likely represent a primitive condition, retained
> by the relatively unspecialized genera, regardless of phylogenetic affinities,
> whereas reduction of the milk teeth is probably an advanced characteristic
> independently attained by the various other lineages.

With the recent advances in our knowledge on the tissues and tissue interactions involved in odontogenesis, the process of tooth reduction may be better understood. Tooth development depends largely on a series of inductive interactions between oral epithelium and a condensed mass of ectomesenchyme. Each of these interactions is dependent upon two major factors: the capacity of one tissue to induce and the capacity of the other tissue to respond appropriately. The occurrence of two types of transient enamel organs provides an interesting example of the complexity of reduction processes. One type of minimal morphological expression of an enamel organ belonging to a vestigial tooth appears to be a fold of epithelium with a mesenchymal papilla projecting *into* it (Fitzgerald, 1973; Harrison, 1901) rather than an invagination of an epithelial structure into mesenchyme and *surrounding* a mesenchymal papilla.

There are several descriptions in the literature on another type of transient enamel organ which does not differentiate beyond the cap stage (Karlsen,

1962; Kindahl, 1959; Kubota and Togawa, 1970). A similar structure was seen in this study. It is clear that we deal here with two types of observations:

(a) A tooth-like structure in which dentine has been deposited, but without prior epithelial invagination to form a distinct enamel organ.
(b) A distinct epithelial invagination forming an enamel organ, but without further odontoblastic differentiation or dentine deposition.

Epithelial invagination and odontoblastic differentiation are two separate events in odontogenesis. The first depends on the capacity of the ectomesenchyme to induce the epithelium to proliferate and on the capacity of the epithelium to make this appropriate response. The second depends on the capacity of the epithelium to induce the differentiation of odontoblasts and on the capacity of the ectomesenchymal cells to respond appropriately. The observations described above strongly suggest that the capacity for either of these inductive interactions may be lost independently of the other.

Whether tooth loss in evolution is the result of a reduced inductive capacity of either tissue or of a reduced capacity of either tissue to respond appropriately—or whether the reduction is predominantly an ectomesenchymal event, as Kollar's data (1972) seem to suggest—there is no question that new information about tooth development will aid in a better understanding of evolutionary tooth loss.

SUMMARY

Some new data were presented on the prenatal development and loss of the vestigial incisor teeth in the upper and lower jaw of the rabbit. These data were compared with earlier observations on similar vestigial teeth in the rat and mouse. An analysis of the homology of incisor teeth in these examples of lagomorphs and rodents was made, based on relevant embryological studies and on some palaeontologic data. This analysis led to the conclusion that all vestigial teeth in these three species are deciduous in nature and that all functional incisors (except the second maxillary incisor in the rabbit) belong to the same deciduous tooth generation. These functional incisors persist during life and are not replaced by a corresponding permanent tooth.

REFERENCES

DE BEER, G. (1958). "Embryos and Ancestors," 3rd edition. Oxford University Press, Oxford.
BERKOVITZ, B. K. B. (1968a). The early development of the incisor teeth of *Setonix brachyurus* (Macropodiae: Marsupialia) with special reference to the prelacteal teeth. *Archs oral Biol.* **13**, 171–190.
BERKOVITZ, B. K. B. (1968b). Some stages in the early development of the post-incisor dentition of *Trichosurus vulpecula* (Phalangeriodea: Marsupialia). *J. Zool., Lond.* **154**, 403–414.

BERKOVITZ, B. K. B. (1972). Tooth development in *Protemnodon eugenii. J. dent. Res.* **51**, 1467–1473.

BERKOVITZ, B. K. B. (1973). Tooth development in the albino ferret (*Mustela putorius*) with special reference to the permanent carnassial. *Archs oral Biol.* **18**, 465–471.

COBB, W. M. (1933). The dentition of the Walrus, *Odobenus obesus. Proc. zool. Soc. Lond.* **3**, 645–668.

FITZGERALD, L. R. (1973). Deciduous incisor teeth of the mouse (*Mus musculus*). *Archs oral Biol.* **18**, 381–389.

FOSSE, G. and RISNES, S. (1972a). Development of the teeth in a pouch-young specimen of *Isoodon obesulus* and one of *Perameles* gunnii (Peramelidae: Marsupialia). *Archs oral Biol.* **17**, 829–838.

FOSSE, G. and RISNES, S. (1972b). Development of the incisors in two pouch-young stages of *Isoodon macrourus. Archs oral Biol.* **17**, 839–845.

FREUND, P. (1892). Beiträge zur Entwicklungsgeschichte der Zahnanlagen bei Nagethieren. *Arch. mikrosk. Anat.* **39**, 525–555.

GAUNT, W. A. (1966). The disposition of the developing cheek teeth in the albino mouse. *Acta anat.* **64**, 572–585.

HARRISON, H. S. (1901). The development and succession of teeth in *Hatteria punctata. Q. Jl microsc. Sci.* **44**, 161–213.

HATT, S. D. (1967). The development of the deciduous incisor in the sheep. *Res. vet. Sci.* **8**, 143–150.

HIRSCHFELD, Z., WEINREB, M. M. and MICHAELI, Y. (1973). Incisors of the rabbit: morphology, histology and development. *J. dent. Res.* **52**, 377–384.

HOROWITZ, S. L., WEISBROTH, S. H. and SCHER, S. (1973). Deciduous dentition in the rabbit (*Oryctolagus cuniculus*). A roentgenographic study. *Archs oral Biol.* **18**, 517–523.

HUXLEY, T. H. (1880). Cited by WOODWARD, M. F. (1894). *Anat. Anz.* **9**, 619–631.

KARLSEN, K. (1962). Development of tooth germs and adjacent structures in the whalebone whale (*Balaenoptera physalus* L.) *Det Norsk Vidensk-Akad, Oslo* **45**, 1–56.

KINDAHL, M. (1959). The tooth development in *Erinaceus europaeus. Acta odont. scand.* **17**, 467–489.

KOLLAR, E. J. (1972). Histogenetic aspects of dermal–epidermal interactions. In "Developmental Aspects of Oral Biology" (Slavkin, H. C. and Bavetta, L. A., eds), Ch. 7, pp. 125–149. Academic Press, New York and London.

KUBOTA, K. (1963). Morphological observations of the deciduous dentition in the fur seal (*Callorhinus ursinus*). *Bull. Tokyo med. dent. Univ.* **10**, 75–87.

KUBOTA, K. and TOGAWA, S. (1970). Development study of the monophyodont teeth in the Northern fur seal (*Callorhinus ursinus*). *J. dent. Res.* **49**, 325–331.

KÜKENTHAL, W. (1891). Das Gebiss von *Didelphys*, ein Beitrag zur Entwicklungsgeschichte des Beuteltiergebisses. *Anat. Anz.* **6**, 658–666.

LESTER, K. S. (1969). The unusual nature of root formation in the molar teeth of the laboratory rat. *J. Ultrastruct. Res.* **28**, 481–506.

MAYER, R. (1969). Recherches au sujet de l'appareil masticateur des Lagomorphes. *Bull. Group Int. Rech. Sc. Stomat.* **12**, 295–333.

MOSS-SALENTIJN, L. (1975). Vestigial lacteal incisor teeth in the rat. *Acta anat.* **92**, 329–350.

OOË, T. (1965). A study of the ontogenetic origin of human permanent tooth germs. *Okaj. Fol. Anat. Jap.* **40**, 429–437.

OWENS, P. D. A. (1974). A light microscopic study of the development of the roots of premolar teeth in dogs. *Archs oral Biol.* **19**, 525–539.

PETERS, S. and STRASSBURG, M. (1967). Zur Morphogenese der Zahnleiste. Histologische und entwicklungsphysiologische Untersuchungen über die frühesten Differenzierungsphasen der Zahnleiste beim Kaninchen. *Dt. Zahnärztl. Z.* **22**, 346–356.

PETERS, S. and STRASSBURG, M. (1969). Zur frage der ersten Dentition bei Kaninchen und Maus. *Z. Säugetierk.* **34**, 91–97.

POUCHET, G. and CHABRY, L. (1884). Cited by Woodward, M. F. (1894). *Anat. Anz.* **9**, 619–631.

ROMANOFF, A. L. (1960). "The Avian Embryo". McMillan N.C.

ROMER, A. S. (1966). "Vertebrate Paleontology," 3rd edition. University of Chicago Press, Chicago.

RÖSE, C. (1892a). Beiträge zur Zahnentwicklung der Edentaten. *Anat. Anz.* **7**, 495–512.

RÖSE, C. (1892b). Ueber rudimentäre Zahnanlagen der Gattung Manis. *Anat. Anz.* **7**, 618–622.

RÖSE, C. (1892c). Ueber die Zahnentwicklung der Beuteltiere. *Anat. Anz.* **7**, 639–650.

RÖSE, C. (1892d). Ueber die Zahnentwicklung der Beuteltiere. *Anat. Anz.* **7**, 693–707.

RÖSE, C. (1892e). Ueber die Zahnleiste und die Eischwiele der Sauropsiden. *Anat. Anz.* **7**, 748–758.

SANTONÉ, P. (1935). Studien über den Aufbau, die Struktur und die Histiogenese der Molaren der Säugetiere. 1. Molaren von *Cavia cobaya*. *Z. mikrosk.-anat. Forsch.* **37**, 49–100.

STRASSBURG, M., PETERS, S. and EITEL, H. (1971). Zur Morphogenese der Zahnleiste. 2. Histologische Untersuchungen über die frühesten Differenzierungsphasen der Zahnleiste bei der Maus. *Dt. Zahnärztl. Z.* **26**, 52–57.

SYCH, L. (1971). Results of the Polish–Mongolian palaeontological expeditions. Part III. Mixodontia, a new order of mammals from the Paleocene of Mongolia. *Palaeontol. Pol.* **25**, 147–158.

WILSON, J. T. and HILL, J. P. (1896). Observations upon the development and succession of the teeth in Perameles: together with a contribution to the discussion of the homologies of the teeth in marsupial animals. *Q. J. microsc. Sci.* **47**, 427–588.

WILSON, R. W. (1949). Early tertiary rodents of North America. *Contr. Paleont. Carnegie Instit. Wash. Publ.* **584**, 67–164.

WOOD, A. E. (1940). The Mammalian Fauna of the White River Oligocene. 3. Lagomorpha. *Trans. Amer. Phil. Soc. N.S.* **28**, 3, 271–362.

WOOD, A. E. (1962). The early Tertiary Rodents of the family Paramyidae. *Trans. Am. Phil. Soc. N.S.* **52**, 1, 1–261.

WOODWARD, M. F. (1894). On the milk dentition of the Rodentia with a description of a vestigial milk incisor in the mouse (*Mus musculus*). *Anat. Anz.* **9**, 619–631.

ZIEGLER, A. C. (1971a). A theory of the evolution of therian dental formulas and replacement patterns. *Q. Rev. Biol.* **46**, 226–249.

ZIEGLER, A. C. (1971b). Dental homologies and possible relationships of recent Talpidae. *J. Mammal.* **52**, 50–68.

3. The Role of the Inner Dental Epithelium in the Formation of the Teeth in Fish

R. P. SHELLIS

M. R. C. Dental Unit,
Bristol, England

INTRODUCTION

In the tetrapods, the principal function of the inner dental epithelium (i.d.e.) is the production of enamel. The dental papilla, rather than the dental epithelium, appears to be responsible for the primary determination of tooth shape (Kollar and Baird, 1969). Nevertheless, the epithelium has an important role in morphogenesis because the distribution and thickness of enamel determine the external shape of the crown.

The available evidence indicates that the coelacanth, *Latimeria chalumnae*, possesses true enamel (Miller, 1969; Grady, 1970; R. P. Shellis and D. F. G. Poole, unpublished). A layer of enamel has also been reported on the teeth of the lungfishes *Ceratodus* by Peyer (1968) and *Lepidosiren* by Schmidt (Schmidt and Keil, 1971). In these fish, therefore, the i.d.e. presumably has the same functions as in tetrapods. The crossopterygians and dipnoans are, however, exceptional. In the vast majority of fish, the place of enamel on the teeth is taken by a tissue known as enameloid (Ørvig, 1967; Poole, 1967) which resembles enamel in being hard, shiny and highly mineralized but differs from it in its finer structure and in its mode of formation.

Enamel formation begins after a thin layer of dentine has been laid down. The protein matrix of enamel has a unique amino acid composition and can be regarded as a gel-like material which is not highly ordered like fibrous proteins such as collagen and keratin (Eastoe, 1965). Even in the early stages of enamel formation, the matrix contains some mineral, the content of which increases progressively with time with concomitant loss of protein and water. The ameloblasts are initially concerned with synthesis and secretion of enamel matrix but, after this has reached its full thickness, the ameloblasts differentiate into cells concerned with resorption of water and protein from, and transfer of mineral to, the maturing enamel (Reith, 1970).

Enameloid forms in a rather different fashion. The matrix of the tissue is laid down at the beginning of tooth development, before any dentine appears. This matrix grows inwards, away from the i.d.e., and contains collagen, which is clearly secreted by the odontoblasts. Only after it has been fully formed does the matrix of enameloid start to mineralize and only then does dentine make its appearance. The mineralization of enameloid entails the loss of all or part of the collagen from the matrix and this distinguishes enameloid from hard tissues such as dentine and bone, where all of the collagen is retained in the mature state. Nevertheless, because of its mode of formation and because of the presence in the matrix of collagen, most workers have regarded enameloid as a form of modified dentine, implying that it is formed entirely by the odontoblasts (see Poole, 1967; Peyer, 1968; Schmidt and Keil, 1971). However, the i.d.e. cells associated with forming enameloid show marked cytological changes (loc. cit.). Because previous work has been almost entirely histological, the significance of these changes and the function of the i.d.e. in enameloid formation have not been elucidated. Solution of these problems is essential if we are to understand the evolutionary origins of true enamel.

In this chapter an outline will be presented of the results of studies of tooth development in fish, using the electron microscope and other techniques. The emphasis will fall on the teleosts, which have been studied more closely than the elasmobranchs. Some of the work has been published previously (Shellis and Miles, 1974; Shellis, 1975) and some of the remainder will be reported in more detail elsewhere.

ENAMELOID FORMATION

The various forms of enameloid can be grouped under three broad headings: cap enameloid, which constitutes the tooth tip in teleosts; collar enameloid, which forms a layer of very variable thickness on the sides of the teeth in teleosts; and elasmobranch enameloid, which, although varying in structure between species, is always uniform in structure within any given species and forms a layer thickest at the functional regions of the tooth, thinning off towards the base. Of these forms of enameloid, the cap enameloid of teleosts seems to be most like true enamel in hardness and degree of mineralization, and the formation of this tissue will be considered first.

Cap Enameloid (Teleosts)

Under the electron microscope, it is seen that in a very young tooth germ, the cells of the inner dental epithelium are short and undifferentiated. As the matrix of the cap enameloid forms, the adjacent i.d.e. cells become tall and acquire the cytology of cells engaged in the synthesis and secretion of protein (Fig. 1). The rough endoplasmic reticulum and Golgi apparatus become

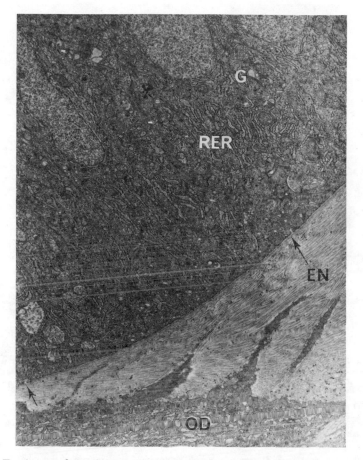

Fig. 1. Tooth germ from the common eel *Anguilla anguilla*, during the formation of the matrix of cap enameloid (EN): electron micrograph of part of the inner dental epithelium. The cells are polarized, the nuclei lying away from the matrix. The cytoplasm contains a large Golgi complex (G) and abundant rough endoplasmic reticulum (RER). Vesicles are seen opening at the cell surfaces in a number of places (arrows). The odontoblasts (OD) have a similar cytology to the i.d.e. cells. × 9000.

highly developed and vesicles are to be seen opening at the surface of the cells near the matrix. This phase of the differentiation of the i.d.e. cells proceeds in parallel with the differentiation of the mesenchymal cells of the papilla into odontoblasts, which are also engaged in protein secretion. The ultrastructural evidence suggests that the odontoblasts produce the collagen component of the matrix, while the i.d.e. secretes additional protein.

After the onset of mineralization of the tooth cap, the odontoblasts are engaged in the formation of dentine. Interesting cytological changes occur in the i.d.e. cells in association with mineralization of the cap. The organelles

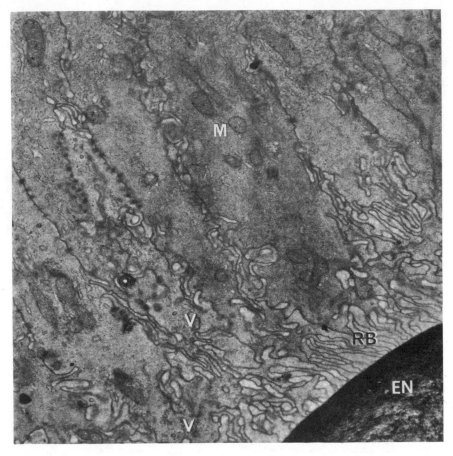

FIG 2. Tooth germ from the common eel, during mineralization of the cap enameloid. Electron micrograph of the i.d.e. cells, which at this stage possess a ruffled border (RB) and contain mainly mitochondria (M) and vesicles (V). × 11 500.

associated with secretion become much reduced and the i.d.e. cells at this stage contain mainly mitochondria, lysosome-like bodies and vesicles (Fig. 2). At the pole next to the mineralizing enameloid, the cell membrane is deeply folded to form a ruffled border. Similar features have been reported in ameloblasts during the later stages of enamel formation in both mammals (see Reith, 1970, for summary) and amphibians (Meredith Smith and Miles, 1971). Mineralization of cap enameloid entails the almost complete loss of the matrix protein, including the collagen, and it seems certain that the protein is extruded from the enameloid, transported into the inner dental epithelial cells by way of the ruffled border and broken down enzymatically inside the cells. In addition, mineral salts in large quantities probably enter the enameloid across the ruffled border at the same time.

Experiments with autoradiography (Shellis and Miles, 1974) have confirmed that the i.d.e. cells secrete matrix protein and have shed light on the properties of the protein. If tritiated proline is injected into teleost fish, newly secreted, labelled protein is detected after 1–2 h in the matrix of cap enameloid next to both the odontoblasts and the i.d.e. At first, the protein of epithelial origin is concentrated near the epithelium but, over a few days, it becomes uniformly distributed throughout the matrix. In contrast, the collagen secreted by the odontoblasts is laid down as a discrete band which persists throughout the experimental period. The diffusive behaviour of the epithelial protein resembles that of newly secreted enamel proteins in mammals (see Greulich and Slavkin, 1965, for summary) and suggests that the protein is relatively labile.

Histochemical studies of cap enameloid matrix show, in tests for amino acids, a high reactivity compared to dentine, especially with methods for tyrosine (Fig. 3), tryptophan and cystine. The results suggest further similarity

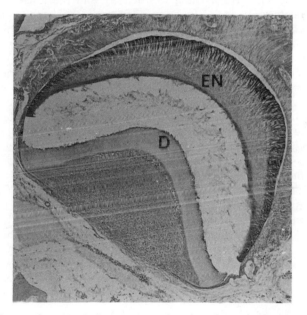

FIG. 3. Tooth germ from the ballan wrasse *Labrus bergylta*, stained with a histochemical method to demonstrate tyrosine. Note the intense reaction in the enameloid matrix (EN) compared to the dentine (D). × 560.

of the epithelial protein to the proteins of developing mammalian enamel (Shellis, 1975).

Collar Enameloid (Teleosts)

Autoradiography (Shellis and Miles, 1974) and electron microscopy reveal that the inner dental epithelium also secretes protein into the matrix of this tissue. This protein is not detected in histochemical tests for amino acids (Shellis, 1975) and is probably present in a lower concentration in collar enameloid than in cap enameloid.

Elasmobranch Enameloid

During enameloid matrix formation in elasmobranchs, the cells of the inner dental epithelium are columnar, their nucleoli are enlarged (Fig. 4) and the cytoplasm towards the enameloid is moderately rich in RNA (Fig. 6). These features suggest that the cells may be active at this stage in the formation and secretion of matrix protein. It may be significant that the cell size and abundance of cytoplasmic RNA are greatest in the regions where the enameloid reaches its greatest thickness.

The i.d.e. cells increase further in height during mineralization of the enameloid (Fig. 5). At the same time, most of the RNA is lost from the cytoplasm (Fig. 6), the cells stain less densely and the nuclei swell. These features indicate a change of function of the cells, perhaps towards matrix resorption and mineral secretion. The picture is complicated by a cycle of accumulation and subsequent loss of glycogen in the i.d.e. cells (see also Kerr, 1955), the significance of which is obscure.

The above suggestions as to the role of the i.d.e. in elasmobranchs are so far unconfirmed. Electron microscopical studies of the cells have not yet been carried out. An autoradiographic study of amino acid utilization similar to that carried out by Shellis and Miles (1974) revealed that the rates of protein synthesis and turnover by the i.d.e. cells are high, but did not yield conclusive evidence that the cells secrete matrix protein. The matrix became labelled more or less uniformly; epithelial and odontoblastic components could therefore not be separately identified (Fig. 7). The enameloid matrix gives weak reactions to histochemical tests for amino acids (Fig. 8). This suggests that the matrix is entirely collagenous but it must be pointed out that the epithelial component of collar enameloid is not histochemically demonstrable either and it is thus possible that an epithelial protein could be present in elasmobranch enameloid in small amounts. Levine *et al.* (1966) analysed mature shark enameloid protein and found it to resemble the protein of mature mammalian enamel rather than collagen in amino acid composition. This adds weight to the concept of the i.d.e. being involved in enameloid formation in this group.

Conclusions

In summary, it is concluded that, in the teleosts, the inner dental epithelium secretes protein into the matrix of enameloid and that it is also responsible for matrix resorption and mineral secretion during mineralization of the tissue. With respect to the elasmobranchs, some evidence points to the i.d.e. having a secretory role during matrix formation but further studies are needed to establish the functions of the i.d.e. in this group with more

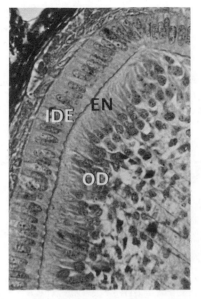

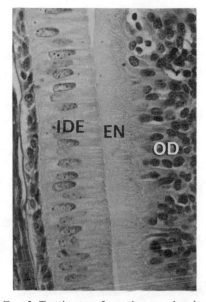

FIG. 4. Part of a tooth germ from the thorn-back ray, *Raia clavata*, showing the forming enameloid matrix (EN), the odontoblasts (OD) and the inner dental epithelium (IDE). The cells of the inner dental epithelium are columnar, with moderately-stained cytoplasm and prominent nucleoli. Heidenhaln's Azan. × 333.

FIG. 5. Tooth germ from the ray, showing the structure of the i.d.e. cells associated with mineralizing enameloid. The cells are taller than in Fig. 4 and show alterations in stainability and nuclear morphology. Masson's trichrome. × 333.

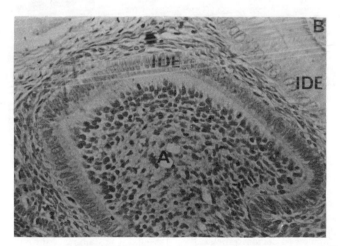

FIG. 6. Two tooth germs from the ray. In the left-hand germ (A) enameloid matrix is forming, while in the right-hand one (B) it is mineralizing. Section stained with methyl green-pyronin to demonstrate RNA. This substance is more abundant in the i.d.e. cells of the younger tooth germ than in those of the more advanced germ. × 210.

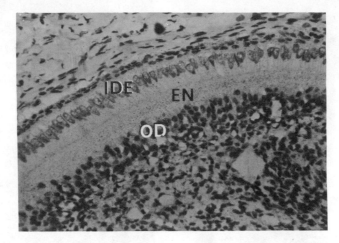

FIG. 7. Tooth germ from the ray, showing enameloid matrix forming. Autoradiograph after injection of ³H-proline. The inner dental epithelium (IDE) odontoblasts (OD) and enameloid are strongly labelled. The enameloid is more or less uniformly labelled and separate epithelial and odontoblastic components of the labelling cannot be identified. × 210.

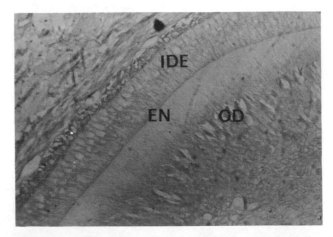

FIG. 8. Tooth germ from the ray, showing enameloid matrix forming. Section stained with histochemical method demonstrating carboxyl groups. The staining of the enameloid (EN) with this and other methods for protein groups is weak. × 210.

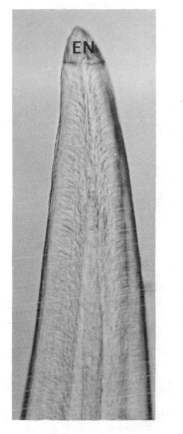

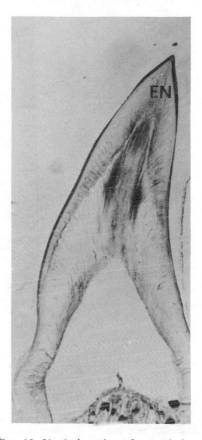

FIG. 9. Whole mount of tooth from the pike, *Esox lucius*, showing the small size of the cap of enameloid (EN). × 165.

FIG. 10. Vertical section of a tooth from the piranha, *Serrasalmus rhombeus*. The enameloid is very thick at the cutting edge (apex of section) and also covers most of the lateral surfaces of the tooth. × 40.

certainty. As a working hypothesis, however, it seems reasonable to believe that, in all fish possessing enameloid, the i.d.e. plays the same part in tooth formation.

In fish possessing enameloid, the i.d.e. does not influence the external shape of the tooth as the ameloblasts do in tetrapods. This is because any matrix protein they secrete does not form an outwardly growing layer on top of a preformed substratum of dentine. The epithelial enameloid protein mixes with a collagenous matrix which is laid down by the odontoblasts and which grows inwards. Therefore, in fish, the final shape of the tooth is exactly the same as that of the boundary between the odontoblasts and the i.d.e. at the start of tooth formation. However, the i.d.e. probably influences tooth morphology in a different way.

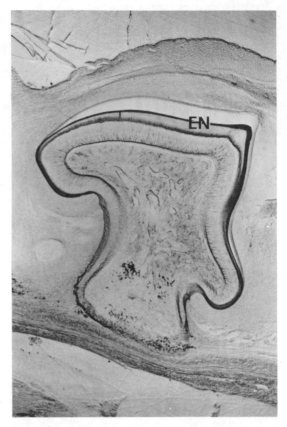

FIG. 11. Vertical section of a tooth from the thornback ray. The enameloid is thickest at the cutting edge and on the upper surface and thins off towards the base. × 57.

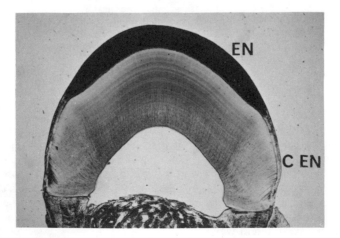

Among fish, the thickness and extent of enameloid and the relative volume of the tooth occupied by enameloid vary considerably from species to species. Systematic studies have not been carried out but, broadly speaking, these features seem to vary according to the function of the dentition. In fish such as the pike and the eel, where the teeth are used in prehension, the amount of enameloid is generally relatively small and it tends to be concentrated at the tip of the tooth (Fig. 9). Where the teeth of a predatory fish are employed as cutting and slicing organs, as in the sharks among the elasmobranchs and the piranha among the teleosts, the cutting edge is covered by a thick layer of enameloid and the tissue tends to be well-developed down the sides of the tooth (Fig. 10). Fishes living off hard materials such as corals and molluscs usually have, in some part of the mouth, flattened or rounded crushing teeth covered on the functional surface with a thick layer of enameloid (Figs 11, 12). In the rays (Fig. 11), the enameloid thins off on the sides of the tooth but in some of the teleosts of this category, collar enameloid reaches its greatest development and forms a substantial layer on the sides of the teeth (Fig. 12).

Assuming that all fish enameloid is formed in the same way as in teleosts, the tissue will arise in a matrix composed partly of collagen and partly of protein arising from the i.d.e. It has been postulated elsewhere (Shellis and Miles, 1974) that these two components interact in such a way that the collagen becomes labile during mineralization with the result that all or part of it can be removed from the tissue rather than remaining in place as it does in dentine, bone and cement. Since the matrix of enameloid is fully formed before undergoing any mineralization, it follows from this hypothesis that in any given tooth, the amount of enameloid and the relative proportions of enameloid and dentine will depend on the amount of collagenous matrix which has been laid down, and become infiltrated by, the epithelial protein at the moment when mineralization begins. This, in turn, will be determined by two factors: the timing of the onset of mineralization and, perhaps more importantly, by the rate and duration of the secretory activity of the cells of the i.d.e. relative to the rate of deposition of collagen by the odontoblasts. The i.d.e. would influence the distribution of enameloid on the tooth in a similar fashion.

ACKNOWLEDGEMENTS

The bulk of the work reported here was carried out for the degree of Ph.D. in the Department of Oral Pathology, London Hospital Medical College, London E1. I wish to thank Professor A. E. W. Miles, my supervisor and head of that Department, for his support and for many useful discussions. I am grateful to Mr J. E. Linder, Mr A. Churchland and Mr J. S. Hart for technical assistance and to Mr M. S. Gillett for preparing the figures.

FIG. 12. Vertical section of a tooth from *Sargus*, showing the extremely thick layer of cap enameloid (EN) and the well developed layer of collar enameloid (C EN) laterally. × 6.5.

REFERENCES

EASTOE, J. E. (1965). Recent studies on the organic matrices of bone and teeth. *In* "Bone and Tooth" (H. J. J. Blackwood, ed.), pp. 269–281. Pergamon Press, Oxford.

GRADY, J. E. (1970). Tooth development in *Latimeria chalumnae* (Smith) *J. Morph.* **132**, 337–388.

GREULICH, R. C. and SLAVKIN, H. C. (1965). Amino acid utilization in the synthesis of enamel and dentine matrices as visualized by autoradiography. *In* "The Use of Radioautography in Investigating Protein Synthesis" (C. P. Leblond and K. B. Warren, eds), Symposia of the International Society for Cell Biology, Vol. 4, pp. 121–132. Academic Press, New York and London.

KERR, T. (1955). Development and structure of the teeth of the dogfish, *Squalus acanthias* L. and *Scyliorhinus canicula* L. *Proc. zool. Soc. Lond.* **125**, 95–112.

KOLLAR, E. J. and BAIRD, G. E. (1969). The influence of the dental papilla on the development of tooth shape in embryonic mouse tooth germs. *J. Embryol. exp. Morph.* **21**, 131–148.

LEVINE, P. T., GLIMCHER, M. J., SEYER, J. M., HUDDLESTON, J. E. and HEIN, J. W. (1966). Noncollagenous nature of the proteins of shark enamel. *Science, N.Y.* **154**, 1192–1194.

MEREDITH SMITH, M. and MILES, M. (1971). The ultrastructure of odontogenesis in larval and adult urodeles: differentiation of the dental epithelial cells. *Z. Zellforsch. mikrosk. Anat.* **121**, 470–498.

MILLER, W. A. (1969). Tooth enamel of *Latimeria chalumnae* (Smith) *Nature, Lond.* **211**, 1244.

ØRVIG, T. (1967). Phylogeny of tooth tissues: evolution of some calcified tissues in early vertebrates. *In* "Structural and Chemical Organization of Teeth" (A. E. W. Miles, ed.), Vol. I, pp. 45–110. Academic Press, London and New York.

PEYER, B. (1968). *In* "Comparative Odontology" (R. Zangerl, trans. and ed.), pp. 114–115. Chicago University Press, U.S.A.

POOLE, D. F. G. (1967). Phylogeny of tooth tissues: enameloid and enamel in recent vertebrates, with a note on the history of cementum. *In* "Structural and Chemical Organization of Teeth" (A. E. W. Miles, ed.), pp. 111–149. Academic Press, London and New York.

REITH, E. J. (1970). The stages of amelogenesis as observed in molar teeth of young rats. *J. Ultrastruct. Res.* **30**, 111–151.

SCHMIDT, W. J. and KEIL, A. (1971). *In* "Polarizing Microscopy of Dental Tissues" (D. F. G. Poole and A. I. Darling, trans.), p. 244. Pergamon Press, Oxford.

SHELLIS, R. P. (1975). Histological and histochemical studies on the matrices of enameloid and dentine in teleost fishes. *Archs oral Biol.* **20**, 183–187.

SHELLIS, R. P. and MILES, A. E. W. (1974). Autoradiographic study of the formation of enameloid and dentine matrices in teleost fishes using tritiated amino acids. *Proc. R. Soc. Lond.* B. **185**, 51–72.

4. Development of the Structure of the Enamel of the Incisor Teeth in the Three Classical Subordinal Groups of the Rodentia

A. BOYDE

Department of Anatomy, University College London

INTRODUCTION

The organization of the prisms in the enamel of the incisors of rodents is sufficiently different between clear-cut representatives of the three suborders (Simpson, 1945) for a diagnosis of affinity to be made on the basis of the examination of a small fragment of this tissue alone (Tomes, 1850; Korvenkontio, 1934–1935). Since enamel is a "fossil" when it erupts, and is in any case the tissue least likely to be altered by fossilization processes, there is an attractive possibility for adding new information leading, perhaps, towards the solution of disputed taxonomic problems. Closer study of variability within species may show to what extent the measurable quantitative parameters may be relied upon. However, the purpose of this chapter is to describe certain qualitative aspects of the development and fine structure of the three major "types" of enamel found in the incisor teeth of hystricomorph, sciuromorph and myomorph rodents, respectively.

MATERIALS AND METHODS

Suborders

A list of the species from which material was obtained and studied in the present investigations is shown in Table I. That which was subjected to structural analysis only was preserved either by drying or by storing in 50–100% ethanol. Specimens for scanning electron microscopy (SEM) were prepared either by fracturing in longitudinal, transverse or oblique–transverse

A. BOYDE

directions, or by polishing and etching facets in the enamel. In most cases, the teeth were embedded in plastic (araldite, methyl methacrylate or poly-ester) to facilitate handling. The desired "planes of section" were exposed by grinding on successively finer grades of wet abrasive paper, using a binocular dissecting light microscope to control and vet progress. The

TABLE I

Species		Number after Morris (1965)	Number of animals	Satisfactory developing enamel surfaces	Good preservation of ameloblasts	
English name	Latin name				For LM and TEM	For SEM
Suborder SCIUROMORPHA						
Grey squirrel	*Sciurus carolinensis*	J 2	4	8	–	–
Finlayson's Siamese squirrel	*Callosciurus finlaysoni*	J 18	1	–	–	–
Bocourt's squirrel	*Callosciurus bocourti*	J 18	1	–	–	–
Prairie marmot	*Cynomys* sp.	J 31	1	–	–	–
Chipmunk	*Tamias striatus*	J 33	1	4	–	4
Smaller flying squirrel	*Pteromys* sp.	J 37	1	–	–	–
Suborder MYOMORPHA						
Common hamster	*Cricetus cricetus*	J 123	4	4	–	–
Smaller gerbil	*Gerbillus* sp.	J 158	1	–	–	–
Jird	*Meriones shawi*	J 165	4	16	–	–
Rat, various strains	*Rattus* sp.	J 207	50+	100	50	16
Mouse, various strains	*Mus* sp.	J 227	12	20	20	4
Arabian spiny mouse	*Acomys* sp.	J 241	2	8	–	8
Suborder HYSTRICOMORPHA						
Brush-tailed porcupine	*Atherurus* sp.	J 305	1	2	–	–
Guinea pig	*Cavia porcellus*	J 311	10	10	2	4
Capybara	*Hydrochoerus hydrochaeris*	J 317	1	–	–	–
Paca	*Cuniculus paca*	J 319	1	–	–	–
Viscacha	*Lagostomus*	J 323	1	–	–	–
Coypu	*Myocastor*	J 330	10	10	20	–

orientation of the prism lamellae can be seen at a magnification of $\times 40$–80, which is important, because, in so far as any standard section direction is required, this is one of them. After grinding to the chosen level and orientation, the facets were polished dry on a very fine abrasive paper. They were then etched for periods of from 20 to 60 s (most commonly 30 s) with 0.05 M H_3PO_4. Each specimen was treated individually and, after etching, was washed in distilled water and dried with Freon 13 gas from an aerosol cannister. Some preparations were stained with Harris haematoxylin before washing and drying; they were then examined by reflected light microscopy. For SEM the specimens were coated either with carbon and gold by vacuum evaporation as described by Boyde and Wood (1969) or with gold by sputtering in a 1·2 kV discharge in an argon atmosphere at 0·15 Torr (Figs 5, 10 and 11).

Developing enamel surface preparations were usually made using incisors dissected out from freshly killed animals. The enamel organ was dissected off with the aid of fine instruments and a thin stream of water. They were dried by the critical point method, air-drying from a volatile solvent or by freeze drying (Boyde and Wood, 1969; Figs 4, 6, 8 and 12).

For light microscopy and transmission electron microscopy (TEM) either 2·5% glutaraldehyde in 0·15 M cacodylate buffer was perfused through the aorta, or the growing incisor apices were dissected free and fixed by immersion. Post fixation was in 1% OsO_4. The specimens were embedded in 2:1 butyl:methyl methacrylate, araldite, Spurr's resin or Isopon.* Sections were cut on diamond knives at 0·5–2 μm for light microscopy (L/M) and 0·05–0·1 μm for TEM. L/M sections were stained with toluidine blue.

Preparations of ameloblasts retained in situ on the developing enamel surface were made in a variety of ways, but the most satisfactory and that which can be recommended to others was as follows: 1% OsO_4 in 0·15 M cacodylate buffer (pH 7·2) was perfused through the aorta after injecting heparin and sodium nitrite and flushing out the blood with the same cacodylate buffer. The osmic acid perfusion was continued intermittently for 1·5 h, following which a solution of 0·5% boric acid in 0·15 M cacodylate (pH 7·0) was used to wash out the osmium. This was followed by ethanol substitution through the same perfusion needle using 30, 50, 70, 80, 90 and 95% ethanol. The jaws were then removed and placed in several changes of absolute ethanol prior to substitution with Freon 113 in successive steps (25, 50, 75 and 100% Freon 113 in ethanol). They were then placed in the critical point bomb† which was filled with liquid CO_2 and left overnight to ensure displacement of the Freon 113. They were then dried by elevating the temperature of the bomb to 35°C. The critical point dried (CPD) specimens were then dissected dry under the binocular light microscope. In the ideal case, the incisor apex was removed with the enamel organ attached, the dental pulp dissected away and the dentine cut with the tip of a new hypodermic needle so that it would fracture easily in the desired, say longitudinal, plane (Fig. 9).

Three SEM models have been used in these studies—the Cambridge Scientific Instruments Stereoscan Marks 1, 600 and 4–10 operated at 10 kV. The TEMs used were Siemens Elmiskop I and Philips EM 300 operated at 60 or 80 kV.

* Isopon InterChemicals, Marylands Avenue, Hemel Hempstead, Herts, England.
† Polaron Ltd., Holywell Industrial Estate, Watford, Herts, England.

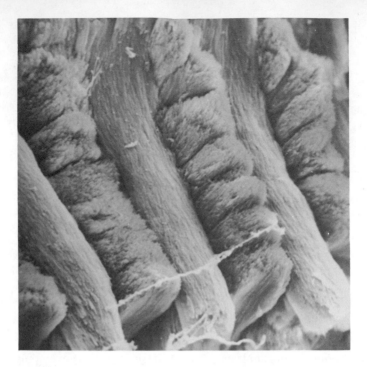

FIG. 1. Longitudinal fracture of grey squirrel lower incisor inner enamel. The break is parallel with one set of prisms and transverse to the alternating rows. Note the absence of an obvious interprismatic phase. EDJ bottom, enamel surface top. SEM. Width of field 20 μm.

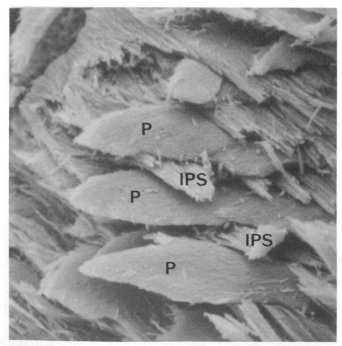

FIG. 2. Obliquely fractured chipmunk upper incisor external enamel. Prisms (P) are separated by interprismatic sheets (IPS) of crystallites which run perpendicularly to the enamel surface which just shows in the top left hand corner of the field. SEM. Width of field 14 μm.

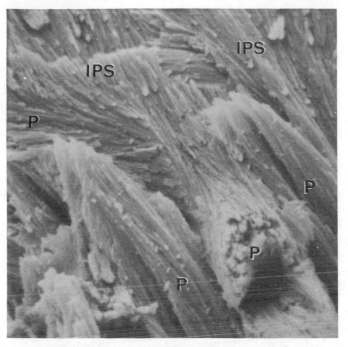

FIG. 3. Longitudinal fractured chipmunk upper incisor showing region of transition from inner (bottom right) to outer enamel (top left). In the inner enamel of sciuromorphs practically all the crystallites can be assigned to prisms. In the transitional zone, roughly half of them bend through approx. 45° to run perpendicular to the surface in the inter-prismatic sheets (IPS) which are present in the outer layer; the other half bend incisally and longitudinally and continue as prisms (P). SEM. Field width 14 μm.

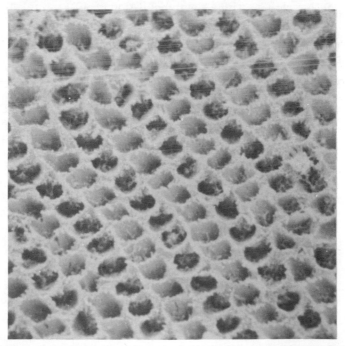

FIG. 4. Surface of developing inner enamel of chipmunk lower incisor showing alternate rows of Tomes' process (ameloblast) pits entering the surface in opposite directions. SEM. Field width 34 μm.

RESULTS

The SEM preparations have been the most significant in terms of being able to understand the complex three-dimensional organization of rodent incisor enamel (see also Boyde, 1969b). Both fractured preparations and those which have been polished and etched reveal structural features, and characteristic appearances are easily related to the orientation and position within the whole specimen, because the latter is retained largely intact. Developing enamel surface preparations showing the pits caused and occupied by the Tomes' (secretory pole) processes of the ameloblasts have an especial value when trying to develop an understanding of this complex situation. The newly developed technique for the preservation of cells in such a condition that they may be dissected dry has played an important part in describing the behaviour of the enamel secretory cells—the ameloblasts. (This technique and the logic behind it is described in more detail elsewhere; see Boyde, 1975, and Fig. 9.)

Sciuromorpha

Structure. The present results confirm those of Tomes (1850) and Korven-kontio (1934–1935) with respect to the pattern of organization of the enamel of the species studied. The prisms decussate in an inner layer which amounts to about one-half of the enamel layer, which is itself very thin in comparison both with the size of the teeth and when compared with absolute values for the thickness of the enamel in the other groups of Rodentia. The decussating layers, lamellae or zones of prisms are one prism wide, and appear to stand at right angles—perhaps with a slight inclination (c. 10°) towards the incisal edge of the tooth—when viewed in longitudinal sections or surfaces (LS). The decussation angle between prisms in adjacent lamellae is roughly 90° (Fig. 1).

There is little structural change to define the mutual borders of prisms within one lamella (Fig. 1). Prisms are nearly parallel bundles of crystals. Prisms in adjacent lamellae are clearly distinguished from one another by the fact that the crystals that they contain are oriented at 90° to each other. In the inner enamel, therefore, all the crystals can be assigned to prismatic bundles. If any interprismatic phase is present, it is exceedingly sparse.

In the outer half of the enamel, roughly half the crystals continue as prisms which incline outwards towards the surface and longitudinally towards the incisive edge (incisally). They all have the same orientation so that there is no decussation. There is a well marked interprismatic phase in the outer enamel, which is formed from crystal bundles and sheets continuous with those in the prisms of the inner enamel. These bend through roughly 45° to course through the gaps between the prisms straight towards the tooth surface (Figs 2 and 3).

Developing surface. These are two main zones to be seen at the developing enamel surface corresponding to the decussating inner layer and the "longitudinal" outer layer. Tracing the pattern incisally from the naked surface of the dentine, the first enamel is evidently secreted between the Tomes' processes so as to form a roughly hexagonal grid over the surface of the dentine. This honeycomb rapidly changes form to show transversely oriented rows of pits with common inter-row walls. The pits enter the surface obliquely and in opposite directions in alternate rows (Fig. 4). The prisms in the internal enamel develop between two ameloblasts, though with a strongly predominant component derived from one of these two cells. This accounts for the absence of an "interprismatic phase" between prisms in one row or lamella. If any sparse interprismatic phase forms it is in relation to the common inter-row, inter-pit walls.

The total length of the developing enamel is very short compared with that seen in myomorph rodents. Roughly half-way along it there is found a transitional zone, where the pits change their direction of entry into the surface (i.e. the ameloblasts change the direction in which they are moving "away" from the surface). Beyond the transitional zone the pits enter the surface from incisal towards apical. The predominating surface appearance is one of narrow longitudinal clefts (the pits). The aspect ratio of these pits is generally greater than 3:1, and their centres are much wider than their tapered ends so that it is difficult to see whether they are organized as rows in one or the other direction. However, the fact that such a high proportion of the total free developing surface is occupied by the inter-pit wall (between Tomes' processes rather than at the end of Tomes' processes) component accounts for the relative abundance of the interprismatic phase in the external layer; the latter contains crystals which grow perpendicular to that surface, which is nearly perpendicular to the surface of the tooth. The crystals in the prisms in the outer zone are roughly parallel with those prisms.

Ameloblasts. The SEM preparations of ameloblasts retained on the developing enamel surface show that transverse rows of cells (corresponding to the transverse rows of pits seen in the developing inner-enamel surface preparations) may be seen just before the honeycomb of pits is evident on the surface of the future enamel–dentine junction (EDJ) and throughout that part in which decussation occurs. Seen in monocular LS views, the cells appear straight and normal to the enamel surface. They are slightly curved as seen in TS projections.

Myomorpha

Structure. The enamel is again organized into two layers; in the inner layer the prisms, in alternate one-prism-thick layers, decussate at roughly 90°, whereas in the external layer they are parallel to one another and inclined incisally (Fig. 5). However, in distinction to the squirrel-like condition, the inner layer occupies about 0·75 of the thickness of the enamel and the lamellae are inclined at angles of roughly 45° to the enamel–dentine junction (EDJ), and are more inclined in the lower than in the upper incisor. The prisms in the external layer are inclined even more strongly against the EDJ so as to lie typically within 15° of being parallel to it (Fig. 5). Thus far the description takes us no further than that of Tomes (1850) and Korvenkontio (1934–1935). These authors both noted that the margins of the prisms in the internal enamel of myomorph rodent incisors appeared serrated. The present SEM and TEM studies make it clear that this is due to the presence of a separate interprismatic phase. This is present as thin sheets or bundles of

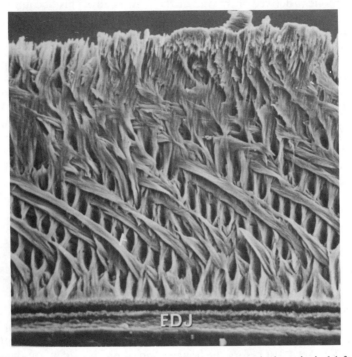

Fig. 5. H_3PO_4 etched longitudinal section of hamster lower incisor: incisal left, enamel surface top, EDJ bottom. In the inner enamel nearly transversely cut prisms have etched more rapidly because of exposure of ends of hydroxyapatite crystals. More longitudinally cut alternating prism rows expose sides of crystals to etching fluid and are removed correspondingly more slowly. Similarly, the interprismatic crystallite bundles which run vertically in this illustration, are more etch resistant. Note continuity of prisms in the approx. 45° tilted prism rows in inner enamel with prisms running at a very shallow angle to the surface in the outer enamel. SEM. Field width 85 μm.

often comparatively strongly curved crystals which penetrate the gaps between the decussating layers of prisms.

There are thus three groups of crystals in the internal layer: namely, the right and left, alternately oriented, decussating prismatic bundles inclined at about 90° to each other, and the penetrating interprismatic slips oriented roughly perpendicular to the surface of the tooth. (From the developmental picture it will be seen that their mean orientation is 90° to the "plane" of the developing surface which is inclined at only a few degrees (say 3–5°) to the completed surface.)

In the external enamel layer, the prisms may show a slight convexity towards the surface, in contrast to the usually slightly concave course of the lamellae seen in longitudinal sections of the internal layer. They are separated by an abundant longitudinal interprismatic phase which is continuous with and contains crystals in the same basic orientation as the highly divided interprismatic phase in the internal enamel. Prisms in the inner-outer transition layer can be traced from one layer to the other (Fig. 5).

The greater thickness of the total enamel layer in myomorph rodents permits study of the most external part of the enamel in more detail and in more cases. The outermost layer of enamel consists of crystals all oriented perpendicular to the surface. A similar prism-free layer has been described in most mammalian enamels examined and is the consequence of the loss of the secretory pole (Tomes') processes at the end of amelogenesis (Boyde, 1964, 1971).

Developing surface. Proceeding incisally from the naked dentine, the future EDJ surface, the first enamel deposited is again organized as a hexagonally packed inter-Tomes' process honeycomb. An arrangement of transverse rows of pits soon takes over. The pits enter the surface obliquely from incisal towards apical—the reverse of the dynamic event of the movement of the ameloblasts— and also obliquely from opposite sides in alternate rows. This beautiful arrangement gives rise to a variety of appearances depending upon the angle from which the surface is viewed in the SEM (Fig. 6).

The interprismatic phase crystals grow in the inter-pit walls, i.e. in an inter-Tomes' process location, in parallel with the plane of the wall and normal to the plane of the developing surface, though with a distinct anti-incisal inclination. The course of individual crystals or small groups of crystals is sinusoidal —they incline to the right or left when growing in lateral inter-pit walls (i.e. when passing between prisms in one lamella) and normal to the surface when growing in incisal-apical inter-pit walls (i.e. when passing from one lamella to the next; see Fig. 7). The prismatic crystals form in relation to single ameloblasts, the single pits filling in from the apical-lateral corners, starting from the corner opposite to the side to which the prisms in the lamella are inclined.

Double rows of pits, as well as rows which end well away from any edge of the developing enamel surface are commonly found in both myomorph and sciuromorph developing inner-enamel surfaces. The existence of these features in both groups implies that ameloblasts and their related prisms may change course in the centre of the developing inner enamel so that they switch from one lamella to the next, and that occasional portions of double lamella will be intercepted in longitudinal sections. In one LS of a mandibular incisor of a 25-day-old rat, the frequency of abnormal lamellae, including part lamellae and partly and wholly doubled lamellae, was 48 per 256, which is equivalent to 3 in every 16.

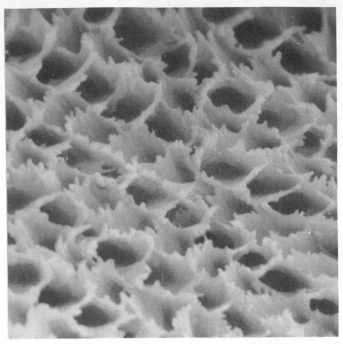

FIG. 6. Developing inner enamel surface of *Meriones shawi* upper incisor, showing alternating transverse rows of Tomes' process pits which enter from alternate sides as well as obliquely from incisal, thus mirroring the movement-during-secretion of the ameloblasts. This is the pattern found in all the myomorph rodents studied in the present series. SEM. Field width 23 μm.

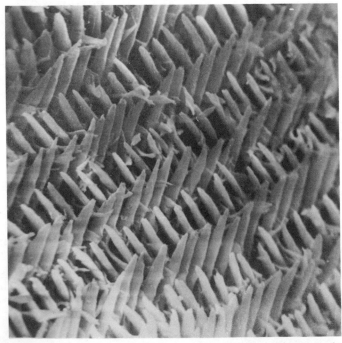

FIG. 7. Developing rat lower incisor inner enamel etched with a combination of trypsin and EDTA (a chelating, calcium phosphate solubilizing agent) to reveal the subsurface developing prisms—these are partially destroyed, but the preparation shows the orientation of the alternating transverse rows. SEM. Field width 40 μm.

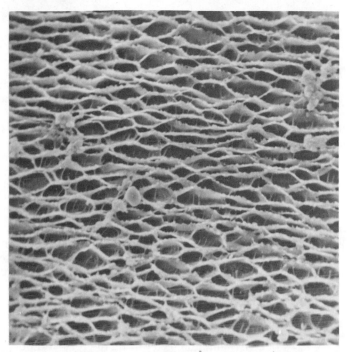

FIG. 8. *Meriones*, developing outer channel surface of upper incisor showing typical appearance found in all rodents, with only minor and probably insignificant differences between suborders. Incisal is to right of this field. Note very oblique entry of pits (exit of ameloblasts which caused them) from right to left. SEM. Field width 66 µm.

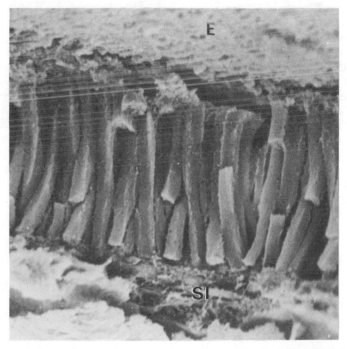

FIG. 9. Rat lower incisor ameloblasts opposite forming inner enamel surface. OsO₄ perfusion fixation; boric acid post-treatment; critical point dried; dissected dry. Note decussating alternate transverse rows of ameloblasts. SEM. Field width 90 µm.

The transitional zone between obviously decussating transverse rows of pits (corresponding to the last of the internal enamel) and obviously longitudinally inclined pits of the external enamel is several pits wide. The incisal portion corresponding to the development of the external layer is hardly to be distinguished between the three groups except that the narrow clefts in the surface which show the location of the Tomes' processes have even higher aspect ratios in the myomorphs than in the sciuromorphs or hystricomorphs. The proportion of the most superficial plane occupied by the inter-pit walls phase is high in all species studied and accounts for the abundant longitudinal sheet type interprismatic phase (Fig. 8).

Ameloblasts. The preparations of osmium fixed, boric acid post-treated critical-point-dried ameloblasts *in situ* show that they are organized as transverse rows opposite those portions of the developing surface which show transverse rows of pits. These rows may be recognized at all levels through the ameloblast layer, i.e. from the junction with the stratum intermedium to the Tomes' processes, and in all appropriate breaks or planes of section. The long axes of the ameloblasts are nearly parallel, but the cells curve slightly and in alternate directions in the alternate rows (Fig. 9).

Transverse rows of cells cannot be seen during the formation of the outer layer of the enamel. The cells may be curved, but they are all, within a limited area, curved in the same sense.

Hystricomorpha

Structure. The enamel of the incisor teeth of hystricomorphis is quite distinct from that of the myomorphs and sciuromorphs. It is again divided into two layers, with prism decussation present only in the internal layer and a strong incisal inclination in the outer layer. As already intimated, there is little to distinguish the structure and development of the outer layer of the enamel between the three groups. The decussating lamellae of prisms in the inner layer are inclined incisally as in the myomorphs, but they are several, typically 3 to 5, prisms wide. A plentiful interprismatic phase is present in both the internal decussating layer and the external layer (Figs 10 and 11): the arrangement of the prisms as longitudinal rows separated by longitudinal inter-row sheets of interprismatic crystals (Pattern 2 in Boyde, 1964) can usually be clearly seen in both inner and outer enamel. The mean orientation of the interprismatic crystals in both layers is perpendicular to the plane of the developing surface, with but little deviation from this mean in the outer layer. The interprismatic crystals in the inner layer form divided sheets whose parts incline to one side or the other according to the lateral inclination of the lamella in which they are sandwiched at a particular level. Any particular group of interprismatic crystals passes from one lamella to the next and thus curves from side to side. This packing arrangement is apparently difficult to fill, and a high proportion of crystal-free spaces—evidently the "cells" of Tomes (1850) and the Räumchen or Kanälchen of Korvenkontio (1934–1935)—characterizes hystricomorph enamel. These spaces are best seen in TEM pictures of thin

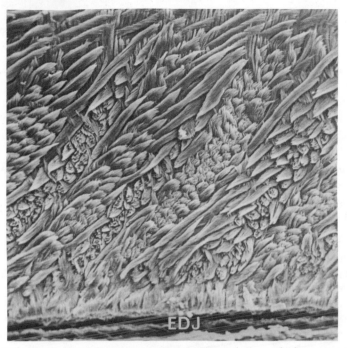

Fig. 10. H_3PO_4 etched longitudinal section of guinea pig lower incisor enamel. Tooth surface top, EDJ at bottom of field. Note zones are a few prisms wide and that these prisms are continuous with those in the external layer towards the top of the field. The orientation of the interprismatic crystals is the same in the inner and outer layers, running vertically in this figure. SEM. Field width 100 μm.

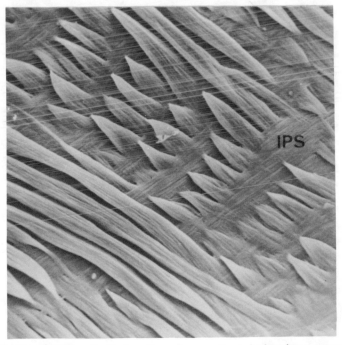

Fig. 11. H_3PO_4 etched longitudinal section of coypu lower incisor inner enamel. In this species, the interprismatic crystals form more clearly marked sheets (IPS) which have a marked anti-incisal inclination. Incisal is left, and the lower edge of the field is parallel with the EDJ. SEM. Field width 50 μm.

sections of immature enamel (see, for example, Fig. 24, p. 173 of Boyde, 1969b).

The continuity of prisms in the inner and outer enamel layers as well as that of the interprismatic phase in these layers at the junction between the two layers can be easily demonstrated in suitable fractured or polished and etched preparations in the SEM (Fig. 10).

Developing surface. The first enamel "honeycomb" formed on the future enamel–dentine junction dentine surface resembles that seen in the other rodent groups and, for that matter, other mammalian orders. The size of the elements of the honeycomb is smaller in the rodents, however (Boyde, 1969a).

The part of the developing enamel surface corresponding to the formation of the internal layer shows longitudinal inter-pit, inter-row walls of a classical Pattern 2 type (Boyde, 1964). The interprismatic sheets evidently form in this location. The bridges that divide the longitudinal troughs into separate pits may not reach to the level of the tops of the walls of the troughs. Each prism in a longitudinal row is formed predominantly by one ameloblast, with a small contribution (to its apical side) from the next cell.

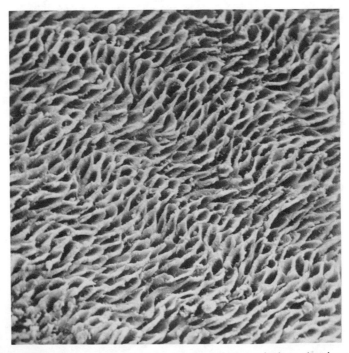

FIG. 12. Developing inner enamel surface of guinea pig lower incisor, showing transverse (top left to bottom right) zones of pits, some 3 to 5 pits wide, facing in alternating directions. SEM. Field width 100 μm.

The pits enter the surface obliquely from incisal towards apical and also from one side or the other according to their location in zones which are usually from 3 to 5 pits wide (Fig. 12).

Ameloblasts. I have not so far been able to demonstrate the existence of the 3 to 5 cell wide rows corresponding to the evident organization of the pits in preparations of hystricomorph incisors with ameloblasts retained on the developing enamel surface.

DISCUSSION

From the examples studied, it is clear that at least three clearly definable patterns of enamel development exist during the formation of the inner layer of the enamel of rodent incisors and that there is a strong correlation between developmental and structural findings. I feel that this evidence is so strong that we may now draw implications from the one regarding the other. If we see the developing inner enamel surface alone then we will know which characteristic structural pattern will form below it; and if we have determined the structural pattern we may develop a picture of what the surface was like during development. We therefore have a basis for future studies of other, even rather fragmentary, rodent incisor material which may assist in the solution of certain classification problems regarding mutual interrelationships in rodent groups.

The organization of the ameloblasts corresponding to the formation of the three types of inner enamel described here is interpreted as indicative of the movement-during-secretion of these cells. The course of the prisms is defined by the course through which the ameloblasts move during the formation of the enamel. The relative arrangements of the prisms are defined by relative movements of neighbouring ameloblasts. It therefore appears that the structure of enamel is determined by factors related to cell movement and/or selective release of secretory product from specialized locations on the surface of the secretory poles of the ameloblasts—these locations corresponding to areas where the relative sliding or shear movement between the surface of the cell and the surface of its secretory product is at a minimum (Boyde, 1964). Genetic factors evidently determine differences in cell behaviour patterns; local geometric factors must be excluded on the basis that the size and the shape of the incisor teeth of the members of these three groups are similar. The conclusion that genetic control of cell behaviour determines the enamel structure explains the strong taxonomic basis found for the structures described here.

SUMMARY

The fine structure of the enamel of the incisor teeth and the development of the structure have been studied in several rodent species all clearly falling within the three classical subordinal groups Sciuromorpha, Myomorpha and Hystricomorpha (Simpson, 1945). The methods used included light microscopy, transmission electron microscopy and scanning electron microscopy. The conclusions of Tomes (1850) and Korvenkontio (1934–1935) that there are basic arrangements of the enamel prisms corresponding to these three groups are confirmed, with the addition of fine structural details and developmental-mechanical explanations for the observed structures. The structure and development of the incisor enamel is very conservative, and it is concluded that it is controlled genetically through the pattern of behaviour of movement and secretion of the ameloblasts. Certain features of the incisor enamel are common to all rodents and not found in other orders—this confirms the unity of the order. The differences confirm the classical subdivisions of the order. Further studies of enamel histology should shed further light on disputed areas of the classification.

ACKNOWLEDGEMENTS

These studies have been indirectly supported by grants from the Medical Research Council and the Science Research Council. The author would like to thank Mrs Elaine Bailey and Mr Philip Reynolds for their technical assistance and Miss Joan Hymans for her secretarial assistance.

REFERENCES

BOYDE, A. (1964). The structure and development of mammalian enamel. Ph.D. thesis, University of London.

BOYDE, A. (1969a). Correlation of ameloblast size with enamel prism pattern: use of scanning electron microscope to make surface area measurements. *Z. Zellforsch.* **93**, 583–593.

BOYDE, A. (1969b). Electron microscopic observations relating to the nature and development of prism decussation in mammalian dental enamel. *Bull Group Int. Rech. Sc. Stomat.* **12**, 151–207.

BOYDE, A. (1971). The tooth surface. *In* "The prevention of periodontal disease" (Eastoe, J. E., Picton, D. C. A. and Alexander, A. G., eds), pp. 46–63. Henry Kimpton, London.

BOYDE, A. (1975). A method for the preparation of cell surfaces hidden within bulk tissue for examination in the SEM. *In* "Scanning Electron Microscopy/1975" (Johari, O., ed.), pp. 295–303. Illinois Institute of Technology Research Institute, Chicago.

BOYDE, A. and WOOD, C. (1969). Preparation of animal tissues for surface-scanning electron microscopy. *J. Microscopie* **90**, 221–249.

KORVENKONTIO, V. A. (1934–1935). Mikroskopische Untersuchungen an Nager-incisiven unter Hinweis auf die Schmelzstruktur der Backenzähne. Histologisch-phyletische Studie. *Annales zoologici Societatis zoologico-botanicae fennicae. Vanamo* **2**, 1.

MORRIS, D. (1965). "The mammals". Hodder and Stoughton, London.

SIMPSON, G. G. (1945). The principles of classification and a classification of mammals. *Bull. Am. Mus. nat. Hist.* **85**, 1–350.

TOMES, J. (1850). On the structure of the dental tissues of the order Rodentia. *Phil. Trans. Roy. Soc. Lond.* **140**, 529–567.

5. Racial Traits in the Dentition of Living Skolt Lapps

PENTTI KIRVESKARI

Institute of Dentistry, University of Turku, Finland

INTRODUCTION

The population is the building block of species, and biologically the most meaningful taxon at the subspecies level. The common use of the term race in a wider sense makes the synonymous use of "population" and "race" impracticable. For instance, the terms geographical, local and micro-race (Garn, 1965) are more accurate and appropriate in the discussion about racial orgins of a given population. "Major race" and "racial stock" are often used instead of geographical race.

None of the better-known dental traits are race-specific. The existing differences are only differences in frequencies. While many trait frequencies vary from population to population only some of them show a clearly unequal distribution between geographical races. Which traits are "racial" must be determined purely empirically as long as the degree of heritability and mode of inheritance are unknown.

The heritability of tooth dimensions is better known than that of the non-metric traits (Lundström, 1948; Alvesalo and Tigerstedt, 1974). However, the range of variation of tooth size in geographical races is too large to be useful for taxonomic purposes. Differences in the raw data between populations are often significant (Selmer-Olsen, 1949), but generally useless in racial comparisons. The "crown-size profile pattern" has recently been demonstrated to be effective in distinguishing between populations (Garn *et al.*, 1968a), and its genetic basis has been demonstrated on related individuals (Garn *et al.*, 1968b).

The question of Lapp origins has long been open. Their dissimilarity from

* The non-metric part of this study is based on the author's doctoral thesis (Kirveskari, 1974).

the neighbouring populations is demonstrable in numerous ways. The present state of knowledge in this respect is comprehensively reviewed by Eriksson (1973). In view of the population bottlenecks and the long isolation the Lapps have survived (Lewin, 1971), we may expect their dental traits to show the original conditions better than the serological factors which are more susceptible to drift.

MATERIAL

Lapps belonging to the Skolt tribe were examined during the IBP–Human Adaptability studies in Finnish Lapland from 1967 to 1970. They numbered 515 in the 1967 census, and well over 90 % of them were examined at least once. Skolts are the eastern-most tribe of Lapps, and they have remained in isolation longer than the other tribes. Their genetic isolation as well as the genealogy of the individuals is well documented (Lewin, 1971). Although marriages between first cousins are very rare among Skolts, kinship in the ancestry of marriage partners is common, and the coefficient of inbreeding is relatively high (Vollenbruck et al., 1974).

Odontometric data for comparative purposes were taken from original literature: Swedes (Seipel, 1946); Norwegian Lapps (Selmer-Olsen, 1949); Medieval Danes (Lunt, 1969); and Finns (Alvesalo, 1970).

METHODS

Dental hard stone casts were made in the field according to standard methods. The casts were subsequently measured and visually examined in laboratory conditions. Only the right side of the dental arches was used for statistics. In cases of missing teeth observations on antimeres, if present, were accepted.

The mesiodistal diameter of the permanent teeth was measured with a sliding calliper according to Moorrees (1957), i.e. the greatest distance between the mesial and distal surface parallel to the occlusal and buccal surfaces. The reading accuracy was 0·05 mm. The T-scores of the crown-size profile patterns were calculated as described by Garn et al. (1968a), using the same reference population, namely Ohio Caucasians, for direct comparability of results. The coefficients of correlation are ordinary Pearsonian product–moment correlation coefficients for 14 pairs of T-scores.

The depth of the lingual fossa was measured at the deepest part of the fossa, at right angles to the surface, and on unworn teeth only. Modified dial gauges with a reading accuracy of 0·01 mm were used, but the readings were rounded off to the nearest 0·05 mm. The non-metric morphological traits were classified according to the standards in the Zoller Laboratory Plaque series (Dahlberg, 1956), whenever possible. The sixth and seventh cusp were classified according to the definitions and standard plaques by Turner II et al. (1969, 1970). The definitions of the deflecting wrinkle of the metaconid and the distal trigonid crest are given by Weidenreich (1937) and Hanihara (1961). These traits were only recorded as present or absent.

Results

Crown-size Profile Pattern

Comparisons of the crown-size profile pattern of Skolt Lapps to that of other Nordic populations is exemplified by five graphs in Fig. 1, and the coefficients of correlation are given in Table I. Medieval Danes and Norwegian Lapps showed patterns very similar to Skolts while Finns and Swedes proved different with considerably lower r_T values. Hybrid Skolts occupied an intermediate position.

TABLE I. Correlation coefficients of the crown-size profile patterns (expressed in T-scores relative to a standard) between Skolt Lapps and other Nordic populations.

	Boys	Girls
Skolt Lapps –Medieval Danes	0·91	0·87
–Norwegian Lapps	0·89	0·71
–Hybrid Skolt Lapps	0·65	0·58
–Swedes	0·49	0·47
–Finns	0·39	0·62

Shovel-shape

The distribution of shovel-shapedness in visual estimation is given in Table II. Fifty-one per cent of the maxillary lateral incisors and 56% of the central incisors were classified as "no shovel." Semi-shovel and shovel forms were rather uncommon, 10% in the lateral and 9% in the central incisor.

The depths of the lingual fossa are given in Table III. The lateral incisor averaged 0 39 mm and the central incisor 0·54 mm

TABLE II. Shovel-shape of maxillary incisors of Skolt Lapps.

	N	No Shovel n (%)	Trace Shovel n (%)	Semi-Shovel n (%)	Shovel n (%)
Lateral	200	101 (51)	79 (40)	18 (9)	2 (1)
Central	223	124 (56)	79 (35)	18 (8)	2 (1)

TABLE III. Depth of lingual fossa of maxillary permanent incisors in Skolt Lapps

	N	Mean Depth (mm)	s.d.	Mean Mesiodistal Diameter (mm)
Lateral	155	0·39	0·25	6·76
Central	173	0·54	0·27	8·68

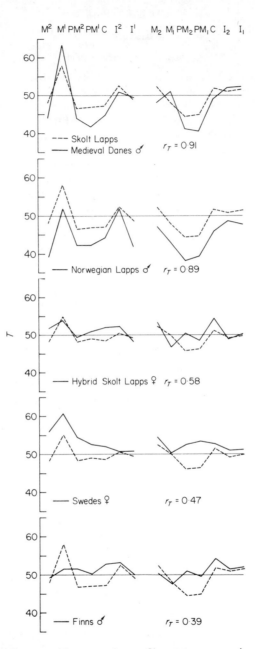

FIG. 1. Examples of sex-specific crown-size profile pattern comparisons. Ohio Caucasians (Garn *et al.*, 1968a) are used as the reference population. Mean $T = 50$, and the standard deviation of $T = 10$.

Carabelli Trait

The frequency of occurrence of the different expressions of the Carabelli trait is presented in Table IV. While 20 % of Skolts showed no trace of the trait, only 2 % possessed cusps. Protuberances without a free tip were present in 14 %, and pits or grooves in 64 %.

Cusp Number of Mandibular Molars

Cusp number of mandibular first and second molars is given in Table V. Four cusps occurred in 22 % of the first molars, and in 90 % of the second molars. Accessory cusps were ignored in counting these frequencies.

TABLE IV. Expressions of the Carabelli trait on the first permanent molar of Skolt Lapps.

N	Absent n (%)	Furrowed n (%)	Protuberance n (%)	Cusp n (%)
182	36 (20)	117 (64)	26 (14)	3 (2)

TABLE V. Number of cusps on mandibular first and second permanent molars of Skolt Lapps.

	N	5-Cusped n (%)	4-Cusped n (%)
M_1	133	104 (78)	29 (22)
M_2	143	15 (10)	128 (90)

Sixth and Seventh Cusp

The occurrence of accessory occlusal cusps the sixth and seventh cusp—on the mandibular first molar is presented in Table VI. A cuspoid expression of the sixth cusp was present in 7 % and of the seventh cusp in 5 %.

Protostylid

The different protostylid expressions of the mandibular first molar are given in Table VII. A buccal pit was present in 22 % while the trait was totally absent in 62 %. A slight prominence of the surface was present in 5 %, but no pronounced expressions were observed.

TABLE VI. Occurrence of sixth and seventh cusp on the mandibular first permanent molar of Skolt Lapps.

	N	Absent n (%)	Furrows only n (%)	Cusp n (%)
c6	113	100 (89)	5 (4)	8 (7)
c7	131	118 (90)	7 (5)	6 (5)

TABLE VII. Expressions of the protostylid on the mandibular first permanent molar of Skolt Lapps.

N	Absent		Pit		Deviation of Groove		Irregularity of Surface		Prominence		Prominence and Furrow		Cusp	
	n	(%)	n	(%)	n	(%)	n	(%)	n	(%)	n	(%)	n	(%)
104	64	(62)	23	(22)	4	(4)	8	(8)	5	(5)	0		0	

TABLE VIII. Occurrence of the deflecting wrinkle and the distal trigonid crest on the first permanent molar of Skolt Lapps.

	N	Absent n (%)	Present n (%)
Deflecting Wrinkle	39	30 (77)	9 (23)
Distal trigonid crest	39	39 (100)	0

Deflecting Wrinkle and Distal Trigonid Crest

Table VIII presents the frequency of occurrence of the distal trigonid crest and of the deflecting wrinkle of the metaconid. The former was not seen in Skolts at all, while the deflecting wrinkle occurred in 23 %.

DISCUSSION

The usefulness of comparing crown-size profiles of populations relative to a standard becomes evident when using sex- and tooth-specific T-scores instead of raw data. Garn et al. (1968a) conclude from their studies on 14 populations that the crown-size profile pattern comparisons provide a numerical measure of genetic similarity.

The almost identical pattern of Skolts and Norwegian Lapps was expected and the degree of similarity between Skolts and hybrid Skolts, Finns and Swedes was also within expectations. But it is very hard to find an explanation for the great similarity between Skolts and medieval Danes, as their genetic and environmental differences are well known. One might suspect that interproximal wear has something to do with the similarity. Modern Skolts eat mainly processed foods, and interproximal wear of their teeth is minimal. The teeth of medieval Danes were considerably more worn.

The Norwegian Lapp material consists of skulls from the eighteenth century. The difference in food quality and consistence that must be rather striking between Norwegian Lapps of the eighteenth century and modern Skolt Lapps did not obscure the similarity of their crown-size profile patterns. Analogically, the differences in measuring techniques are not helpful in solving the dilemma.

Recalling the similarity between Norwegian Lapp and Thule Eskimo patterns (Garn *et al.*, 1968a) and the fact that a difference of correlation coefficients of less than $0 \cdot 5$ in 14 pairs of scores is not statistically significant, one can but draw this conclusion: the crown-size profile pattern cannot be given much weight in racial comparisons. Garn *et al.* also make a reservation as to the taxonomic value of the crown-size profile pattern.

Shovel-shape of the anterior teeth is one of the most reliable traits in distinguishing between Mongoloid and other racial stocks (Hrdlička, 1920; Dahlberg, 1949; Tratman, 1950; Moorrees, 1957; Carbonell, 1963; Hanihara, 1967; Zubov, 1973: 101–104). In Hrdlička's four-degree scale the dividing line is best placed between the trace shovel and semi-shovel classes; trace shovel is not uncommon in Caucasoid populations while semi-shovel and shovel are. The latter are a little more frequent in Skolts than is usual in Caucasoid populations, but the frequency is within the Caucasoid range. This result is unmistakably the same in the comparison of the depths of the lingual fossae: Skolts have a slightly larger mean depth of fossa than Caucasoid populations in general, while Mongoloid populations show considerably deeper fossae.

A high frequency of Carabelli's cusp is commonly accepted as a Caucasoid racial trait. It also seems that a relatively high frequency of total lack of the trait is typical of the Caucasoid race. A high frequency of intermediate or "negative" expressions (pits and grooves) together with a low frequency of the absence of the trait is typical of the Mongoloid race (Kraus, 1959). The very low frequency of Carabelli's cusps in Skolts is particularly conspicuous, and possibly speaks of genetic drift during the long isolation. On the whole, the distribution of the expressions is clearly reminiscent of that of Mongoloid populations.

Cusp number of lower molars has proven a rather powerful discriminator between the Caucasoid and other races. The fissure pattern is commonly reported together with the cusp number, but it is the latter that differs most between races (Jorgensen, 1955; Suzuki and Sakai, 1973). In spite of the inclusion of faint expressions of a cusp, Skolts showed a high degree of cusp number reduction. They undoubtedly fall within the Caucasoid range in this respect.

The frequencies of the sixth and seventh cusp are difficult to use for comparative purposes because of the common lack of definitions. A standardized method is now available (Turner II *et al.*, 1969, 1970), and it was followed in the present study. The racial diagnostic value of the seventh cusp is unclear, perhaps excepting the American Negroes, who show an exceptionally high frequency (Hellman, 1928). The sixth cusp appears to be less common in Caucasoids than in other racial groups (Remane, 1960; Suzuki and Sakai, 1973).

Neither the seventh nor the sixth cusp was very common in Skolts, even if the faintest expressions were included. However, it is probable that the frequency of stronger expressions is better comparable with more previous reports. With this in mind, Skolts would appear to be closer to the Caucasoid than to the Mongoloid pattern.

In the evaluation of the protostylid expressions care was taken to include the low-degree expressions, and to exclude the paramolar cusps, as suggested by Dahlberg (1950). The interrelationship between the low-degree expressions (buccal pit and distal deviation of the buccal groove) and the strong expressions is not fully clear. Likewise, the racial distribution of the low-degree expressions in particular is poorly known. There is some indication, however, that the protostylid tends to be more common in the Mongoloid than in the Caucasoid populations (Hanihara, 1967). At this stage of knowledge about the protostylid it is perhaps fair to say only that Skolts seem to differ from both of the major stocks.

The deflecting wrinkle of the metaconid has received considerable attention as a racial trait in recent years (Suzuki and Sakai, 1956; Hanihara, 1961; Zubov, 1973: 144). It is commonly believed that Caucasoid populations show the deflecting wrinkle less often than other populations. However, the distribution of the trait is not too well known in populations other than Mongoloid. For instance, orthodontic patients in Gothenburg, Sweden, displayed the deflecting wrinkle in 29 % in a random sample of 70 individuals (Kirveskari, unpublished data). Nevertheless, in view of the data available in the literature, the frequency of the deflecting wrinkle in Skolts seems clearly higher than in Caucasoid populations in general.

The lack of an uninterrupted distal trigonid crest in Skolts was perhaps unexpected in view of the relatively high frequency of the deflecting wrinkle. These two traits are supposed to be morphologically related, but they do not seem to be so genetically. The lack of the crest conforms with the Caucasoid pattern; Mongoloids and some populations of India show frequencies of up to 46 % (Zubov, 1973: 142).

Drawing racial conclusions from the distribution of a single dental trait can be misleading. The use of trait complexes is more useful. However, the diagnostic value of each trait of a complex is not likely to be the same; therefore a simple count of 'Caucasoid" and "Mongoloid" traits may give a biased picture of the racial background of the population in question. It is also a fact that variations of trait frequencies are relatively well known only in the Mongoloid stock, including Eskimo and American Indian.

Summarizing, two "strong" or "reliable" traits, the shovel-shape of the anterior teeth and the reduction of mandibular molar cusps, occur in "Caucasoid" frequencies in Skolts. The low frequency of Carabelli's cusps can be interpreted as a "strong" Mongoloid trait. Of the "weaker" traits, the sixth cusp and the distal trigonid crest indicate Caucasoid, and the deflecting wrinkle Mongoloid affinities in Skolts. Their dental trait complex is clearly different from both of the major stocks, and calling Skolts (and other Lapps) a race of their own appears justified. If the origin of Skolts is traceable to one of the major stocks, their teeth suggest a Caucasoid origin.

SUMMARY

The permanent dentition of living Skolt Lapps from northern Finland is studied from a racial viewpoint. By means of the so-called crown-size profile pattern comparisons, odontometrics is shown to be of little value in tracing the racial origins of the population. Both the visual estimation of shovel-shape of the anterior teeth, and the metric depth of the lingual fossa place the Skolts close to the Caucasoids. Also the high degree of mandibular molar cusp reduction, low frequency of the sixth cusp and lack of the distal trigonid crest conform to the Caucasoid pattern. The very low frequency of Carabelli's cusp and the relatively high frequency of the deflecting wrinkle represent Mongoloid features in the Skolt dentition. They are judged to be different from both of the major races, but closer to the Caucasoids than to the Mongoloids.

REFERENCES

ALVESALO, L. (1970). The influences of sex-chromosome genes on tooth size in man. *Suom. Hammaslääk. Toim.* **67**, 1–54.

ALVESALO, L. and TIGERSTEDT, P. M. A. (1974). Heritabilities of human tooth dimensions. *Hereditas* **77**, 311–318.

CARBONELL, V. M. (1963). Variations in the frequency of shovel-shaped incisors in different populations. *In* "Dental Anthropology" (Brothwell, D. R., ed.), pp. 211–234. Pergamon Press, London.

DAHLBERG, A. A. (1949). The dentition of the American Indian. *In* "Papers on the Physical Anthropology of the American Indian" (Laughlin, W. S., ed.)' pp. 138–176. The Viking Fund, New York.

DAHLBERG, A. A. (1950). The evolutionary significance of the protostylid. *Am. J. phys. Anthrop.* **8**, 15–25.

DAHLBERG, A. A. (1956). "Materials for the establishment of standards of classifications of tooth characters, attributes and techniques in morphological studies of the dentition." Zoller Laboratory of Dental Anthropology, University of Chicago, U.S.A.

ERIKSSON, A. W. (1973). Genetic polymorphisms in Finno-Ugrian populations. *Israel J. med. Sci.* **9**, 1156–1170.

GARN, S. M. (1965). "Human Races." 2nd edition, pp. 12–22. Charles C. Thomas, Springfield, Illinois.

GARN, S. M., LEWIS, A. B. and WALENGA, A. J. (1968a). Crown-size profile pattern comparisons of 14 human populations. *Archs oral Biol.* **13**, 1235–1242.

GARN, S. M., LEWIS, A. B. and WALENGA, A. J. (1968b). Genetic basis of the crown-size profile pattern. *J. dent. Res.* **47**, 1190.

HANIHARA, K. (1961). Criteria for classification of crown characters of the human deciduous dentition. *Zinruigaku Zassi* **69**, 21–45.

HANIHARA, K. (1967). Racial characteristics in the dentition. *J. dent. Res.* **46**, 923–926.

HELLMAN, M. (1928). Racial characters in human dentition. *Proc. Am. phil. Soc.* **67**, 157–174.

HRDLIČKA, A. (1920). Shovel-shaped teeth. *Am. J. phys. Anthrop.* **3**, 429–465.

JØRGENSEN, K. D. (1955). The Dryopithecus pattern in recent Danes and Dutchmen. *J. dent. Res.* **34**, 195–208.

KIRVESKARI, P. (1974). Morphological traits in the permanent dentition of living Skolt Lapps. *Proc. Finn. dent. Soc.* **70**, Suppl. II.

KRAUS, B. S. (1959). Occurrence of the Carabelli trait in Southwest ethnic groups. *Am. J. phys. Anthrop.* **17**, 117–123.

LEWIN, T. (1971). Genealogy of the Skolt Lapps. *Suom. Hammaslääk. Toim.* **67**, Suppl. I, 55–62.

LUNDSTRÖM, A. (1948). "Tooth Size and Occlusion in Twins," 2nd edition. S. Karger, Basle and New York.

LUNT, D. A. (1969). An odontometric study of mediaeval Danes. *Acta odont. scand.* **27**, Suppl. 55.

MOORREES, C. F. A. (1957) "The Aleut Dentition." Cambridge, Massachusetts: Harvard University Press, Cambridge, Massachusetts.

REMANE, A. (1960). Zähne und Gebiss. *In* "Primatologia" (Hofer, H., Schultz, A. H. and Starck, D. eds), Handbuch der Primatenkunde III, pp. 637–846. S. Karger, Basle and New York.

SEIPEL, C. M. (1946). Variation of tooth position. *Svensk Tandläkare-Tidskrift* **39**, Suppl.

SELMER-OLSEN, R. (1949). An odontometrical study on the Norwegian Lapps. *Skrifter utgitt av Det Norske Videnskaps-Akademi i Oslo*, Mat.-Naturv. Klasse, No. 3.

SUZUKI, M. and SAKAI, T. (1956). On the "deflecting wrinkle" in recent Japanese. *Zinruigaku Zassi* **65**, 49–53.

SUZUKI, M. and SAKAI, T. (1973). Occlusal surface pattern of the lower molars and the second deciduous molar among the living Polynesians. *Am. J. phys. Anthrop.* **39**, 305–316.

TRATMAN, E. K. (1950). A comparison of the teeth of people; Indo-European racial stock with the Mongoloid racial stock. *Dent. Rec.*, 70: 63–88.

TURNER II, C. G., SCOTT, G. R. and ROSE, T. A. (1969). "Mandibular Molar Cusp 6 Plaque and Definitions of Variation." Dept. Anthropology, Arizona State University, Arizona 85281, U.S.A.

TURNER II, C. G., SCOTT, G. R. and LARSEN, M. (1970). "Mandibular Molar Cusp 7 Plaque and Definitions of Variation." Dept. Anthropology, Arizona State University, Arizona 85281, U.S.A.

VOLLENBRUCK, S., LEWIN, T. and LEHMANN, W. (1974). Inbreeding pattern of the Skolt Lapps. *Nordic Council for Arctic Medical Research Reports* No. 9.

WEIDENREICH, F. (1937). The dentition of Sinanthropus pekinensis. *Palaeontol. Sinica* New Series D. No. 1.; Whole Series No. 101.

ZUBOV, A. A. (1973). *Etničeskaja odontologija*. Moskva: Izdatelstvo "Nauka."

6. Uto-Aztecan Premolar: the Anthropology of a Dental Trait

D. H. MORRIS

Department of Anthropology, Arizona State University, Arizona, U.S.A.

S. GLASSTONE HUGHES

Cambridge, England

and

A. A. DAHLBERG

Department of Anthropology and Zoller Memorial Dental Clinic, University of Chicago, Illinois, U.S.A.

INTRODUCTION

In the preface to *Dental Anthropology* (Brothwell, 1963), "dental anthropology" and "dental variability" appear to be synonymous and it seems often to be the case that the terms are considered as identical. In America, "anthropology" has a considerably different meaning, serving to join together physical anthropology (or human biology), cultural anthropology (or social anthropology), archaeology and linguistics. It is in this wider sense that the term is used in this chapter. We believe that the maxillary first premolar trait which we identify in this chapter as the Uto-Aztecan premolar has biological, cultural and archaeological significance. "Uto-Aztecan" is the name of an American Indian language stock whose speakers linguistically dominated western North America at the time of European contact. We hypothesize that the trait is limited to certain North American Indians who are linked together as members of the same broad speech community. The hypothesis may serve as a useful tool to apply to long-standing anthropological problems in the American Southwest.

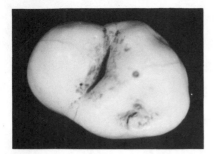 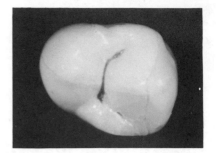

FIG. 1. Uto-Aztecan premolar, left, and normal maxillary first premolar, right. Note the relative size of the buccal cusp on the affected tooth, distal fossa and large ridge connecting the apex of the buccal cusp with the distal border.

UTO-AZTECAN PREMOLAR

We propose the name "Uto-Aztecan premolar" for the trait which was originally reported as a maxillary premolar variation among the Papago Indians of the southern Arizona desert (Morris, 1967). It is characterized by marked buccolingual expansion of the buccal cusp, the paracone, of the first premolar. The paracone is much broadened distally and the distal portion possesses a large, characteristic fossa (Fig. 1). A lobular ridge, at times equal in size to the paracone's distal occlusal border, connects the paracone apex with the distal occlusal border, intersecting the border at the distal terminus of the sagittal sulcus. This ridge could be thought of as a hypertrophied medial occlusal paracone ridge if not for its distal positioning. The fossa lies between the latter ridge and the true distal occlusal border of the paracone.

The trait is not known to occur outside of North American Indians and does not occur in all groups of them even in the Southwest (Table I). It reaches its highest known frequencies (7·1–5·0%) in the prehistoric Sinagua Indians of northern Arizona at sites N.A. 10806 and N.A. 405. Its highest known frequency among living peoples (1·6%) is among the Papago Indians of southern Arizona. As Table I shows, the trait was not seen in 2793 non-North American Indians. Our survey has not been exhaustive but has included peoples from northern and southern Africa, Europe, Asia and Oceania, as well as the American Eskimo. We did find four anomalous maxillary first premolars in the survey, two in the Africans and one each in the Hawaiian and Solomon Islands' samples and include illustrations of them (Fig. 2) because here, as with the Uto-Aztecan premolar, the second premolars are unaffected by the presence of an unusual form in the first premolar.

The genesis of the trait is unknown. It apparently does not influence occlusion. It occurs in both sexes and is often unilateral as well as bilateral in its expression. In one Papago family all four siblings of the propositus had one maxillary first premolar missing although the remaining teeth were unaffected. Recollections were too vague to implicate the absent teeth with the trait. In the only other family for which data could be gathered, neither

TABLE I. Uto-Aztecan premolar:
its occurrence among North American Indians and
among other groups.[a]

Group	N	Affected	%
North American Indians			
[b]N.A. 10806, Arizona[c]	14	1	7·1
[b]Wupatki Pueblo (N.A. 405), Arizona[c]	40	2	5·0
[b]Gran Quivira, New Mexico[c]	71	2	2·8
Papago, Arizona[c]	190	3	1·6
[b]Casas Grandes, Chihuahua[c]	94	1	1·06
Hopi–Tewa, Arizona[c]	162	1	0·6
Pima, Arizona[d]	200	0	0·0
Navajo, Arizona and New Mexico[e]	400	0	0·0
[b]Pecos Pueblo, New Mexico[f]	84	0	0·0
[b]Zuni, New Mexico[c]	21	0	0·0
[b]Montezuma's Castle, Arizona[c]	12	0	0·0
Non-North American Indians			
[b]Eskimo, North America[c]	54	0	0·0
Whites, United States[c]	63	0	0·0
Whites, South Africa[c]	175	0	0·0
Central Sotho, South Africa[c]	252	0	0·0
Bantu, South Africa[g]	1200	0	0·0
Bushmen, Botswana[c]	174	0	0·0
[b]Nubians, North Africa[c]	153	0	0·0
Asiatic Indians, South Africa[c]	200	0	0·0
Solomon Islands[c]	281	0	0·0
Easter Island[c]	119	0	0·0
[b]Hawaiians[c]	98	0	0·0
Yaps[c]	24	0	0·0

[a] The trait is also known in a Bannock Indian from the American West (Hrdlička 1921) and in individuals from three prehistoric sites in Arizona. It is also illustrated by Diamond (1952).
[b] sample from prehistoric site
[c] sample at Dental Anthropology Laboratory, Arizona State University
[d] sample at University of Chicago
[e] personal communication, G. Richard Scott
[f] sample at Peabody Museum, Harvard University
[g] field notes, Shirley Glasstone Hughes

sibling of the propositus was affected. Parents were unavailable in either family.

DISCUSSION

The maxillary premolars have not been given a great deal of attention by morphologists probably because their form usually is relatively simple. Uto-Aztecan premolar is a striking polymorphism: to Diamond, who thought

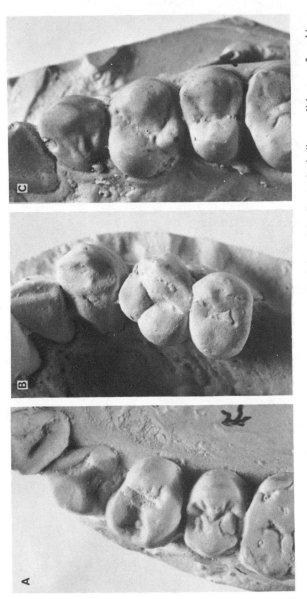

Fig. 2. Unusual maxillary first premolar forms found in (A) a Bushman; (B) a Bantu (a similar condition was found in a Hawaiian); and (C) a Solomon Islander. Note that the second premolar is unaffected.

that it resembled a molar, it "(was) a very unusual specimen" (Diamond, 1952: 200). Diamond's example is unidentified but quite plausibly is from an American Indian. Stanley Garn thought it "caniniform" in a Papago example. Hrdlička's 1921 example from a Bannock Indian is paired with an anomalous "three-cusped" antimere which he referred to as a "tricuspid premolar". Thus the trait has impressed various observers quite differently.

Anthropology can help us to understand the distribution of the trait in only certain groups of the American Indian geographical race (Fig. 3). Beginning with those prehistoric sites where the trait reaches its highest known frequencies, Wupatki Pueblo (N.A. 405) was occupied from 1080 to 1225 A.D. after vulcanism in 1066–1067 had deposited a layer of water-holding ash over a 1000 square mile area of northern Arizona (Stanislawski, 1964). Site N.A. 10806 is 20 miles from Wupatki. Traditionally the occupants of this region at this time period are referred to as "Sinagua" Indians, i.e. "without water." There are seven prehistoric sites in the Southwest at which the trait is known to occur and all these occurrences fall nominally into the time period shortly before European contact. Five occurrences are in Arizona, one in New Mexico and one in Chihuahua, Mexico. The five in Arizona all fall broadly into the prehistoric Pueblo Indian area (including Sinagua, see Figs 3 and 4). Gran Quivira Pueblo, New Mexico, lies at the southeastern limit of the Pueblo area. The site of Casas Grandes, Chihuahua, is not normally considered to be "Pueblo," and lies slightly south of the Pueblo area.

The living Hopi–Tewa, among whom the trait occurs, are modern Pueblo Indians; thus the trait was widely distributed in the prehistoric Pueblo region and it occurs among modern western Pueblos in Arizona. The trait is also known in a Bannock Indian and in the Papago Indians. When one looks for a device to tie these latter three groups together, language is immediately suggested: Bannock and Hopi both speak Shoshonean languages, a branch of the Uto-Aztecan stock, and Papago are members of the Sonoran Branch of the same stock (Figs 3 and 4). Unfortunately archaeologists cannot reconstruct speech from teeth and bones; however, the prehistoric occurrences of the trait in Arizona are in sites culturally affiliated with the modern western Pueblo Hopi. The very wide distribution of Uto-Aztecan speakers in western North America at the time of European contact also argues for Uto-Aztecan speech at the prehistoric sites at which the trait occurs. The Navajo Indians, who do not possess the trait (Table I), are an enclave of Athapaskan speakers who moved into the Southwest shortly before European contact. The trait is also lacking at Pecos Pueblo (Table I) where Towan, a Tanoan language was spoken. Again, while our data are not exhaustive, they do support the hypothesis that the trait is limited to members of a single speech stock.

A potential exception to the hypothesis that the trait is limited to Uto-Aztecan speakers is its occurrence at Gran Quivira Pueblo, New Mexico, where the inhabitants possibly spoke Piro, an extinct Tanoan language. One must add that the occurrence of the trait among Hopi–Tewa (both Hopi and Tewa live in the same village) might be another possible exception since

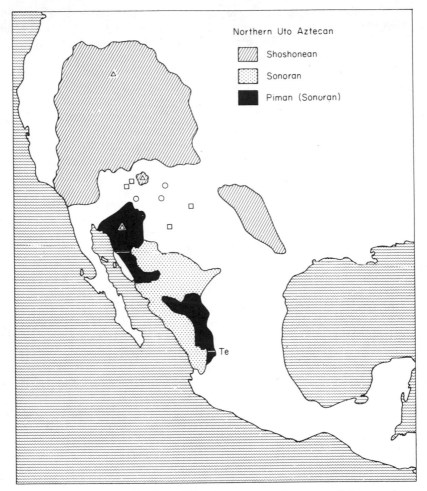

FIG. 3. Map showing distribution of Uto-Aztecan premolar among living peoples, pre
historic peoples and in isolated instances in which it has not been possible to pinpoint the
precise prehistoric site from which an affected individual comes. Triangles, living peoples:
top, Bannock; middle, Hopi; lower, Papago. Squares, Wupatki Pueblo (N.A. 405) and
N.A. 10809 west and Gran Quivira and Casas Grandes east. Circles, affected individuals
from unlocated prehistoric sites. All occurrences are shown in relation to the northern
Uto-Aztecan linguistic branches, Shoshonean and Sonoran. The symbol "Te" identifies
the location of the southern Piman language, Tepehuan. Nahuatl, or Aztecan, the third
major branch of Uto-Aztecan, lies south and southeast of Sonoran. Map is adapted from
Kroeber (1934).

Tewa is another Tanoan language. However, since the trait is absent at
Tanoan Pecos Pueblo (and archaeologists believe that Gran Quivira may
have had a heterogeneous population) and because it is present in Bannock
and Papago, Uto-Aztecan is pointed to more surely than both Uto-Aztecan

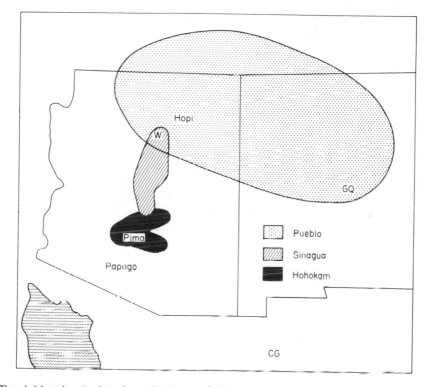

Fig. 4. Map showing locations of living Hopi, Pima, and Papago Indians and the prehistoric sites of Wupatki Pueblo (W), Gran Quivira Pueblo (GQ) and Casas Grandes (CG) in relation to the prehistoric Pueblo, Sinagua and Hohokam regions. The Pima, who do not have the premolar trait, occupy the core of the old Hohokam area.

and Tanoan. The issue is not acute; the linguistically determined time of divergence of the two branches of Uto-Aztecan, Shoshonean (Bannock and Hopi) and Sonoran (Papago), is estimated to be 32 minimum centuries (Hale, 1958). This would place the origin of the trait somewhat before that time to account for its presence in members of both branches, at a time of pre-agricultural hunting-and-gathering adaptation to a generally desert habitat. However, the estimated time of divergence of Uto-Aztecan and Tanoan is only 48 minimum centuries (Swadesh, 1960), roughly 1500–2000 years earlier than the split in the northern Uto-Aztecan branches, i.e. at a somewhat greater remove Tanoan and Uto-Aztecan themselves diverged from a common stock. Plausibly the trait appeared as a mutation in a member of a small band of hunter–gatherers in the American West, and because it neither affected occlusion nor was especially caries-susceptible, continued to be carried along in low frequency in subsequent generations, becoming ultimately dispersed over a wide geographical region. Our data does indicate that the trait is lacking in the Navajo, the largest American Indian tribe in western North America, whose linguistic congeners trace to northwestern Canada.

Our hypothesis of a "Uto-Aztecan premolar" can be tested as other language stocks and other divisions of the Shoshonean and Sonoran branches of Uto-Aztecan are sampled, and as work progresses to include the great southern Uto-Aztecan branch, Nahuatlan or Aztecan, which extends the length of Mexico. The first test of the hypothesis is already present. The neighbours of the Papago, the Pima Indians of southern Arizona, do not possess the trait (Table I) yet they too are Uto-Aztecan speakers, both tribes being traditionally allied within the Piman division of the Sonoran branch. Dahlberg has worked with the Pima for many years and never seen the trait among them. The fact that the Pima live between the Papago and the Pueblo area gives rise to the following questions. How does one account for the trait's absence among the Pima when their neighbours possess it? Why should a trait that is relatively common in the area be absent among the Pima? The prehistoric and historic distribution of the trait, and especially its occurrence among the Papago, make its absence in the Pima truly remarkable.

To place the problem in perspective, a brief consideration of past speculative attempts to reconstruct the origin of the Papago and Pima genotypes will be given. On the one hand they are considered to be closely related (Sofaer et al., 1972) yet elsewhere the Pima genotype is hypothesized as being 40% Athapaskan and 60% Yuman (Brown et al., 1958). "Yuman" refers to yet another distinctive speech stock. The first study to attempt to use known blood group gene frequencies to relate the present with the past inhabitants of the Pima–Papago area was that of Hanna et al. (1953) in which it was estimated that the Papago genotype was composed of 99% Hohokam genes and 1% Caucasoid genes (through admixture), and the Pima genotype was 47–57% Hohokam, 6–7% Caucasoid, 1–3% Salado, and 35–45% of unknown American Indian derivation. Both "Salado" and "Hohokam" refer to prehistoric archaeological cultures in the Pima–Papago area. More than half a century ago Hrdlička wrote:

> Being closely related in language to the Pima, the Papago were supposed to be physically identical with them, but such is not the case, although there is considerable blood relationship between the two tribes, due to intermarriage (Hrdlička, 1908: 10).

If the two tribes are closely related, why is the trait fairly common in one and unknown in the other? There are no known influences on the Pima population's history that would account for this differential loss and neither "selection" nor "genetic drift" are satisfying alternatives. Ezell emphasizes that the proposal that the Pima are actually an Athapaskan–Yuman mix is "incongruent with historical and ethnographical information on the relations of the Pimas and adjacent populations" (Ezell, 1961: 15). It is with the last estimates, those that depend heavily upon the Hohokam, that we wish to deal. Probably shortly before the time of Christ, irrigation agriculture was introduced into the desert river valleys of southern Arizona as a highly efficient technique for coping with the harsh land. Its practitioners are called 'Hohokam" by the archaeologist and they have remained a continuing source of interest to him because their cultural remains have the heavy stamp of Mexico upon them (Fig. 4). They lie outside the indigenous Southwestern cultural traditions. The Hohokam flourished for 1500 years in southern Arizona but at contact time most of their irrigation canals had been abandoned and filled in by the passage of time. As luck would have it, the physical remains of the Hohokam are lost to us because they cremated their dead. When Jesuit missionaries contacted the Pimas in the 1600s the Pimas inhabited the Hohokam core area and practised irrigation agriculture. Tantalizing as this is, it has nevertheless been impossible to tie the Pima directly to the Hohokam through either ethnographical or archaeological means (Ezell, 1963).

What the foregoing does do is provide us with a simple explanation for the occurrence of the premolar trait in the Papago and elsewhere in the Southwest and its absence in the Pima. We hypothesize that the Pima are in fact the descendants of the Hohokam, the Uto-Aztecan speakers from Mexico who migrated into the Arizona desert river valleys about the time of Christ, bringing irrigation agriculture with them. They moved into a Uto-Aztecan area in which the premolar trait was fairly common, and they did not possess the trait themselves. Appealing as this hypothesis is it has a flaw: Papago and Pima languages are mutually intelligible and their linguistic nearness presents a problem to the view that one group is indigenous to the Southwest and the other group is descended from the Mexican Hohokam. We see these linguistic relationships as serious obstacles even though they have seldom influenced previous arguments about Pima and Papago origins.

There are dialect differences within each language and between the two. As previously mentioned there is some intermarriage between the two tribes although their contacts are limited by ecological considerations: the Pima live in the Gila River valley and the Papago live in the desert south of the Pima. Traditionally the Pima are called the "river people" and the Papago the "desert people." From time to time Papago visit the Pima to trade their desert products for the agricultural produce of the Pima and to help harvest the crops of the Pima (Russell, 1908). Father Balthasar has put it this way: "The Papagos are a poor people whom circumstances force to work for the Pima . . ." (Dunne, 1957: 82). Using lexicostatistical techniques, Hale (1958) calculated the minimum time of divergence of the two languages as 198 years.

Before we prematurely abandon our hypothesis that the Pima are descendants of the Mexican Hohokam and that the Papago are indigenous Southwesterners, we believe that the linguistic consequences of 2000 years of such associations need to be considered. In particular we suggest that consideration be given to the view that rather than diverging, Pima and Papago are actually converging. Over-dependence upon lexicostatistics should be cautioned. Papago, Pima and Tepehuan (Fig. 3) together form the Piman subdivision of Sonoran Uto-Aztecan and Hale has calculated the minimum time of divergence of Papago and Tepehuan as only 427 years. Tepehuan is spoken at the southernmost extension of Piman in west coast Mexico. Consider that the Hohokam may have come to the Southwest about 2000 years ago from west coast Mexico and that their speech might have been similar to Tepehuan. Further, consider the possibility that the Pima and Papago are both descended from the Hohokam (which is believed by many archaeologists): then the lexicostatistical time of divergence of less than 500 years is a very poor estimate of a 2000-year time of divergence. It is certainly possible that Pima and Papago both entered the southwest within the last 500 years and this would accord with the lexicostatistical dates; however, this is not a popular view and would not help us to understand why the Papago have the dental trait and the Pima lack it. We maintain that a Mexican origin of the Pima is the simplest explanation for our observed distribution of Uto-Aztecan premolar.

We realize that we leave questions unanswered but we believe that we make an important first step. We have identified a morphological trait of restricted distribution and proposed a testable explanation for its distribution based upon anthropological considerations. We have attempted to go from description to understanding. We believe that our view makes excellent use of biological data on living and skeletal samples and archaeological data, and recognizes the realities of linguistic relationships while not exceeding what is actually known of them.

Acknowledgements

Dr Mahmoud El-Najjar collected data on affected Papago families, aided by genealogical information provided by the Bureau of Ethnic Research, Tucson, Arizona. He also gathered data on Sinagua samples. Dr Jane Hainline Underwood made available the Yap material, Dr Howard Bailit the Solomon Islands material, and Major Alexander G. Taylor and Dr Stanley C. Skoryna the Easter Island material. The Hawaiian, Casas Grandes and Gran Quivira samples were provided by Dr William Bass, Dr Charles C. Di Peso, and Mr Alden C. Hayes, National Park Service, respectively. The Eskimo and Nubians were studied through the courtesy of Dr. Charles C. Merbs, and Dr Christy G. Turner, II, made the Hopi–Tewa available. Professor J. F. van Reenen, South Africa, aided our work in many ways. Ms Susana Berdecio provided the photographs. Arizona State University generously made available a faculty grant-in-aid for the Papago genealogical study.

References

BROTHWELL, D. R. (ed.) (1963). "Dental Anthropology", Symposia of the Society for the Study of Human Biology, Vol. 5. Pergamon Press, New York.
BROWN, K. D., HANNA, B. L., DAHLBERG, A. A. and STRANDSKOV, H. H. (1958). The distribution of blood group alleles among Indians of southwest North America. *Am. J. hum. Genet.* **10**, 175–195.
DIAMOND, M. (1952). "Dental Anatomy". Macmillan, New York.

DUNNE, P. M. (1957). "Juan Antonio Balthasar: Padre Visitador to the Sonora Frontier 1744–1745." Arizona Pioneers Historical Society, Tuscon.

EZELL, P. (1961). "The Hispanic Acculturation of the Gila River Pima". *Am. Anthrop. Assoc. Mem. Menasha.* no. 90.

EZELL, P. (1963). Is there a Hohokam–Pima culture continuum? *American Antiquity* **29**, 61–66.

HALE, K. (1958). Internal diversity in Uto-Aztecan. *Int. J. Am. Ling.* **24**, 104–107.

HANNA, B. L. DAHLBERG, A. A. and H. H. STRANDSKOV. (1953). A preliminary study of the population history of the Pima Indians. *Am. J. Hum. Genet.* **5**, 377–388.

HRDLIČKA, A. (1908). Physiological and Medical Observations Among the Indians of Southwestern United States and Northern Mexico. *Bur. Am. Ethnol. Bull.* **34**.

HRDLIČKA, A. (1921). Further studies on tooth morphology. *Am. J. Phys. Anthrop.* **4**, 141–182.

KROEBER, A. L. (1934). Uto-Aztecan Languages of Mexico. *Ibero-Americana,* Berkeley **8**.

MORRIS, D. H. (1967). Maxillary premolar variation among the Papago Indians. *J. dent. Res.* **46**, 736–738.

RUSSELL, F. (1908). The Pima Indians. *Bur. Am. Ethnol. 26th A. Rep., Wash.* 3–390.

SOFAER, J. A., NISWANDER, J. D., MACLEAN, C. J. and P. L. WORKMAN. (1972). Population studies on Southwestern Indian tribes. V. Tooth morphology as an indicator of biological distance. *Am. J. phys. Anthrop.* **37**, 357–366.

STANISLAWSKI, M. (1964). Wupatki Pueblo: a Study in Culture Fusion and Change in Sinagua and Hopi Prehistory. *Diss. Abst.* **25**, 24–25.

SWADESH, M. (1960). Estudios sobre Lengua y Cultura. *Acta Antropologica (Mexico City)* **2**, No. 2.

7. Anthropological and Family Studies on Minor Variants of the Dental Crown

A. CAROLINE BERRY*

Royal Free Hospital School of Medicine, London.

INTRODUCTION

Minor variations of the skull and skeleton have been widely used by anthropologists to determine distances and relationships between human populations (summarized by Corruccini, 1974). The method assumes a considerable genetical control over the variants used, which, although well documented for mice (Grüneberg, 1963) is nearly impossible to demonstrate in human skeletons. Minor variations of the dental crown seemed to offer themselves both for investigation of their inheritance and possibly as anthropological markers in their own right.

The present study was designed to throw light on the degree of genetical control over the variants but there were also anthropological significances which will only briefly be touched upon, being more fully reported elsewhere (Berry, 1976).

Animal studies on the genetics of crown cusp variation have been described by Grüneberg (1965) and Sofaer (1969a, b, c). They show that, for the cusp variants they describe, the effect of the gene responsible for the appearance of the variant is modified by several factors, one of the most important of which is the genetical background of the individual. Even in inbred laboratory animals we have evidence of a complex genetical situation.

Human studies are inevitably of a somewhat superficial nature. Family and twin studies have been quoted to demonstrate a very strong genetical control of major variants such as missing teeth (Bachrach and Young, 1927; Schultz, 1932; Keeler, 1935; Dahlberg, 1937; Montagu, 1940) and general dental

* Present address: Paediatric Research Unit, Guy's Hospital Medical School, London.

arch and tooth configuration (Goldberg, 1929; Asbell, 1957). In fact it was generally assumed that twins had completely identical mouths (Korkhaus, 1930a, b) so that dental variation has been used for zygosity determination by Lundstrom (1963).

More recently population approaches using incidences and the Hardy–Weinberg law have been used to claim single gene control of some variants, in particular shovelling of the incisors (Turner, 1967; Devoto *et al.*, 1968): Kraus (1951) using pedigree analysis considered the Carabelli trait to be due to two autosomal alleles of intermediate inheritance, while Tsuji (1958) believed the inheritance to be dominant.

This type of method has been extremely successful in unravelling single gene effects, such as that of blood groups and the like. These genetical markers, however, are very intimately related to the primary products of the genes controlling them and their expression is unaffected by any other factors (genetical or environmental) and hence they are suitable for a simplistic Hardy–Weinberg type analysis. The final dental crown appearance is far removed from the primary action of the genes controlling it. This allows other influences to operate and affect the final outcome, making the Hardy–Weinberg law too clumsy a tool for the elucidation of putative genetical factors. Shovelling, for example, has been claimed to be controlled by a single dominant gene (Turner, 1967) or more recently by an autosomal gene of intermediate inheritance (Portin and Alvesalu, 1974).

Sofaer (1970) has exposed the fallacies of the single-factor genetical approach. Mating type studies by Goose and Lee (Goose and Lee, 1971; Lee and Goose, 1972) for several recognized dental crown variants contradict any single gene hypotheses and support the idea of multifactorial control. Recently Suarez and Spence (1974) have analysed family data on hypodontia and have shown that they fitted a polygenic model much better than a single gene one.

The present work aims to investigate a wide spectrum of minor dental variants to determine to what extent and in what ways their expression is genetically determined, by the use of twin and family studies. An indication of the amount of variation available for study is given by Kraus and Furr (1953), who describe 17 variants of the lower first premolar.

MATERIALS AND METHODS

Twin Study

Casts from 56 monozygous twin pairs (MZ) and 57 dizygous twin pairs (DZ) from Professor Korkhaus's collection in Bonn and 35 MZ pairs and 32 DZ pairs from Professor Ritter's collection in Heidelberg were studied. In Bonn, zygosity was determined by assessing developmental history, several body measurements and facial photographs from three aspects, while in Heidelberg blood groups were used in addition. Both these collections were made before the large range of current serological markers was available but it is unlikely that errors of zygosity determination of any significance have crept in.

Method. Each cast was scored for the presence or absence of 45 minor variants. These are listed in Table I and illustrated in Figs 1–4. Dahlberg's reference plaques were used as standards, though the term "shovel" has been applied where Dahlberg's plaque used "semi-shovel" as full shovel shape is rare in the European samples studied. A cusp was defined as having an independent apex, however small. Concordance values were calculated for

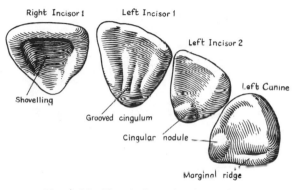

FIG. 1. Maxillary incisors showing variants.

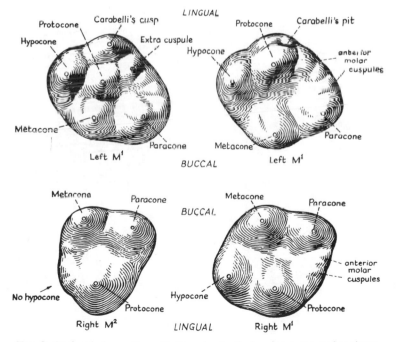

FIG. 2. Occlusal views of maxillary molar teeth showing cusps and variants.

TABLE I. Concordance rates for individual dental characters for monozygous twin pairs, dizygous twin pairs and pairs of unrelated children. Actual number of occurrences of each variant and number of teeth scored also shown. I = incisor; C = canine; PM = premolar; M = molar.

Character	Monozygous		Dizygous		Unrelated	
	Number of occurrences	Concordance	Number of occurrences	Concordance	Number of occurrences	Concordance
Maxilla						
1. Shovelling of I¹	163/304	79·1	135/284	57·0	152/300	36·9
2. Shovelling of I²	117/252	64·8	104/252	46·5	95/236	30·1
3. Grooved cingulum on I¹	87/302	61·1	83/290	31·7	85/302	16·7
4. Grooved cingulum on I²	69/254	43·8	69/254	38·0	68/236	25·9
5. Cingular nodule present on I¹	1/304	–	6/294	–	3/300	–
6. Cingular nodule present on I²	25/258	47·1	38/256	15·2	37/234	8·8
7. Cingular nodule present on C	50/180	66·7	48/172	33·3	33/142	26·9
8. Marginal ridges on C	122/182	74·3	115/174	74·2	104/150	57·6
9. Extra labial cusp on PM¹	0/222	0	0/218	0	0/204	0
10. Extra labial cusp on PM²	2/192	0	6/180	20·0	0/158	0
11. Extra lingual cusp on PM¹	0/218	0	0/218	0	0/206	0
12. Extra lingual cusp on PM²	0/190	0	0/108	0	0/158	0
13. Labial marginal ridges on PM¹	33/216	22·2	34/214	9·7	33/198	6·5
14. Labial marginal ridges on PM²	109/188	57·9	115/182	47·4	94/158	46·9
15. Lingual marginal ridges on PM¹	40/214	42·9	40/218	17·6	40/204	11·1
16. Lingual marginal ridges on PM²	73/182	37·3	90/180	42·9	86/156	38·7
17. Cusp number other than 4 on M¹	35/328	75·0	23/204	35·3	12/296	20·0
18. Cusp number other than 4 on M²	105/120	90·9	62/82	77·1	19/62	0
19. Carabelli's pit present	123/326	59·7	102/316	30·8	96/310	18·5
20. Carabelli's cusp present	64/326	68·4	88/316	51·7	83/310	15·3
Carabelli's phenomenom present		76·4		62·4		36·6
21. Anterior molar cuspules on M¹	122/276	58·4	116/300	41·5	96/260	37·1

Mandible

22. Shovelling of I	12/642	71·4	1/570	0	7/626	0
23. Marginal ridges on C	93/208	60·3	99/178	50·0	110/208	46·7
24. Extra labial cusp on PM_1	0/230	0	0/192	0	0/170	0
25. Extra labial cusp on PM_2	14/192	55·6	3/152	0	8/144	0
26. Extra lingual cusp on PM_1	9/230	50·0	13/202	18·2	14/180	7·7
27. Lingual groove on PM_1	29/230	45·0	24/202	26·3	20/180	17·6
28. Extra lingual cusp on PM_2	74/186	68·2	62/146	34·8	67/142	28·8
29. Lingual groove on PM_2	0/180	0	0/146	0	0/142	0
30. Labial marginal ridges on PM_1	93/222	55·0	74/194	29·8	94/202	30·0
31. Labial marginal ridges on PM_2	67/178	63·4	57/136	39·0	56/132	30·2
32. Lingual marginal ridges on PM_1	1/224	0	9/190	0	8/170	0
33. Lingual marginal ridges on PM_2	39/176	44·4	30/140	15·4	23/134	4·5
34. Reduced lingual cusp on PM_1	131/228	79·5	119/200	58·7	126/208	38·5
35. Furrow instead of pits on PM_1	37/218	76·2	46/196	39·4	46/202	21·1
36. Pits instead of furrows on PM_2	22/186	69·2	17/146	30·8	12/144	0
37. Cusp number other than 5 on M_1	72/282	71·4	60/254	33·3	56/252	9·8
38. Cusp number other than 4 on M_2	4/136	100·0	6/98	0	1/80	0
39. Groove pattern X on M_1	9/166	0	22/170	29·4	9/160	0
40. Groove pattern Y on M_1	65/156	54·8	59/170	43·9	60/160	33·3
41. Groove pattern + on M_1	92/166	59·3	89/170	45·9	83/160	45·6
42. Groove pattern X on M_2	14/84	40·0	15/78	15·4	8/44	14·3
43. Groove pattern Y on M_2	8/84	100·0	0/78	0	0/44	0
44. Groove pattern + on M_2	62/84	75·7	61/78	74·3	36/44	71·4
45. Protostylid present	3/298	50·0	0/280	0	1/254	0

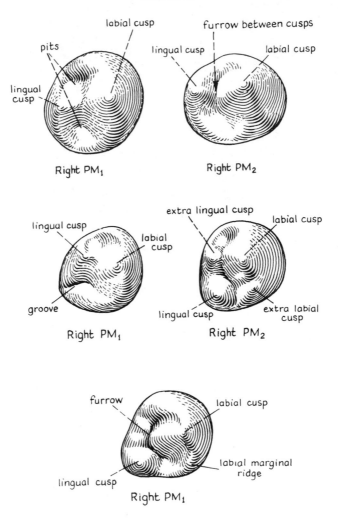

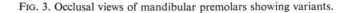

FIG. 3. Occlusal views of mandibular premolars showing variants.

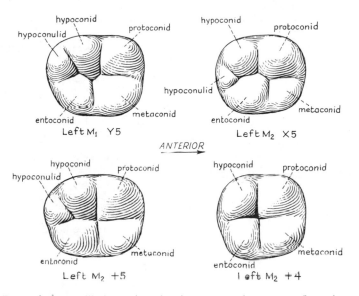

FIG. 4. Left mandibular molars showing cusps and groove configuration.

each variant using the formula for MZ twins, DZ twins and unrelated pairs (i.e. pairs taken at random).

$$\text{Concordance} = \frac{C}{C + D} \times 100$$

where C = no. of concordant pairs and D = no. of discordant pairs. Individual tooth scorings were used in the determination.

Family Study

Casts from members of 122 Caucasian Liverpool families were used. They had originally been collected for an investigation of the heritability of tooth and mouth size by Bowden and Goose (1969). Goose and Lee have used the same material for a mating type study of Carabelli's cusp (see below).
Method.   Scoring for presence or absence of the variants was carried out as above. However, during the scoring of the twin material and other samples described elsewhere it became clear that a number of the variants listed in Table I were unsuitable for use either because they occurred so rarely in the European samples under consideration or because they seemed chiefly to occur in newly erupted teeth and therefore probably were quickly eradicated by wear. Failure of reproducibility on repeat scoring was a further source of elimination. These 20 eliminated variants, together with their reason for elimination and MZ concordance value, are listed in Table II. The family study material was therefore scored only for the remaining 25 variants.

TABLE II. Showing 20 variants excluded, with reasons for their abandonment

Variant		Reason	MZ Concordance (%)
Maxilla			
2. Shovelled I^2	Combined with I^1 to become "Shovelled Incisors"	High correlation for shovelling between I^1 and I^2	65
8. Marginal ridges on C ⎫			74
13. ⎫ Lingual and labial		Lack of consistency	22
14. ⎬ marginal ridges on	Abandoned	in scoring	58
15. ⎭ PM^1 and PM^2			43
16. ⎭			37
21. Anterior molar cuspules, on M^1	Abandoned	Probably only scorable on newly erupted teeth	58
Mandible			
23. Marginal ridges on C ⎫			60
30. ⎫ Lingual and labial			55
31. ⎬ marginal ridges on	Abandoned	Lack of consistency	63
32. ⎭ PM$_1$ and PM$_2$		in scoring	0
33. ⎭			44
34. Reduced lingual cusp on PM$_1$	Abandoned	Too subjective	80
39. ⎫			0
40. ⎪			55
41. ⎪ *Dryopithecus* pattern	Abandoned	Lack of consistency	59
42. ⎬ on molars		in scoring,	40
43. ⎪		particularly newly	100
44. ⎭		erupted teeth	76
45. Protostylid present	Abandoned for present study	Very rare in Europe	50

For the actual calculation of within family correlations only variants having quite a high population incidence could be used. Variants occurring only occasionally in the sample could contribute nothing to the family study particularly as the relevant teeth in the family members of any "propositus" would frequently be missing, decayed or filled and thus unscorable. Thus only 9 individual variants could be used for the calculation of correlation coefficients between different family members. Correlation coefficients were calculated for the following pairings: father:child; mother:child; sib:sib; and mother:father. The correlation coefficient r was calculated from the following formula:

$$r = \frac{ad - bc}{\sqrt{(a + b)(c + d)(a + c)(b + d)}}$$

where a, b, c and d are derived from a 2×2 table:

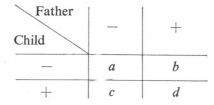

	Father −	Father +
Child −	a	b
Child +	c	d

In this case the occurrence or non-occurrence of a variant in the mouth rather than on individual teeth was scored. The significance of r was derived from the expression $\chi^2 = r^2(a + b + c + d)$ for 2 degrees of freedom. The population incidences were also calculated. Mating type tables were constructed for families where both parents and at least one child could be scored for any particular variant.

RESULTS

Table I lists the variants used for the twin study together with their concordance rates between MZ, DZ and unrelated pairs. The distribution of these concordance figures is shown graphically in Fig. 5.

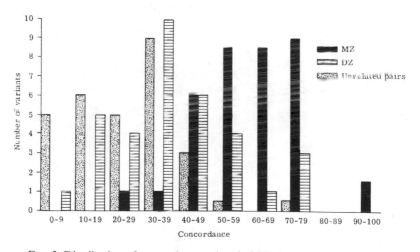

FIG. 5. Distribution of concordance values in MZ, DZ and unrelated pairs.

Correlation coefficients between family members are shown in Table III. Population incidence and twin concordance rates are also shown for comparison. No mother:father correlation coefficients are shown in the table, since there was no evidence whatsoever of any correlation.

TABLE III. Family Studies

Variant	Interfamily Correlations			Population Incidence (%)	Twin Concordances (%)	
	Father/child	Mother/child	Sib/sib		MZ	DZ
Shovelled upper incisors	0·26**	0·28**	0·43**	42	79	57
Sagittal furrow on PM_1	0·54**	0·21*	0·32**	20	76	39
Carabelli phenomenon	0·28*	0·40**	0·10	59	76	62
Cingular nodule on I^2	0·20*	0·14	0·31**	21	47	15
Extra lingual cusp on PM_1	0·03	0·06	0·31**	10	50	18
Extra lingual cusp on PM_2	0·15	0·25	0·30*	54	68	35
Grooved lingual cusp on PM_1	0·16	0·23*	0·19	53	45	26
Cingular nodule on upper canine	0·15	0·21*	0·08	32	67	33
Carabelli pit	0·14	0·08	0·14	42	60	31
Carabelli cusp	-0·05	0·24	-0·06	25	68	52

* Significant at 5% level
** Significant at 1% level

TABLE IV. Showing numbers and phenotype of children born to parents of each phenotype.

		Parents			
		++	+−	−−	
Children	+	2	8	9	Cingular nodule on I^2
	−	0	13	40	
	+	11	16	10	Shovelled incisors
	−	5	12	25	
	+	8	19	5	Grooved lingual cusp on PM_1
	−	4	17	10	

The progeny of the various mating types are given in Table IV. Only three variants are shown. The other six variants used in the family study give very similar results.

DISCUSSION

Twin Study

Figure 5 shows clearly that MZ twins have in general higher concordance values than DZ pairs and that these in turn have higher values than for unrelated pairs. It can be seen from Table I that this remains so for every individual variant. More unexpected, however, is the small number of variants having MZ concordance values approaching 100 %, only molar cusp number frequently reaching this exalted state. In general, MZ concordances tend to lie between 50–70 %. This is at variance with other twin studies such as those of Korkhaus (1930a, b). These earlier works were concerned with fairly large variations such as occlusion pattern and abnormalities of the teeth. Kraus (1957) and Ludwig (1957) found higher concordance values for MZ twins than those reported here for their 16 independent premolar variants but even they remark on the lack of complete concordance. Unfortunately numerical comparisons of concordance values are not possible because of the method of presentation of these authors' data. It would seem that where finer variations in the crowns of individual teeth are considered there is greater scope for the action of non-genetical influences.

It remains, however, that the present concordance figures are lower than those reported by Kraus and by Ludwig. This may be partly due to the fact that different variants were under consideration and also to the small samples of 12 and 17 MZ pairs used respectively by the aforementioned workers. Some of the less common variants were unlikely to have occurred at all in those small samples. The present results also differ from those of Kraus in that concordance figures for DZ twins are higher than those for unrelated random pairs. Although fraternal twins would share a common environment unshared by the unrelated pairs, it would seem more likely that the higher fraternal concordance rates indicate a degree of genetical control over the variants' incidence. Kraus believed that his figures showed no significant difference between concordance rates for DZ twins and unrelated pairs but these findings were based on only 14 and 8 pairs respectively.

The use of dental variants in twin zygosity determinations assumes a high degree of concordance in monozygous twins. In his large study Lundstrom (1963) found that zygosity determined by dental variation agreed with that made on the basis of anthropological determinations (including blood groups) in 117 pairs out of 124 (94 %). He used a large number of dental variants which would enable a discordance in one minor feature to be over-ruled by consistent concordance in other features. Wood and Green (1969) used only seven traits of the mandibular second premolar. In 18 pairs of monozygous and 14 dizygous twins the dental diagnosis agreed with the anthropological one in 88 % of the comparisons. The greater discordance is probably due to the smaller number of traits employed. The lack of complete concordance in monozygotic twins is not entirely surprising in view of the asymmetrical occurrence of so many of the variants.

Biggerstaff's (1970) twin study of mandibular first molars which included consideration of the problem of dental asymmetry, led him to conclude that hypotheses for simple modes of inheritance were untenable, and he favoured a polygenic type of control. The findings of the present study would be in agreement with this though non-genetic factors would seem to be implicated as well since Bailit *et al.* (1970) have shown dental asymmetry to be related to both genetic and environmental stress.

Discarded Variants

In general the reasons for this are clear from Table II. The *Dryopithecus* pattern has been accepted as useful in evolutionary studies but other workers have remarked on its unsatisfactory nature (Robinson and Allin, 1966; Biggerstaff, 1968; Morris, 1970; Sofaer *et al.*, 1972b).

Family Study

The interfamily correlation figures given in Table III show that though these correlations are not uniformly high there is a consistent pattern of significant positive correlation, and that provided Carabelli's cusp and pit are considered together (Carabelli trait), significant correlation is found for every variant considered. Correlation values of 0·50 are to be expected between one parent and child if a trait is controlled by a number of genes such as height is. Since this value is reached only once in the present series of correlations it would seem likely that other non-genetical factors are also involved, though non-additive inherited factors would produce the same effect.

The present correlation figures are, however, larger than those reported by

Sofaer *et al.* (1972a) in a similar study of the inhabitants of Bougaineville. Why genetic influences should act more strongly in Liverpool than Bougaineville is hard to assess. It is possible that there is more inbreeding in Bougaineville which could produce the effect or it may be that the population is under environmental stress and reacting in a way similar to that mentioned above (Bailit *et al.*, 1970) when increased asymmetry was associated with increased stress. Goose and Lee (1973) have reported evidence for a lesser degree of inheritance of tooth size in the Chinese population of Liverpool than for the native Liverpudlian population. Presumably the immigrant Chinese are under greater "genetical" stress as they have to adapt to a new environment.

If the order in which the variants occur in Table III is considered, shovelled incisors top the list. Saheki (1958) found shovelling to be the most highly heritable variant of his ten variants in a twin study. Sofaer *et al.* (1972a) found Carabelli's cusp to have the highest interfamilial correlations although Biggerstaff's (1973) twin study led him to the conclusion that the variant was not strongly inherited. However, it is not clear whether his concordance scoring separated different degrees of cusp formation and pit development. The low correlations for cusp and pit taken separately and the high correlation, if they are considered as one, was an unexpected and unexplained finding in the present study, particularly in view of the comparatively high value for MZ concordance for Carabelli's cusp. For the other variants the MZ concordance figure seems to accord reasonably well with the degree of interfamily correlation.

An important factor that should be considered when treating individual variants as separate entities is whether or not there is any tendency for certain variants to occur together within the same mouth since high within family correlations would then merely be a reflection of the fact that the variant was strongly associated with some other variants with high inter family correlations. A search for associations between variants has been carried out as part of another project (Berry, 1976). In two large English samples a significant association was discovered between shovelling of the incisors and the occurrence of cingular nodule on incisor 2. No other relevant statistical associations were found but it could be that the incisor cingular nodule has ranked too high on Table III because of its association with incisor shovelling. Its unspectacular MZ concordance rate would concur with this suggestion.

The mating tables drawn up in Table IV are comprised of small numbers of families as both parents had to have teeth scorable for the variant concerned. However they firmly renounce any trend towards a simple dominant and recessive type of inheritance as there is no evidence of any type of couple succeeding in "breeding true" as would be expected if both parents showed the recessive character. More detailed mating tables have been made by Goose and Lee (1971) for Carabelli's cusp from the material used for this work and for several other crown variants in a Chinese sample from Liverpool (Lee and Goose, 1972). These authors also concluded that a multifactorial inheritance is demonstrated by their findings.

Thus the twin, family and mating type approach lead independently to the conclusion that minor variants of the dental crown are indeed controlled by genetical mechanisms but that these mechanisms are complex and likely to be influenced by environmental factors. What the factors are is as yet by no means clear. Work on the occurrence or non-occurrence of the third molar tooth of the mouse has thrown some light on the problem. Grüneberg (1951) showed that tooth size was inherited on a multifactorial basis, and both he and Grewal (1962) noted that absence of the tooth tended to occur in some but not all litters of certain matings, suggesting a maternal environmental effect. Searle (1954a, b) showed that both first litters and poor maternal diet were associated with third molar loss, results that were confirmed by Deol and Truslove (1957). A summary of the numerous factors affecting third molar development in the mouse is shown in diagrammatic form in Fig. 6, which indicates the complexity of the situation.

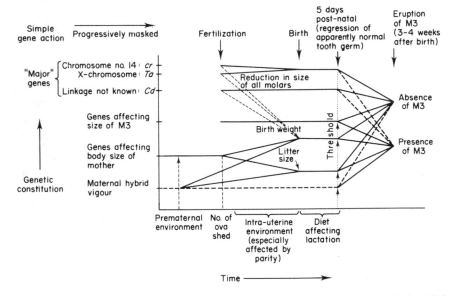

FIG. 6. Interaction of genetical and developmental factors in the occurrence of the third molar in the mouse. From Berry (1968).

In humans Keene (1965) has shown hypodontia in American naval recruits to be associated with low birth weight, first-born children and low maternal age. However, an earlier investigation by Grahnén (1956) did not reveal any effect either of birth order or of maternal age on hypodontia in Swedish families. In Australia, Davies (1967) has reported hypodontia to be more common in females than males, and a similar trend was observed by Barnes (1968) in a large Iteso population. Although the effect may be related to the smaller tooth size in girls, there does seem to be some evidence linking factors affecting tooth development in the mouse with those in the human.

Anthropological Considerations

Although it is likely that non-genetical factors play a part in determining the occurrence or non-occurrence of these minor variants, a definite and moderately strong genetical influence has also been shown to be present.

If a broad spectrum of non-correlated variants are used the genetical element should be strong enough to make these variants a useful means for differentiating populations. Work supporting this has already been published (Jacob, 196n; Greene, 1967; Sofaer *et al.*, 1972b; Kirveskari, 1977) and an attempt to use a single distance statistic to distinguish population samples scored from a large number of dental variants is in progress (Berry, 1976) employing a technique similar to that which was previously used for distance determinations using minor skull variants (Berry and Berry, 1967). Dental variants therefore show considerable promise as useful anthropological markers.

There is, however, one practical problem of overriding importance and that is the modern scourge of caries. Since many of the variants described involve pits or grooves on the dental crown it could be that certain variants are more liable to succumb to caries than others. When this occurs the tooth soon becomes unscorable. Thus differing incidences between populations could be accounted for by differing caries rates; a caries-prone variant being rare in a population with a high incidence of caries and commoner in a caries-resistant population. Until it has been shown which, if any, variants are particularly susceptible or resistant this factor must be borne in mind. In more primitive regions where caries are no problem the teeth tend to be subjected to much wear which is likely to make scoring of many variants difficult.

CONCLUSIONS

The twin and family studies presented here show that even very minor variations in the dental crown have a strong element of genetical control. This genetical control appears to be complex and environmental factors are likely to have some influence. There is sufficient genetical control to make the variants potentially useful in anthropological work but caries and tooth wear are possible factors limiting this usefulness.

SUMMARY

The occurrence of a large number of minor variants of the dental crown have been studied with a view to elucidating the degree of genetical control governing their expression.

Ninety-one pairs of monozygous and 89 pairs of dizygous twins showed that, for each variant, the MZ concordance value was higher than the DZ concordance, although even among MZ pairs 100% concordance values were rare. Using material from 122 families, correlations between the various family members were calculated for nine different variants, and the offspring from various parental combinations considered. In either case multifactorial rather than single gene control was favoured, and environmental factors were thought likely to participate.

The nature of these factors and the anthropological significance of minor dental variants were also discussed.

ACKNOWLEDGEMENTS

I am grateful to Professor Korkhaus of Bonn and Professor Ritter of Heidelberg for permission to study their large collections of twin models, also to Mr Denys Goose of Liverpool Dental School for giving me access to collections of family group casts. Dr J. Sofaer helped with statistical advice and the figures were made by Mr A. J. Lee and the Department of Medical Illustration, Guy's Hospital. The Royal Society European programme provided travelling expenses.

REFERENCES

ASBELL, M. H. (1957). A study of the family line transmission of dental occlusions. *Am. J. Orthod.* **43**, 265–285.

BACHRACH, F. H. and YOUNG, M. A. (1927). A comparison of the degree of resemblance in dental characters shown in pairs of twins of identical and fraternal types. *Br. dent. J.* **48**, 1293–1304.

BAILIT, H. L., WORKMAN, P. L., NISWANDER, J. D. and MACLEAN, C. J. (1970). Dental asymmetry as an indicator of genetic and environmental stress in human populations. *Hum. Biol.* **42**, 626–638.

BARNES, D. S. (1968). Variations in tooth morphology in the Iteso. *J. dent. Res.* **47**, 971–972.

BERRY, A. C. (1976). The anthropological value of minor variants of the dental crown. *Am. J. phys. Anthrop.* **45**, 257–268.

BERRY, A. C. and BERRY, R. J. (1967). Epigenetic variation in the human cranium. *J. Anat.* **101**, 361–379.

BERRY, R. J. (1968). Biology of non-metrical variation in mice and men. *In* "The Skeletal Biology of Earlier Human Populations", Symposia of the Society for the study of Human Biology, Vol. 8, pp. 103–133. Pergamon, Oxford.

BIGGERSTAFF, R. H. (1968). On the groove configuration of mandibular molars: the unreliability of the "*Dryopithecus* Pattern" and a new method for classifying mandibular molars. *Am. J. phys. Anthrop.* **29**, 441–444.

BIGGERSTAFF, R. H. (1970). Morphological variations for the permanent mandibular first molars in human monozygotic and dizygotic twins. *Archs oral. Biol.* **15**, 721–730.

BIGGERSTAFF, R. H. (1973). Heritability of the Carabelli cusp in twins. *J. dent. Res.* **52**, 40–44.

BOWDEN, D. E. J. and GOOSE, D. H. (1969). Inheritance of tooth size in Liverpool families. *J. med. Genet.* **6**, 55–58.

CORRUCCINI, R. S. (1974). An examination of the meaning of cranial discrete traits for human skeletal biological studies. *Am. J. phys. Anthrop.* **40**, 425–445.

DAHLBERG, A. A. (1937). Inherited congenital absence of 6 incisors, deciduous and permanent. *J. dent. Res.* **16**, 59–62.

DAVIES, P. L. (1967). Agenesis of teeth: A sex limited trait. *J. dent. Res.* **46**, 1309.

DEOL, M. S. and TRUSLOVE, G. M. (1957). Genetical studies of the skeleton of the mouse. XX. Maternal physiology and variation in the skeleton of C57BL mice. *J. Genet.* **55**, 288–312.

DEVOTO, F. C. H., ARIAS, N. H., RINGUELET, S. and PALMA, N. H. (1968). Shovel shaped incisors in a Northwestern Argentine population. *J. dent. Res.* **47**, 820–823.

GOLDBERG, S. (1929). Biometrics of identical twins from dental viewpoint. *J. dent. Res.* **9**, 363–409.

GOOSE, D. H. and LEE, G. T. R. (1971). The Mode of Inheritance of Carabelli's trait. *Hum. Biol.* **43**, 64–69.

GOOSE, D. H. and LEE, G. T. R. (1973). Inheritance of tooth size in immigrant populations. *J. dent. Res.* **52**, 175.

GRAHNÉN, H. (1956). Hypodontia in the permanent dention. *Odont. Revy.* **7**, Supplement 3.

GREENE, D. L. (1967). Dentition of meroitic, X-group, and Christian populations from Wadi Halfa, Sudan. University of Utah Anthropological Papers No. 85. University of Utah Press, Salt Lake City, U.S.A.

GREWAL, M. S. (1962). The development of an inherited tooth defect in the mouse. *J. Embryol. exp. Morph.* **10**, 202–211.

GRÜNEBERG, H. (1951). The genetics of a tooth defect in the mouse. *Proc. R. Soc. Lond.* B. **138**, 437–451.

GRÜNEBERG, H. (1963). "The Pathology of Development." Oxford.

GRÜNEBERG, H. (1965). Genes and genotypes affecting the teeth of the mouse. *J. Embryol. exp. Morph.* **14**, 137–159.

JACOB, T. (1967). Racial identification of the Bronze Age human dentitions from Bali, Indonesia. *J. dent. Res.* **46**, 903–910.

KEELER, C. E. (1935). Heredity in dentistry. *Dent. Cosmos.* **77**, 1147–1163.

KEENE, H. J. (1965). The relationship of maternal age, parity and birthweight to hypodontia in naval recruits. *Am. J. phys. Anthrop.* **23**, 330.

KIRVESKARI, P. (1977). Racial traits in the dentition of living Skolt Lapps. Chapter 5 in this volume.

KORKHAUS, G. (1930a). Die Vererbung der Kronenform und -grösse menschlicher Zähne. *Z. Anat. EntwGesch.* **91**, 594–617.

KORKHAUS, G. (1930b). Anthropologic and odontologic studies of twins. *Int. J. Orthod.* **16**, 640–647.

KRAUS, B. S. (1951). Carabelli's anomaly of the maxillary molar teeth. *Am. J. hum. Genet.* **3**, 348–355.

KRAUS, B. S. (1957). The genetics of the human dentition. *J. forens. Sci.* **2**, 420–428.

KRAUS, B. S. and FURR, M. L. (1953). Lower first premolar, Part 1. *J. dent. Res.* **32**, 554–564.

LEE, G. T. R. and GOOSE, D. H. (1972). The inheritance of dental traits in a Chinese population in the United Kingdom. *J. med. Genet.* **9**, 336–339.

LUDWIG, F. J. (1957). The mandibular second premolars: morphological variation and inheritance. *J. dent. Res.* **36**, 263–273.

LUNDSTROM, A. (1963). Tooth morphology as a basis for distinguishing mono and dizygotic twins. *Am. J. hum. Genet.* **15**, 34–43.

MONTAGU, A. M. F. (1940). The significance of the variability of the upper lateral incisor teeth in man. *Hum. Biol.* **12**, 323–328.

MORRIS, D. H. (1970). On deflecting wrinkles and the *Dryopothecus* pattern in human mandibular molars. *Am. J. phys. Anthrop.* **32**, 97–104.

PORTIN, P. and ALVESALO, L. (1974). The inheritance of shovel shape in maxillary central incisors. *Am. J. phys. Anthrop.* **41**, 59–62.

ROBINSON, J. T. and ALLIN, E. F. (1966). On the Y of the *Dryopithecus* pattern of mandibular teeth. *Am. J. phys. Anthrop.* **25**, 323–324.

SAHEKI, M. (1958). On the heredity of the tooth crown configuration studied in twins. *Jap. J. Anat.* **33**, 456–470.

SCHULTZ, A. H. (1932). The hereditary tendency to eliminate the upper lateral incisors. *Hum. Biol.* **4**, 34–40.

SEARLE, A. G. (1954a). Genetical studies on the skeleton of the mouse. IX. Causes of skeletal variation within pure lines. *J. Genet.* **52**, 68–102.

SEARLE, A. G. (1954b). Genetical studies on the skeleton of the mouse. XI. The influence of diet on variation within pure lines. *J. Genet.* **52**, 413–424.

SOFAER, J. A. (1969a). Aspects of the tabby-crinkled-downless syndrome. I. The development of tabby teeth. *J. Embryol. exp. Morph.* **22**, 181–205.

SOFAER, J. A. (1969b). Aspects of the tabby-crinkled-downless syndrome. II. Observations on the reaction to changes of genetic background. *J. Embryol. exp. Morph.* **22**, 207–227.

SOFAER, J. A. (1969c). The genetics and expression of a dental morphological variant in the mouse. *Archs oral. Biol.* **14**, 1213–1223.

SOFAER, J. A. (1970). Dental morphologic variation and the Hardy-Weinberg Law. *J. dent. Res.* **49**, 1505–1508.

SOFAER, J. A., MACLEAN, C. J. and BAILIT, H. L. (1972a). Hereditary and morphological variation in early and late developing human teeth of the same morphological class. *Archs oral. Biol.* **17**, 811–816.

SOFAER, J. A., NISWANDER, J. D., MACLEAN, C. J. and WORKMAN, P. L. (1972b). Population studies on Southwestern Indian tribes. V. Tooth morphology as an indicator of biological distance. *Am. J. phys. Anthrop.* **37**, 357–366.

SUAREZ, B. K. and SPENCE, M. A. (1974). The genetics of hypodontia. *J. dent. Res.* **53**, 781.

TSUJI, T. (1958). Incidence and inheritance of Carabelli's cusp in a Japanese population. *Jap. J. hum. Genet.* **3**, 21. (English summary quoted by Greene, 1967b.)

TURNER, C. G., II. (1967). Dental genetics and microevolution in prehistoric and living Koniag Eskimo. *J. dent. Res.* **46**, 911–917.

WOOD, B. F. and GREEN, L. J. (1969). Second premolar morphologic trait similarities in twins. *J. dent. Res.* **48**, 74–78.

8. The Dentitions of Tabby and Crinkled Mice (an upset in mesodermal: ectodermal interaction)

WILLIAM A. MILLER

Department of Oral Biology, State University of New York, Buffalo, New York, U.S.A.

INTRODUCTION

Grüneberg (1965) described in some detail the dentition of mice which were hemizygous for the semidominant sex-linked gene Tabby (*Ta*) and also the mosaic of dental morphological features which is associated with the heterozygous female (*Ta/+*). In the following year these mosaic features were used for a detailed analysis to assess the validity of the Lyon hypothesis of X-chromosome inactivation in the female in terms of large numbers of animals instead of individuals (Grüneberg 1966a, b). Part of his argument ranged around the similar dental abnormalities found in an autosomal mutant crinkled (*cr*). While the tabby dentition was described in detail that of crinkled was indicated to be identical. Sofaer (1969a, b) has described the embryological and genetic variation of morphological features associated with these dentitions as well as another similar autosomal mutant, downless (*dl*).

It is not the intent of this chapter to discuss the Lyon hypothesis, for the evidence presented by Grüneberg in these and subsequent papers (Grüneberg, 1966b, 1969, 1971a, b) is very persuasive. It is the intent to describe and compare the two dentitions and use this, with information from other murine dental abnormalities, as a starting point in considering some of the factors which might be involved in these unusual dentitions and other abnormalities associated with the mutations.

METHODS AND MATERIALS

Tabby and crinkled material was all on a C_3Hf background and originally obtained from the Institute for Cancer Research, Philadelphia through the courtesy of Dr Beatrice Mintz. Ten tabby male hemizygotes ($Ta/-$), ten tabby female heterozygotes ($Ta/+$) and 10 C_3Hf controls were used in the initial investigation. Thirty-one crinkled homozygotes (cr/cr) and six heterozygotes ($+/cr$) were also studied.

Most animals were killed around 42 days of age, by which time both M^3 and M_3 had erupted and were in occlusion but occlusal wear was minimal (Gaunt, 1961). The $Ta/-$ males were killed at 30 days. The breeding crinkled stock was killed around 14–18 months. Skulls were defleshed and macerated in 5% ammonia in water and stored dry.

Jaw bones and teeth were examined at $\times 25$ magnification and their morphology recorded by *camera lucida* (Wilde M6) and photography. Separated mandibles and upper toothbearing bones were radiographed at 9 mA, 70 kV for 2·5 min at 75 cm using fine grain photographic film which gives exceptionally fine detail of bone structure (Miller and Radnor, 1970). Three times magnification prints of the radiographic image were made to examine variations in incisal shape and molar root morphology *in situ*.

RESULTS

Tabby and crinkled dentitions are remarkably similar. In the small sample examined tabby was the most severely affected, particularly in the root.

Incisor teeth were perhaps the most severely affected—60% of the $Ta/-$ upper incisors were missing or abnormal and likewise for 45% of the lower incisors. This is in contrast to Sofaer (1969a) who found that in his sample the

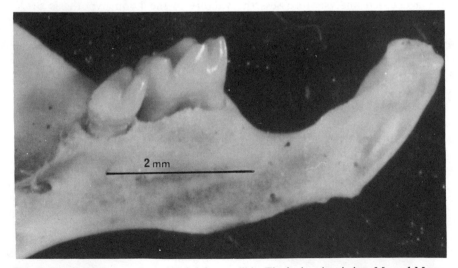

FIG. 1. Tooth-bearing portion of $Ta/-$ left mandible. The incisor is missing. M_1 and M_2 are reduced in size as is their associated alveolar bone; line is 2 mm in length.

lower incisors were more frequently affected. As a consequence the anterior portion of the mandible (Fig. 1) and the premaxillae were much reduced in size. When compared to controls the incisors of both tabby and crinkled mice were much less pigmented. The addition of the iron-containing pigment to the rodent incisor enamel is a very late occurrence in amelogenesis (Miller *et al.*, 1968, unpublished data) which implies that the abnormality is affecting not only organogenesis of the teeth but also the quality of the tissues forming them. Falconer *et al.* (1951) also noted this anomaly in crinkled. The rate of incisor growth appeared slower than normal in both mutants, for at comparable ages, teeth were smaller than those of the controls. In cases of missing incisors, the opposing one had over-erupted and frequently still retained its initial tapering point. In a few animals the curvature of the upper incisors was reduced (Fig. 2). This was found in both old and young animals. In the

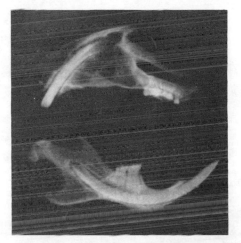

FIG. 2. Radiograph of left mandible and upper jaw for *cr/cr* of 14 months. Note the abnormal upper incisor. The head of the mandibular condyl is abnormal in shape.

older animals some association with age changes, as described by Robins and Rowlatt (1971), might be invoked, however in the younger animals this is unlikely and a more probable explanation is an abnormal relationship between labial and lingual internal dental epithelia at the proliferating distal end of the tooth.

The molar abnormalities of tabby have been described by Grüneberg (1965, 1966a, b). In both mutants the molar teeth are smaller and distinctly bulbous. In both upper and lower jaws the cusps of M1 and M2 stand more erect than in control animals. The phenotype is quite characteristic (Figs 3 and 4). In describing it the cuspal terminology of Gaunt (1955) will be used. The three central cusps of M^1 were present. On the buccal aspect B1 was missing and B2 enlarged and more closely aligned to cusp 2 than in the

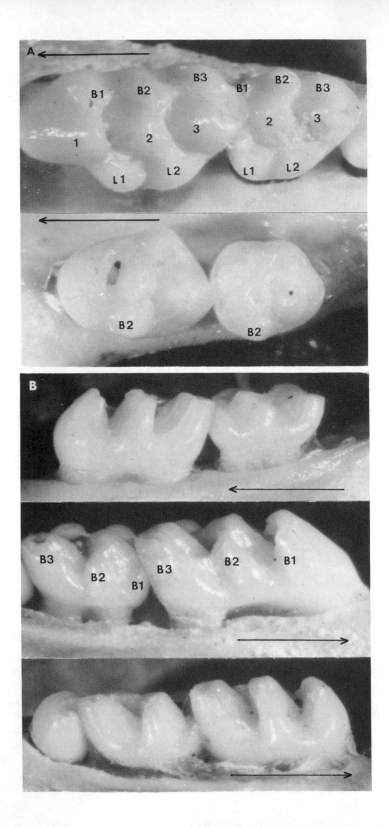

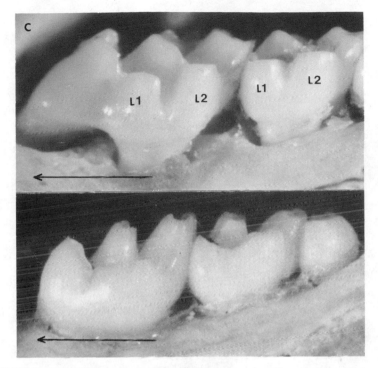

FIG. 3. Maxillary teeth *in situ*. A. Occlusal C₃Hf above, *cr/cr* below; B. buccal *cr/cr* above, C₃Hf middle, *Ta/–* below; C. palatal C₃Hf above, *Ta/–* below. Arrows pointing anteriorly are 1 mm in length. Cusps numbered as Gaunt (1955).

control. B3 was missing or blended into cusp 3. On the palatal side L1 was reduced and semi continuous with a sometimes enlarged L2. In M^2 B_1 was enlarged or continuous with L1 by a rampart around the anterior part of cusp 2. (Cusp 1 in normal mice is missing on M^2.) Again, B2 was larger than normal and closely aligned to cusp 2 while B3 was missing. Cusp 3 was larger than normal. The variations in M^3 have been described by Grüneberg (1965, 1966a, b); in these tabbies all M^3 were present. In crinkled mice, 25% M^3 were missing. In each of the upper molars the roots were fused together or tended to be, and were shorter than normal.

In the lower jaw the first molar is composed normally of an anterior complex of four cusps and a posterior group of three. In tabby and crinkled a combined anterior cusp with a hint of the original cusps was found while there was a single posterior cusp placed more in the midline. In some of the crinkled mice this was found to be a rim of enamel with a centrally placed depression with exposed dentine forming an enlarged and greatly distorted enamel-free area. The cusps of M_2 were similarly changed so that M_1 and M_2 were remarkably similar, both in size and shape. In this tabby mutant ($Ta/–$)

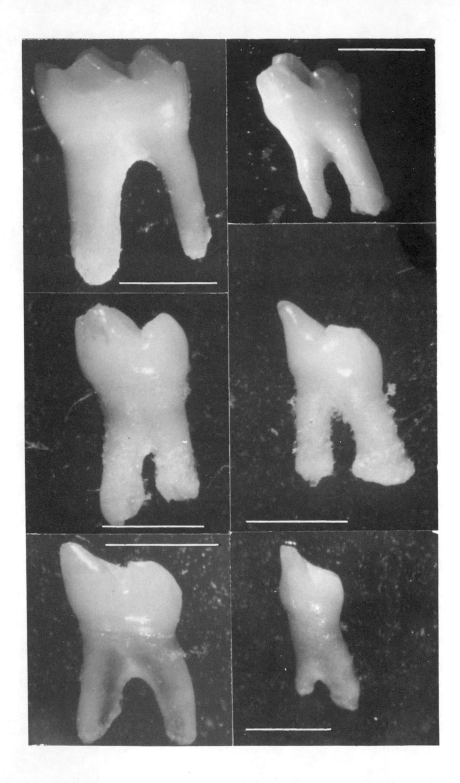

M_2 was found to be more affected than the M_2 of crinkled (cr/cr). The roots were very slight again with tabby more affected than crinkled (Fig. 4). In some animals an abnormal root sheath had resulted in taurodontism. In tabby all M_3 were missing and in crinkled 92% were.

The changes in crown morphology, particularly in M_1 and M_2, had produced an abnormal occlusion with the combined central cusps of the lower teeth occluding directly and traumatically with the central cusps 1, 2 and 3, and 2 and 3 of M^1 and M^2 respectively. In the older crinkled stock abnormal wear patterns had developed and alveolar bone loss was severe. This phenomenon has been described and discussed in detail elsewhere (Miller, 1976).

DISCUSSION

There is clearly a range of defects in the tabby syndrome (Grüneberg, 1971a, b) with teeth and other structures smaller or missing. The threshold phenomenon invoked by Grüneberg (op. cit.) certainly is apparent. However, if we look at the nature of the reduced size another fact becomes apparent.

In the adult the incisors may be missing or reduced, but when they are reduced the enamel is observed to wrap further around the dentine than in a normal tooth. In the bulbous molar teeth the enamel again wraps around a somewhat reduced dentine "core". Similar shapes are observed during the development of teeth associated with this syndrome (Sofaer, 1969a). The general conclusion is that the mesoderm or its product—dentine—is more reduced than the enamel and that there appears to be a discrepancy in relative proportions of the two tissues. The mutant crooked tail (Cd/Cd) has slightly smaller teeth than normal but they are slightly bulbous and certain cusps more erect (Grüneberg, 1965). It would appear to be part-way towards the reduced tooth size of tabby and crinkled.

If we turn to the pelage effects similar considerations seem to apply. Other than the mystacial whiskers, whiskers or guard hairs are reduced or absent. The largest body hairs (awls) are missing as well as the smallest (zig-zags). If the mesoderm directs their morphology (Cohen, 1961, 1969) then it appears that there is a general decrease in the mesodermal component (dermal papilla). It is not certain whether the whiskers form an autonomous group but an awl (the largest of the body hairs) in the site of a missing whisker would be very difficult to identify.

A wide variety of glands are reduced or missing (Grüneberg, 1971a) and although mesodermal "ghosts" have been observed in glands which failed to develop at the time of their initiation some disturbance in their mesodermal component might be looked for. The "solid bud" concept as described by Grüneberg (op cit.) may well also have a mesodermal component.

When the original tooth bud is established too little ectomesenchyme may well result in the last cusp of the original trigon B_3 not developing. One of the

---

FIG. 4. Mandibular molar teeth of C_3Hf above, cr/cr middle, $Ta/-$ below; M_1 on left, M_2 on right; lines 1 mm.

problems in the tabby syndrome has been to explain why cusps 2 and B2, the other members of the trigon, should be near normal while B_3 is abnormal. We cannot agree with Sofaer (1969b) that B3 has migrated and that the tabby cusp 3 is homologous with normal B3. The cusp is still clearly identifiable as 3 and does not have any obvious mixed morphological features as one might expect if homology were the case. Further proliferation of both dental papilla and internal dental epithelium from an already abnormal trigon with associated abnormalities in tension within the internal dental epithelium (Butler, 1956) could then explain subsequently developed abnormalities. If epithelium proliferates less abnormally than decreased mesoderm, variations such as bulbosity and the anterior rampart on M^2 can be understood. The meristic effect between M1 and M2 then becomes related to similar developmental processes, associated in both teeth with similar factors. Failure of M3 could be explained in terms of insufficient ectomesenchyme to initiate or maintain the tooth germ. Although when M^3 does not develop there is some ectodermal proliferation initially (Grewal, 1962; Sofaer, 1969a) but see below and Osborne (1971).

One further point should be raised. What is meant by a threshold in morphogenetic terms? It is established that the teeth are smaller or do not develop and that the colliculi piliferi are smaller (Grüneberg, op. cit.; Dun, 1959). What needs to be established is whether we are discussing a volume or mass of cells, be it ectodermal or mesodermal (ectomesenchyme) or the area of the interface between two interacting cell populations. As yet this is not clear. Implants from various sources apparently need to be of a critical mass before they will be maintained (Cohen, 1969; R. M. Browne, W. A. Miller and R. Oliver, in preparation).

There is also the consideration of the maintenance of the length of the tooth row but, although in morphological terms this is real, the feedback mechanism when none of the components is fully formed in any dimension is difficult to visualize because individual tooth differences can be of the order of only 10% in length.

It is generally agreed that the development of teeth, as shown experimentally in urodeles and presumed in mammals, is initiated by neural crest cells which migrate into the head region (Sellman, 1946; Horstadius, 1950). Odontoblasts or at least some of them are considered to be of neural crest origin and hence ectomesenchyme.

Although epithelial proliferation is not evident until 12–13 days postconception (Cohn 1957) it can be demonstrated that the presumptive molar region is established by 10 days and that of the incisors by 10·5 days (Miller, 1969, 1971). This corresponds temporally to an increase (influx) of RNA-rich, alkaline-positive, glycogen-positive cells postulated by Milaire (1959) and Pourtois (1961) to be migrating neural crest cells. By 14 days postconception the morphogenic information resides in the mesoderm of the presumptive tooth-bearing areas (Kollar and Baird, 1969). Studies on migrating melanoblast populations into the head region (Miller, 1970) show that by 9·5 days post-conception mystacial whiskers will develop and contain melanocytes. At 10 days occasional mandibular melanocytes are visible in explants grown for 10 days on the chick chorioallantois but cannot be identified regularly and with certainty, until 11 days post-conception. The identification of whisker germs is also uncertain.

These are clearly several factors that have to be taken into account in understanding the tabby syndrome. If the mesodermal component—possibly derived from neural crest—is reduced, why might this be so? It has been shown in some genetic mutations that melanoblast migration is slower than normal and abnormalities of pigmentation are more manifest at the points most distant such as the distal parts of limbs (Auerback, 1954). If other neural crest cell migrations can be disturbed then distant regions such as the incisors would be affected and this is the situation in tabby and crinkled. If a certain amount of neural crest material arrived in the molar region, subsequent proliferation distally, in association with dental lamina, might be disturbed with failure of development of M3.

Delayed migration would result in a potential mismatch with ectoderm having increasing competence to respond. This increasing competence of ectoderm in dental development has been discussed by Osborne (1971), in relation to the development of its dentition, in *Lacerta vivipara*, and Grewal (1962) has described an initial ectodermal response in third molar tooth germs at the bud stage prior to their regression and hence non-development of the tooth. There are also the differences (Sofaer, 1973, 1974) between the apparent site of the defect in relation to tail skin of downless (a mutant similar to crinkled) and tabby. In downless the defect lies in the epidermis while there is "no evidence of a primary epidermal effect in tabby" (Sofaer, 1974). Identification of the mechanism of abnormality in this fascinating syndrome has yet to be accomplished.

ACKNOWLEDGEMENTS

The author is indebted to Dr Beatrice Mintz, Institute for Cancer Research, Philadelphia, for a gift of tabby and crinkled mice. The technical assistance of Mona Everett, Malcolm McCuaig and Jeffrey Cramer is also readily acknowledged. This research has been supported in part by NIDR Grant DE02908 and General Research Support Grant 5 S01 RR 05330. I thank my wife Karen for much helpful discussion during this investigation.

REFERENCES

AUERBACH, R. (1954). Analysis of the developmental affects of a lethal mutation in the house mouse. *J. exp. Zool.* **127**, 305–324.

BUTLER, P. M. (1956). The ontogeny of molar pattern. *Biol. Rev.* **31**, 30.

COHEN, J. (1961). The transplantation of individual rat and guinea pig whisker papillae. *J. Embryol. exp. Morph.* **9**, 117–127.

COHEN, J. (1969). Dermis, epidermis and dermal papillae interacting. *Adv. Biol. Skin* **9**, 1–18.

COHN, S. A. (1957). Development of the molar teeth of the albino mouse. *Am. J. Anat.* **101**, 295–320.

DUN, R. B. (1959). The development and growth of vibrissae in the house mouse with particular reference to the time of action of the tabby (*Ta*) and ragged (*Ra*) genes. *Aust. J. biol. Sci.* **12**, 312–330.

FALCONER, D. S., FRASER, A. S. and KING, J. W. B. (1951). The genetics and development of "crinkled", a new mutant of the house mouse. *J. Genet.* **50**, 324–344.

GAUNT, W. A. (1955). The development of the molar pattern of the mouse, *Mus musculus. Acta anat.* **24**, 249–268.

GAUNT, W. A. (1961). The presence of apical pits on the lower cheek teeth of the mouse. *Acta anat.* **44**, 146–158.

GREWAL, M. S. (1962). The development of an inherited tooth defect in the mouse. *J. Embryol. exp. Morph.* **10**, 202–224.

GRÜNEBERG, H. (1965). Genes and genotypes effecting the teeth of the mouse. *J. Embryol. exp. Morph.* **14**, 137–159.

GRÜNEBERG, H. (1966a). The molars of the tabby mouse and a test of the single active X-chromosome hypothesis. *J. Embryol. exp. Morph.* **15**, 233–244.

GRÜNEBERG, H. (1966b). More about the tabby mouse and about the Lyon hypothesis. *J. Embryol. exp. Morph.* **16**, 569–590.

GRÜNEBERG, H. (1969). Threshold phenomena versus cell heredity in the manifestation of sex-linked genes in mammals. *J. Embryol exp. Morph.* **22**, 145–179.

GRÜNEBERG, H. (1971a). The glandular aspects of the tabby syndrome in the mouse. *J. Embryol. exp. Morph.* **25**, 1–19.

GRÜNEBERG, H. (1971b). The tabby syndrome in the mouse. *Proc. R. Soc. Lond.* B. **179**, 139–156.

HORSTADIUS, S. (1950). "The Neural Crest." Oxford University Press, Oxford.

KOLLAR, E. J. and BAIRD, G. R. (1969). The influence of the dental papilla on the development of tooth shape in embryonic tooth germs. *J. Embryol. exp. Morph.* **21**, 131–148.

KOLLAR, E. J. and BAIRD, G. R. (1969). The influence of the dental papilla on the development of tooth shape in embryonic tooth germs. *J. Embryol. exp. Morph.* **21**, 131–148.

MILAIRE, J. (1959). Prédifferentiation cytochimique de diverses ébauches cephaliques de l'embryon de souris. *Archs Biol., Liége,* **70**, 587–730.

MILLER, W. A. (1969). Inductive changes in early tooth development. I. *J. dent. Res.* **48**, 719–725.

MILLER, W. A. (1970). Migration of pigment cells into the jaws of C_{57} B1/6 mice. Abstract No. 578 IADR Annual meeting.

MILLER, W. A. (1971). Early dental development in mice. *In* "Dental Morphology and Evolution" pp. 31–44. University of Chicago Press, U.S.A.

MILLER, W. A. (1976). Genetic traumatic occlusion in the mouse. *J. Perio. Res.* **12**, 64–72.

MILLER, W. A. and RADNOR, C. J. P. (1970). Tooth replacement patterns in young *Caiman sclerops. J. Morph.* **130**, 501–510.

MILLER, W. A. DRINNAN, A. J. and EICK, J. D. Microprobe analysis for Ca, P, Mg and Fe of mouse enamel in normal and genetically anaemic animals (unpublished data).

OSBORN, J. W. (1971). The ontogeny of tooth succession in *Lacerta vivipara* Jacquin (1787). *Proc. R. Soc. Lond.* B. **179**, 261–289.

POURTOIS, M. (1961). Contribution à l'étude des bourgeons dentaires chez la souris. I. Périodes d' induction et de morphodifferenciation. *Archs Biol., Liége* **72**, 17–95.

ROBINS, M. W. and ROWLATT, C. (1971). Dental abnormalities in aged mice. *Gerontologia* **17**, 261–272.

SELLMAN, S. (1946). Some experiments on the determination of larval teeth in *Ambystoma mexicanum*. *Odont. Tidskr.* **54**, 1–128.

SOFAER, J. A. (1969a). Aspects of the tabby–crinkled–downless syndrome. I. The development of tabby teeth. *J. Embryol. exp. Morph.* **22**, 181–205.

SOFAER, J. A. (1969b). Aspects of the tabby–crinkled–downless syndrome II. Observations on the reaction to changes of genetic background. *J. Embryol. exp. Morph.* **22**, 207–227.

SOFAER, J. A. (1973). Hair follicle initiation in reciprocal recombinations of Downless homozygote and heterozygote mouse tail epidermis and dermis. *Devl Biol.* **34**, 289–296.

SOFAER, J. A. (1974). Differences between tabby and downless mouse epidermis and dermis in culture. *Genet. Res.* **23**, 219–225.

WESTON, J. A. (1970). The migration and differentiation of neural crest cells. *Adv. Morphogen.* **8**, 41–114.

9. Dental Morphological Variations associated with Murine Chondrodystrophies (with a comment on the histology of the cartilage disturbances)

KAREN L. FLYNN-MILLER

and

WILLIAM A. MILLER

Department of Oral Biology, State University of New York, Buffalo, New York, U.S.A.

INTRODUCTION

In 1968, Lane and Dickie reported on three genetically distinct recessive mutations, achondroplasia (*cn*), brachymorphic (*bm*) and stubby (*stb*), which produce disproportionate dwarfing in the house mouse (*Mus musculus*). The most obvious defect in all three was shortening of those bones towards whose final form endochrondral ossification contributes. This chapter will deal briefly with the relation of these animals to analogous human conditions, and with their pertinent histology and radiology, and describe in some detail the dental and cranial abnormalities associated with the mutations.

In the past a wide range of human micromelic dwarfism associated with cranial deformities has been grouped under the name of "achondroplasia". Their gradual separation into a variety of distinct chondrodystrophies has been summarized by Maroteaux and Lamy (1963) and Rimoin *et al.* (1970).

The achondroplastic mouse, on the basis of preliminary radiographic and histologic findings (Lane and Dickie, 1968) is considered to be an animal model analogous to the human condition (Rimoin *et al.*, 1970).

Brachymorphic and stubby present, in that order, decreasing degrees of dwarfism from achondroplasia. Histologically, we have found stubby to be similar to achondroplasia, although abnormal to a lesser degree. Brachymorphic is somewhat different and cannot as yet be assigned to an analogous human condition.

METHODS AND MATERIALS

We have examined 11 achondroplastics, 6 brachymorphics and 8 stubbies, and appropriate littermate controls for each, making 47 animals in all. These somewhat rare animals were aged between 5 and 6 weeks, with a few animals around 8–10 weeks, and were obtained from the Jackson Memorial Laboratory in Bar Harbor, Maine. None of the findings include cross references between litters, and all litters were from inbred lines.

On receipt of the specimens, whole body radiographs of skinned specimens were taken at 75 cm at 70 kV, 9 mA using Kodak fine grain professional photographic film and an exposure of 2·5 min. The heads were removed and sectioned just off the midline in the sagittal plane, and radiographs taken of each half head.

Histological material was prepared from the thicker side of the head in the sagittal plane to examine the synchondroses of the base of the skull and the cranial sutures. Other histological material was prepared in an oblique frontal plane parallel to the long axes of M_1 and M^1 and so also transverse to the lower incisor.

Serial 8-μm sections were cut from 10 % formic acid dimineralized, paraffin-embedded material and stained with haematoxylin and eosin, haematoxylin and van Gieson or Alcian blue (Lison, 1950).

Split-head radiographs were analysed for incisal curvature with a standard metric-circle template on three-times enlarged photographs from the radiographic image. Appropriate growth controls were included. The angles of the base of the skull and otic capsule were also examined. The tooth-bearing bones were then separated, defleshed, dried and mounted on glass slides. Cusps on each tooth were identified and numbered according to the system employed by Gaunt (1955), and drawings of each tooth made from occlusal, buccal and lingual views under a dissecting microscope at ×25 magnification with a *camera lucida*. The teeth were left *in situ*, so only crown morphology was considered. Comparisons were made only between littermates.

RESULTS

Bones

Whole body radiographs (Fig. 1) showed the general smallness of the affected animals. Limbs were obviously shorter, as was the tail. In radiographs shortened tail vertebrae of normal width were particularly obvious although body vertebrae were similarly abnormal. Dwarfing of the abdominal contents was less so that the abdomen tended to be distended. The achondroplastic animals were the most affected and the stubbies the least.

The base of the skull was shortened producing retrusion of the maxilla in relation to the mandible, and subsequent malocclusion. Malocclusion is a common finding in the human condition as well, for similar reasons, and patients often show an anterior open bite (King 1972; Shafer *et al.*, 1973). With the incisors in a normal relationship (Fig. 2) the upper molars were at least one, and sometimes two, cusp units displaced to the distal from a normal relationship. An occasional finding was the mandible in a protruded position, possibly in an effort to relieve the breathing difficulties which have been reported to occur (Lane and Dickie, 1968).

Brachymorphic was usually retruded one cusp unit. Stubbies were relatively equally divided between normal and displaced molar relationships. Their maxillary growth retardation, less than that in *cn/cn* and *bm/bm*, may place the molars in a cusp-to-cusp relation which in function slides distally or mesially into a full intercuspal position.

The angle between the occlusal plane, which establishes a form of horizontal reference plane, and the common crus of the vestibular apparatus was measured to further assess the degree of abnormality of the skull. In *cn/cn* this was invariably 5–12° larger than control and the whole otic capsule was positioned at a lower level (Figs 2 and 3).

There are two synchondroses in the base of the skull (Fig. 4), the anterior basispheno: presphenoid synchondrosis and the posterior basispheno: occipital synchondrosis. In the heterozygotes (+ /cn) the cartilages and their conversion to bone form an orderly spacial sequence (Fig. 5). A central cartilage was present with columns of aligned chondroblasts on either side which underwent hypertrophy, calcification and subsequent remodelling to form a joint with a smooth external outline. This was particularly well seen in the basispheno: occipital synchondrosis. The cancellous bone adjacent to the marrow space had slight and evenly arranged trabeculae. In the achondroplastic (*cn/cn*) littermate much of the joint architecture had been lost (Fig. 6). The central cartilage was all but gone although a few, frequently quite well aligned, columns of cartilage cells were still apparent. The ossification sites were closer together and were almost quiescent. The width of the joint was much greater and projected in an angular fashion into the surrounding soft tissues. Periosteal bone remodelling was disrupted over the cartilage itself which resulted in this appearance. The basispheno: presphenoid synchondrosis was similarly distorted although in a less dramatic way.

Stubby homozygotes gave similarly disturbed cartilaginous growth although to a lesser degree. In brachymorphic animals (*bm/bm*) the cartilaginous disturbance was rather more severe in that the columns of chondrocytes were disrupted to a greater extent earlier in the life of the animal (Fig. 7) and the outline of the joint showed an even more irregular relationship between cartilage and periosteal bone. The line of proliferation was also uneven across the joint resulting in variations in cartilage thickness. In spite of this, the dwarfing in this mutation is relatively less than that reported for achondroplasia although more than stubby (Lane and Dickie, 1968).

Similar cartilaginous disturbances were found in the cervical and caudal vertebrae and the long bones. The bossing of the skull also produced characteristic changes in the shape of the cranial sutures which became butt joints instead of overlapping ones. This was particularly pronounced in the

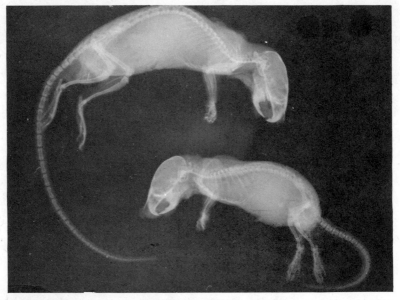

FIG. 1. Whole body radiographs of skinned siblings: $+/cn$ above, cn/cn below. Note the generally smaller body size of the homozygote, which has disproportionate dwarfing of the limbs and tail in particular. The shorter vertebrae of almost normal width are particularly visible in the tail but may also be observed in the trunk.

parietal–postparietal suture. Casual examination of the bone marrow showed a great number of macrophages containing haemosiderin crystals. The animals are reported to be frequently cyanotic (Lane and Dickie, 1968), and these heart failure cells were a likely result. The histology of these disturbances has been described in detail (Miller and Flynn-Miller, 1976).

Dentition

The curvature of the incisors was measured in radiographs of the bones by superimposing a metric circle template over $\times 3$ magnification prints. Although the growth pattern of rodent incisors has long been known to follow a logarithmic spiral (Thompson, 1966), measurements of this sort, admittedly somewhat of an estimation, offered a convenient means for observing gross discrepancies in these patterns between mutant and control animals. In cn/cn lower incisors it was found that the curvature changed, being smaller caudally, below the region of the mesial root of the lower first molar (Fig. 8). The control lower incisor followed the same circle along its entire length. Upper incisors followed the same curvature as controls in cn/cn, bm/bm and stb/stb. The lower incisors in neither bm/bm nor stb/stb showed any changes in curvature. In no animal was there a significant difference between right and left sides indicating that the slight parasagittal orientation of the division of the head did not affect this measurement.

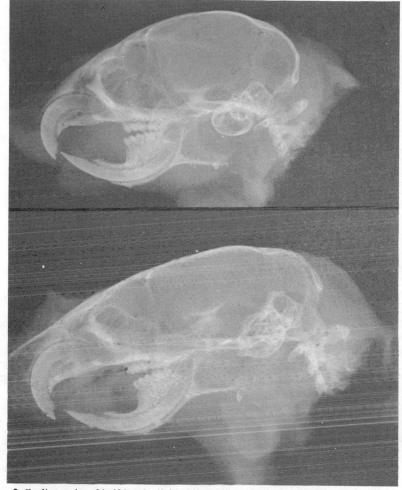

FIG. 2. Radiographs of half heads divided just off the mid-sagittal plane. Note the smaller head with the shortened base of the skull and cranial bossing. Protrusive malocclusion is also visible in the homozygote.

In order to test if this change was partly due to the smaller size of the animals a radiographic series was made of the mandibles and premaxillae of a litter of C_3Hf mice to determine whether incisor curvature, i.e. the diameter of the circle followed by an incisor, was related to growth, or to the final adult size of the animal. It was found that the diameter of curvature in both the upper and lower incisors increased only up to 21 days of age, after which the curvature remained constant while the length of the arc occupied by the incisor increased. This was subsequently found to be true in material up to 14 months of age.

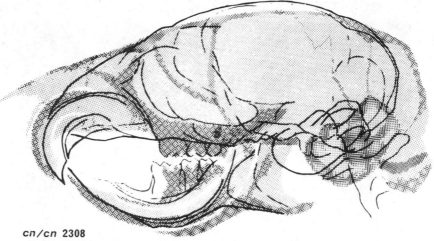

cn/cn 2308
Control 2309

FIG. 3. *cn/cn* (Outline) and its control (hatched) radiographs superimposed with first molar mesial surfaces aligned and occlusal planes horizontal. A line through the common crus of the vestibular apparatus (used as the long axis of the otic capsule) made a 5–12° greater angle with the horizontal in *cn/cn*.

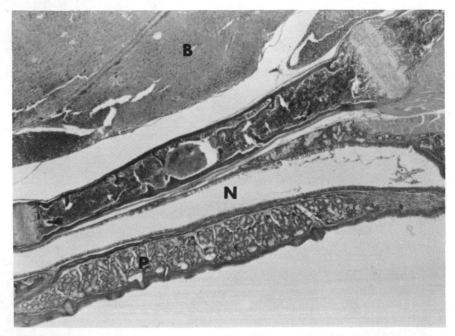

FIG. 4. Low power micrograph of the basispheno: presphenoid and basispheno: occipital synchondroses sectioned in the parasagittal plane. B: brain; N: nasal cavity; P: posterior part of hard and the soft palate.

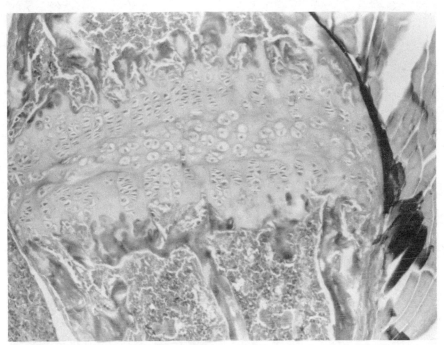

FIG. 5, Basispheno : occipital synchondrosis of a $+/cn$ animal. The proliferative, hypertrophic and calcifying regions of the cartilage are even and the primary ossification is regular. Haematoxylin and van Gieson. ×100.

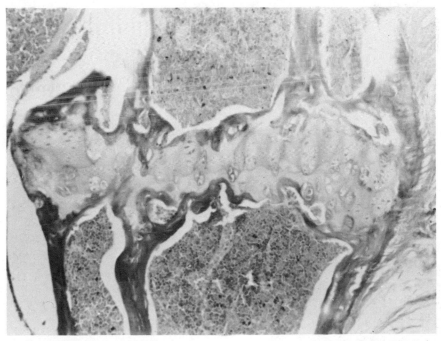

FIG. 6. Basispheno : occipital synchondrosis of a cn/cn animal. As compared to Fig. 5 the joint is wider and the external surface irregular. There is no periosteal bone formation on the remains of the joint cartilage. A few regular chondroblast columns are visible.

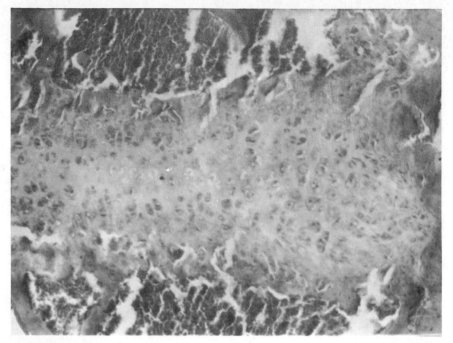

FIG. 7. Basispheno : occipital synchondrosis of *bm/bm*. The irregular orientation of the chondroblast columns is apparent. The width of the joint is increased. Haematoxylin and eosin. ×100.

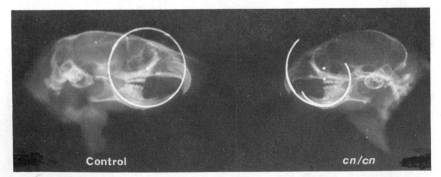

FIG. 8. Radiographs of half-heads of *cn/cn* and control. The circle outlines have been superimposed to demonstrate the change in curvature of the achondroplastic lower incisor.

A |1mm

cn/cn

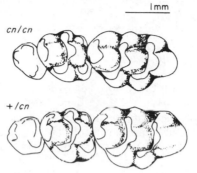

+/cn

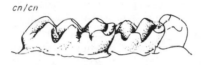

B |1mm

cn/cn

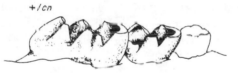

+/cn

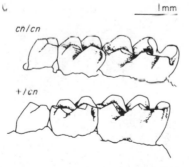

C |1mm

cn/cn

+/cn

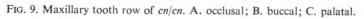

FIG. 9. Maxillary tooth row of *cn/cn*. A. occlusal; B. buccal; C. palatal.

Grüneberg (1965) has demonstrated the essentially identical morphology of all molars within a given inbred strain of the mouse. The animals in this study showed a number of differences which are admittedly subtle but which indicate a particular trend. Figure 9 shows typical right maxillary tooth rows from a *cn/cn* animal and its control in occlusal views. All of the *cn/cn* teeth were shorter mesiodistally, and narrower bucco-lingually, and accordingly the whole tooth row was shorter. The tooth row followed a curve which was concave towards the palate as compared to the alignment in the control, which was straight.

The variations between the achondroplastic and normal teeth all occurred either in the cusp complex at the disto-buccal corner of M^1 (3 and B3), or in the region of B2. The disto-buccal complex in all *cn/cn* M^1 and M^2 appeared to be simplified over that in the control. This simplification took the form either of a diminished B3, resulting in a more acute angle to that corner of the tooth when seen from the occlusal (Fig. 9) or a blurring and rounding of the grooves separating the two cusps, which resulted in a more massive, but less defined complex. This change always appeared meristically in M^1 and M^2. A common finding in the control strains was the division of B2 of M^1 into two cusps, separated from each other by a groove and from the surrounding cusps by varying degrees of notching. In such teeth, the control showed a much more pronounced groove than the *cn/cn*—again a trend towards simplification. These simplifying characteristics were present in achondroplastic teeth regardless of the genetic background, and therefore molar morphology, against which they appeared. Certain other changes were variable and perhaps not attributable to *cn/cn*.

The alignment of the mandibular tooth row showed no change but the entire tooth row was shortened, because all of the *cn/cn* teeth were slightly smaller in both dimensions (Fig. 10). The changed maxillary v. mandibular intercuspation would, in older animals than these, warrant careful distinction between atypical wear patterns and true morphological differences. In the

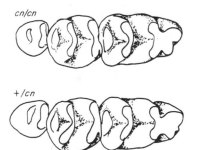

FIG. 10. Mandibular tooth row of *cn/cn*.

mandibular teeth, changes, which could be attributed to achondroplasia, always occurred in specific regions of the teeth. In M_1 the complex formed by the four anterior cusps was an area of variation, and in M_2 the anterior complex was formed by the first major buccal and lingual cusps plus a small accessory buccal cusp. The two buccal and two lingual cusps forming the anterior M_2 complex in the controls often were augmented by accessory grooves, notches and ledges (Fig. 10). These were eliminated in the achondroplastics. In the *cn/cn* M_2 the small first buccal cusp was often blended into the cusp behind and was indistinguishable occlusally. The mandibular molars therefore also showed a meristic effect as in the maxillary teeth.

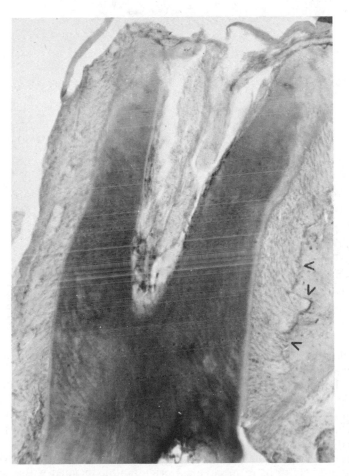

FIG. 11. Longitudinal section of the anterior root of M^1 in *cn/cn*. The root structure and morphology are normal. Increased bone remodelling is visible on the palatal side (arrows). Haematoxylin and eosin. ×100.

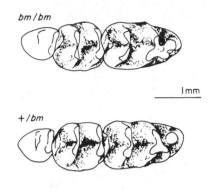

FIG. 12. Mandibular tooth row of *bm/bm*.

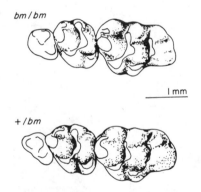

FIG. 13. Maxillary tooth row of *bm/bm*.

Histological examination of the roots of M^1 in frontal section showed that in both $+/cn$ and cn/cn, the morphology of the roots was similar. However, in the achondroplastic there was considerable bone resorption on the palatal aspect indicating that the tooth was moving in a palatal direction (Fig. 11). This was no doubt related to the curved upper molar tooth row. In M_1 this bone remodelling was less pronounced. Similar excessive bone resorption was observed on the lingual side of the lower incisors. These features indicate that the shape of the maxillary tooth row along with the variation in the lower incisor are likely to be of mechanical origin and associated with the relative shortening of the upper jaw.

The brachymorphic molars, as a group, are not distinctly smaller than those of their controls. The simplification process, however, does appear to have functioned in the *bm/bm* molars, in many of the same areas where these changes were found in the *cn/cn* teeth.

The anterior cusp complex of the *bm/bm* M_1 (Fig. 12) shows the fusion of L1 with the L2–B1–B2 group, while it is a quite independent unit in +/*bm*. A small island of enamel, however, often remains in the centre of the enamel-free occlusal surface of the complex even in *bm/bm*. The trend continues in the *bm/bm* maxillary molars (Fig. 13). Cusps B3 and 3 in both M^1 and M^2 are fused and show a continuous enamel-free area, while in +/*bm* they are separate. A buccal view of these teeth shows shallower grooves separating the cusps in *bm/bm*, as well as a more upright cuspal orientation.

In the small number of stubbies examined no obvious differences were noted between *stb/stb* and +/*stb*, except that in the homozygotes M_3 was noticeably delayed in eruption as compared with the heterozygotes.

DISCUSSION

One question which is raised by data such as these which associate the occurrence of some degree of dental morphological variation with faulty cartilage growth and development of various kinds is: what might be the common factor between teeth and cartilage? Or, more specifically, does a common developmental mechanism operate on both tissues?

Konyukhov and Ginter (1966) and Konyukhov and Paschin (1967) have investigated the effect of two different genes, brachypodism-H and achondroplasia, on cartilage growth. They found that a tissue extract of brachypod-H embryos inhibits growth of normal cartilage cells undergoing hypertrophy. Assuming that the effect of *cn/cn* on cartilage cells could also be specified they conducted a series of subcutaneous homotransplantations of bone between 7- or 14-day *cn/cn* and +/*cn* siblings. Humeri of +/*cn* transplanted to *cn/cn* showed decreased growth compared to humeri transplanted from +/*cn* to +/*cn*, indicating a humoral effect of the *cn* gene. The radii of *cn/cn* transplanted to +/*cn* grew less well than transplants between controls, indicating an effect on the chondrocytes themselves. These results show that the growth inhibition of the cartilaginous skeleton of *cn/cn* mice is due to both the primary *cn* gene effect on the chondrocytes and a secondary effect through a hypothesized growth-inhibiting factor in the serum, but they were not able to identify this substance as a protein fraction nor as any serum mucopolysaccharide (Konyukhov and Paschin, 1967). It may well be that the dental defect in these mutants is invoked by the serum factor. This obviously needs to be tested although other explanations are possible.

Oblation of appropriate head neural crest in urodeles (Sellman, 1946; Horstadius, 1950) disturbs both head cartilage and dental development. However, neural crest has been found not to make any direct contribution to trunk cartilage (Weston, 1970). If a humoral factor in achondroplasia can in fact be reasonably postulated, it may be possible, with the aid of studies which accurately time the action of the *cn* gene, to tie in with neural crest cells both an indirect or inductive influence on body cartilage, and to provide some further information of the role of the neural crest in the dental development of mammals.

Histologically, there is a spectrum of disturbed growth of chondral bones—from achondroplasia to brachymorphic, stubby and normal. Whether this is a temporal shortening of an otherwise normal process in *cn/cn* and *stb/stb*, with stubby becoming affected slightly later than achondroplastic, as has been suggested to occur in humans with true achondroplasia (Rimoin *et al.*, 1970), or is the result of a structurally abnormal growth site *per se* can only be determined from the examination of an extended series of timed specimens. Histologically, brachymorphic appears to be a distinct entity with the cartilaginous growth site definitely abnormal in structure, particularly in its cartilaginous part. Subsequent studies are likely to result in this genetic abnormality being placed in a separate category from achondroplasia.

ACKNOWLEDGEMENTS

We should like to thank Dr A. J. Drinnan, Department of Oral Medicine, State University of New York at Buffalo, for making initial material available to us and Mrs P. W. Lane, Jackson Laboratory, for help in obtaining the bulk of our specimens. The excellent technical assistance of Mrs Stephanie Pryshlak and Miss Mona Everett is readily acknowledged. Photographic assistance came from Mr M. McCuaig and Mr H. Velasco.

Supported in part by NIDR General Research Support Grant 5 S01 RR 05330 to W.A.M. and a United Way of Buffalo, New York Summer Fellowship to K.L.F-M.

REFERENCES

GAUNT, W. A. (1955). The development of the molar pattern of the mouse (*Mus musculus*) *Acta anat.* **24**, 244–268.
GRÜNEBERG, H. (1965). Genes and genotypes affecting the teeth of the mouse. *J. Embryol. exp. Morph.* **14**, 137–159.
HORSTADIUS, S. (1950). "The Neural Crest." Oxford University Press, London and New York.
KING, K. J. (1972). Clinical dental findings in achondroplastics. *Int. Assoc. dent. Res.*, annual meeting abstract No. 283.
KONYUKHOV, B. V. and GINTER, E. K. (1966). A study of the action of the brachy-podism-H gene on development of the long bones of hind limbs in the mouse. *Folia. biol, Praha* **12**, 199–206.
KONYUKHOV, B. V. and PASCHIN, Y. V. (1967). Experimental study of the achondro-plastic gene effects in the mouse. *Acta biol. hung.* **18**, 285–294.
LANE, P. W. and DICKIE, M. M. (1968). Three recessive mutations producing disproportionate dwarfing in mice: achondroplasia, brachymorphic, and stubby. *J. Hered.* **59**, 300–308.
LISON, L. (1950). *In* "Handbook of Histopathological Technique" (Culling, C. F. A., ed.), p. 234. Butterworth, London.

MAROTEAUX, P. and LAMY, M. (1963). Achondroplasia in man and animals. *Clin. orthoped.* **33**, 91–103.

MILLER, W. A. and FLYNN-MILLER, K. L. (1976). Achondroplastic, brachymorphic and stubby chondrodystrophies in mice. *J. Comp. Pathol.* **86**, 349–363.

RIMOIN, D. L., HUGHES, G. N., KAUFMAN, R. L., ROSENTHAL, R. E., McALISTER, W. H. and SILBERBERG, R. (1970). Endochondral ossification in achondroplastic dwarfism. *New Eng. J. Med.* **283**, 728–735.

SELLMAN, S. (1946). Some experiments on the determination of larval teeth in *Ambystoma mexicanum. Odont. Tidskr.* **54**, 1–128.

SHAFER, W. G., HINE, M. K. and LEVY, B. M. (1973). "A Textbook of Oral Pathology". W. B. Saunders, Philadelphia, U.S.A.

THOMPSON, D'A. W. (1966). *In* "On Growth and Form" (Bonner, J. T., ed.), pp. 214–216. Cambridge University Press, Cambridge.

WESTON, J. A. (1970). The migration and differentiation of neural crest cells. *Adv. Morphogen.* **8**, 41–114.

10. Differences in Sexual Dimorphism in Dental Morphology among Several Human Populations

KAZURO HANIHARA

Department of Anthropology, The University of Tokyo, Japan

INTRODUCTION

Differences in tooth size between males and females are usually known to be larger in the fossil hominids than in the modern man. For instance, it is well known that the tooth size of the Peking man shows a wide range of variation, and it is believed that this trend is caused by a large difference between sexes. This fact may lead us to an assumption that, even in the recent man, the differences in tooth size between sexes are larger in the populations which still retain some archaic physical characteristics than in those who show more progressive form.

Some years ago, I noticed that between-sex difference in tooth size was smaller in Japanese than in other populations such as Caucasians, American Indians etc. In 1969 when I visited the University of Adelaide, Australia, I was surprised to find that the between-sex difference was rather small in the Aborigines, because I had expected a much larger sexual dimorphism in this population. When I returned home, I compared the data from several populations, and realized that the between-sex differences in tooth size seemed to be correlated neither with the general tooth-size nor with archaic morphology of the teeth and other physical characteristics, at least so far as recent populations were concerned. At the same time, I suspected that the pattern of difference between sexes might have varied from population to population. For example, the difference might have been particularly large in the front teeth in some populations, but in the back teeth in the others. The present study was carried out with a view to analyse the basic factors which give rise to between-sex difference in the tooth-crown size, and their variations among different populations.

Materials and Methods

The data used in this study were mesiodistal crown diameters of the permanent dentition, and the populations compared were Japanese, Caucasians in Chicago, Pima Indians, American Negroes in Washington D.C. and Australian Aborigines settled in Central Australia (Table I). These materials

TABLE I. Materials used.

Population	No. of Samples			Depository
	Male	Female	Total	
Japanese	50	50	100	University of Tokyo
Caucasians	47	34	81	University of Chicago
Pima Indians	60	60	120	University of Chicago
American Negroes	40	40	80	Howard University
Australian Aborigines	80	58	138	University of Adelaide

were dental casts made of artificial stone, the measurements of which were recorded personally. The number of the teeth used for analysis was eight—I^1, C, PM^2, M^2, I_2, PM_1, M_1 and M_2—because the other teeth showed much higher correlations with these teeth.

The calculations for multivariate analysis were processed by the HITAC OS-7 system of the University of Tokyo Computer Centre using FORTRAN programs contained in program libraries PLAS* and HSAP†.

Distances between Male and Female Groups

First of all, Mahalanobis's D-squares, or the so-called generalized distances, between males and females were computed in every population. This calculation was carried out on the basis of the pooled dispersion matrix of the five populations involved, or ten groups if the male and female groups were counted separately. In other words, D-squares shown in Table II are distances between male and female groups in each population scattered in a nine-dimensional space which is common to the ten groups, so that the distances are able to be directly compared with each other.

It is quite evident that between-sex distances are smaller in Japanese and Aborigines, and much larger in the other three populations. However, the distances themselves are significant in every population. Difference in the distances may be more evidently seen in Fig. 1. In Caucasians, Pimas and American Negroes, the distances between male and female groups are more than twice as large as those in Japanese and Aborigines.

* Program library for anthropological statistics
† Hitachi statistical analysis program

TABLE II. Generalized distance between males and females.

Population	D^2 (Unbiased)	Probability
Japanese	0·6285	$p < 0·01$
Caucasians	1·5410	$p < 0·01$
Pima Indians	1·8196	$p < 0·01$
American Negroes	1·6776	$p < 0·01$
Aborigines	0·6850	$p < 0·01$

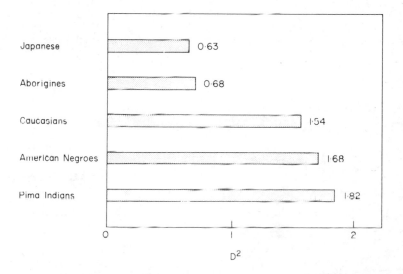

Fig. 1. Generalized distance between males and females (unbiased D^2).

In the second step of the analysis, the canonical variates in Table III were calculated according to C. R. Rao's method (see "Advanced Statistical Methods in Biometric Research", 1952. John Wiley and Sons, New York). The purpose of this procedure was to make relationship between groups more evident. As mentioned above, the generalized distances obtained are those in the nine-dimensional space, because ten groups are being compared in combination, so that the location of each group in such a space is almost impossible to recognize in reality. However, it is possible to project all the groups to a space of reduced dimensions by means of canonical variates.

In the present case, if the first and second canonical variates are taken into account, they may contain about 77% of the total information which could be obtained from the samples. This means that a figure drawn on the basis of these two sets of canonical variates may be equivalent to a projection of the ten groups to a two-dimensional space with a loss of 23% of total variance (Fig. 2).

K. HANIHARA

TABLE III. First and second canonical variates.

Population	Sex	Z_1	Z_2
Japanese	Male	−0·8485	0·5198
	Female	−1·2250	0·1360
Caucasians	Male	−0·0140	−0·5132
	Female	−1·2583	−0·7073
Pima Indians	Male	1·0443	1·3519
	Female	0·1646	0·5879
American Negroes	Male	0·4531	−0·2556
	Female	−0·6069	−0·5492
Aborigines	Male	1·4192	−0·2268
	Female	0·8717	−0·3435

Contribution rate for total variance = 76.72%

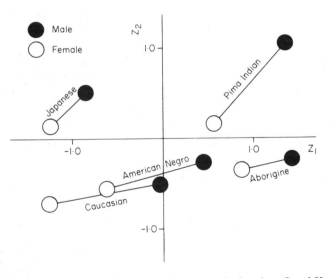

FIG. 2. Between-sex difference based on canonical variates I and II.

The results seem to be quite suggestive. For the first place, the distances between males and females are relatively short in Japanese and Aborigines, and longer in the other three populations. This agrees quite well with the results obtained from the direct comparison of the D-squares. Secondly, it may be realized that the inclination of the lines connecting male and female groups varies from population to population, i.e. the inclination is relatively steep in Japanese and Pimas, but much more gentle in the other populations. In other words, between-sex difference is almost the same in both directions of the first and second canonical variates in the former two populations, but the difference is particularly large in the direction of the first canonical variate in the latter populations. This seems to mean that the between-sex difference is not the same in all the populations, because the two sets of canonical variates represent different factors which are concerned with the tooth-crown size, and they are uncorrelated.

The next step of the study is to interpret the significance of the canonical variates. For this purpose, the factor analysis was applied to the same samples from the five populations.

Factor Analysis of the Tooth Crown Size

Table IV shows factor loadings after the orthogonol rotation. Factor I represents significantly higher correlation with the lower molars, and less

TABLE IV. Factor loadings after rotation.

Tooth	Factor I	Factor II
I^1	0·1373	0·8264[a]
C	0·2007	0·5334
PM^2	0·1658	0·2632
M^2	0·3811	0·1261
I_2	0·2237	0·8332[a]
PM_1	0·2754	0·1629
M_1	0·8191[a]	0·2760
M_2	0·8198[a]	0·1212

[a]Showing high correlations with the related teeth.

but still significant correlation with the upper molar. On the other hand, factor II shows higher correlation with the incisors, and less with the upper canine. The relationship may be realized more evidently on Fig. 3. Even though, after rotation, factors I and II become to correlate with each other to some extent, it is quite evident that the molars largely contribute to the factor I, and the incisors to the factor II. On the other hand, the premolars show almost no correlation with both factors. This means that the premolars could be explained by some other factors.

Next to this, the mean factor scores were calculated for each group on the basis of the rotated factor loadings (Fig. 4). The pattern of Fig. 4 looks somewhat different from that of Fig. 3, but if looked at in detail, it becomes apparent that both figures are essentially the same. For example, the distance between male and female groups are smaller in Japanese and Aborigines than in the other three populations, and the inclination is a little bit steeper in Japanese and Pimas than in the others. However, discrepancy in the angles

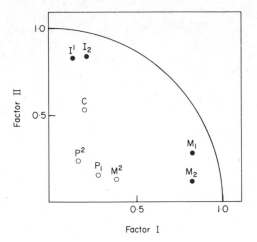

Fɪɢ. 3. Factor loadings after rotation.

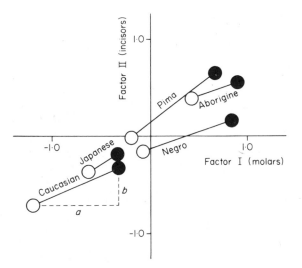

Fɪɢ. 4. Between-sex difference based on factors I and II.

of inclination in Fig. 4 is not so apparent when compaⅰed with Fig. 3. In this regard, a ratio of b to a (see lower left part of Fig. 4), or in a simple word tangent b, was calculated (Table V).

The values of tangent b are apparently larger in Japanese and Pimas than in the other populations. In other words, angle b is about 32° for Japanese and 39° for Pimas, but only 24° for Caucasians and 20° for both American Negroes and Aborigines. This fact is likely to prove that the inclination is

TABLE V. Ratio b/a (tangent b) — ratio between
sex differences on factor scores I and II.

Japanese	0·6186
Caucasians	0·4499
Pima Indians	0·7981
American Negroes	0·3648
Aborigines	0·3729

somewhat steeper in Japanese and Pimas as we have already recognized in Fig. 3 based on the canonical variates.

CONCLUSION

From what has been mentioned above, it seems to be quite evident that the difference in tooth-crown size between males and females may be relatively large in some populations but relatively small in others. In some populations the difference is particularly large in size of the molar teeth, but not in the other populations. In addition, I should like to emphasize that the between-sex difference may be relatively small even in a population which retains some archaic physical characteristics such as the Aborigines; contrary to this, the difference may be relatively large in a population which shows a progressive type of jaw such as that of the Caucasians.

In general, it seems likely that the sexual dimorphism in the tooth size of the modern man does not positively correlate with reduction of the chewing apparatus, but with other factors which are still unknown.

ACKNOWLEDGEMENTS

I should like to express my sincere gratitude to Dr A. A. Dahlberg of the University of Chicago, Dr L. A. Altemus of Howard University and the late Dr M. J. Barrett of the University of Adelaide who gave me opportunities to study a large number of dental casts from various populations.

11. Analysis of Developmental Processes possibly related to Human Dental Sexual Dimorphism

MELVIN L. MOSS

Department of Anatomy, Columbia University, New York, U.S.A.

INTRODUCTION

It is agreed generally that the human permanent dentition exhibits a statistically significant dimensional sexual dimorphism, characterized most clearly in the canine teeth, with male values exceeding those of females (Alvesalo, 1971; Furuhata and Yamamoto, 1967; Garn *et al.*, 1966, 1971; Goose, 1963; Gustafson, 1966; Lunt, 1969; Moorrees, 1959; Schranze, 1964; Stähle, 1959). It has been suggested that a similar dimorphism exists in the deciduous dentition (Meredith and Knott, 1968; see Aryn *et al.*, 1974, for a recent review).

Data exist suggesting that human canine dimorphism is not an isolated phenomenon but may be only the greatest reflection of a similar, but less statistically significant, event in adjacent tooth groups (Ebeling *et al.*, 1973; Horowitz *et al.*, 1958; Garn *et al.*, 1965; Osborne *et al.*, 1958; Osborne, 1962). Other papers imply that dental dimorphism is but one reflection of more widespread somatic sexual differences, such as body size (Garn *et al.*, 1967a) or stature (Garn *et al.*, 1968a, b).

The existence of canine sexual dimorphism is based almost exclusively on data obtained by coronal odontometric techniques. As such, these same data provide no insight into the developmental processes possibly related to the formation of larger male canine teeth. From our knowledge of odontogenetic processes it is possible, theoretically, that the dimorphism could be due to a dimensional increase of the thickness of coronal enamel, dentine, or pulp chamber, either simply or in any combination. The data to answer this question do not now exist, and for reasons discussed below, will be extremely difficult to obtain in the future. Despite this fact, it is possible to critically analyse available information, and to suggest that the dental dimorphism of human permanent canine teeth reflects a greater enamel thickness alone, and further that this is the result of a longer period of amelogenesis in males than in females. The subsequent sections of this chapter present the argument in detail.

QUANTITATIVE DATA

In the literature, permanent canine sexual dimorphism is presented in a variety of ways: absolute values, percentage differences, coefficients of variation and t scores. A review of the data permits certain reasonably acceptable generalizations to be made, with the explicit understanding that variations about these values are expected when any particular population sample is examined. The absolute size differences in the customary coronal diameters (mesio-distal, bucco-(labio-) lingual) generally approximate 0·4– 0·5 mm (Goose, 1963; Moorrees, 1957). Of interest are the reports that sexual dimorphism may be reflected in tooth shape, as well as tooth size (shape defined here as a ratio of mesio-distal (M-D) and labio-lingual (La-Li) measurements). Garn et al. (1967b, 1968a) find greater dimorphism for La-Li diameters than for M-D, and note further their feeling that sexual differences of shape exceed those of size. However, neither coronal dimension seemingly demonstrates a greater metrical dimorphism than the other, when many different human populations are studied (Lunt, 1969). In percentage differences male canine dimensions exceed female ones by values ranging from 3–9% (Garn et al., 1966, 1971; Frisch, 1963; Moorrees, 1957, 1959), while the coefficient of variation (V) of this difference ranges between 4·2 and 11% (Moorrees, 1959; Lunt, 1969; Alvesalo, 1971). Finally, when reported as t scores (or alternatively given as "critical ratios") male teeth exceed female teeth significantly by values that may reach as high as 7·3 for maxillary canines and 12·4 for mandibular canines (Stähle, 1959; also Lunt, 1969; Moorrees, 1957).

DENTAL DIMORPHISM IN NON-HUMAN PRIMATES

Sexual dental dimorphism is exhibited by many species, while the teeth affected and the quantity of the differences vary between species (Almquist, 1974). Some possible functional implications of this condition are reviewed by Zingesser (1968a, b), and we note, in passing, the report of the lack of canine dimorphism in *Macaca nemestrina* (Sirianni and Swindler, 1973).

Although beyond the scope of this chapter, it is pertinent to note that some workers are properly concerned about the possible role that the quantitative decrease in primate canine dimorphism may play in understanding hominid evolution (Greene, 197o; Wolpoff, 1971; see also Sofaer, 1973).

METHODOLOGICAL PROBLEMS

Despite agreement than human canine dimensional sexual dimorphism exists, and despite relative abundant odontometric studies of many populations, we do not yet understand the developmental mechanisms responsible. Further, we continue to be beset by apparently unresolved problems relating to the roles of "genetic" (intrinsic) and "environmental" (extrinsic) factors in such odontogenetic processes. Superficially it appears that the problem should yield to relatively simple methods of study; for example, the careful sectioning of canine teeth and the accurate determination of the absolute dimension of coronal enamel, dentine and pulp chamber. Further analysis, however, shows this approach to be overly simplistic. First, no such data are available at present, to my knowledge. Second, such a study requires relatively large numbers of canine teeth that are completely unabraded, of itself a problem of major proportions. Third, available odontometric data suggest strongly that if such unworn teeth were available, they should be carefully categorized not only by racial group (or better still, "breeding population") but, even more importantly, by experience of the group studied to environmental fluoridation of the drinking water (see below). Finally, and of the greatest significance are the data of Taylor (1969a, b) who notes that in New Zealand children there is no typical form to the maxillary canines. Obviously, meaningful comparisons can be made between the absolute or relative diameters of the three components of canine crowns only for teeth of essentially similar shapes. When all of these factors are considered, it seems that any present attempt to resolve the problem of the processes related to the production of canine sexual dimorphism should be done by indirect analysis of available data, for a considerable period of time may well elapse before the necessary direct data become available, if ever they do.

Since this chapter will suggest that a differential duration of amelogenesis is responsible for canine dimorphism, it will be well to review briefly the possible intrinsic and extrinsic factors possibly operative in the regulation of the rate, duration, or both, of enamel formation.

Aspects of Genetic Regulation of Dental Dimorphism

At present there is consensual agreement, in the broadest, non-specific sense, that both genetic and environmental factors play some role in the regulation of dental dimorphism (Ebeling et al., 1973; Garn et al., 1960, 1967a, c, 1968; Grüneberg, 1965; Horowitz et al., 1958; Kraus, 1962; Lewis and Grainger, 1967; Ludwig, 1947; Lundström, 1948, 1949, 1963; Osborne et al., 1958; Osborne, 1962; Riesenfeld, 1970). This topic has been well reviewed recently by Alvesalo (1971). However, beyond this generalization little data are available to indicate either the primary site or the specific developmental processes being so regulated by some presumed combination of intrinsic and extrinsic factors.

Reviewing available data clearly indicates a lack of knowledge concerning the possible gene loci implicated in the intrinsic contribution to sexual dimorphism of permanent canine teeth. Some hold for the X-chromosome (Garn et al., 1968b; Grüneberg, 1965; Lewis and Grainger, 1967), the

Y-chromosome (Kraus, 1962; Garn et al., 1967a) and for both X and Y sites, as well as for polygenic autosomal linkage (see Alvesalo, 1971, for a review).

Extrinsic (non-genetic) factors obviously are involved in the regulation of dental dimorphism. Ebeling et al. (1973) note a secular increase in La-Li dimensions of almost all permanent teeth in Scandinavian populations and attribute this to extrinsic (diet, trace elements) factors, as well as to intrinsic ones. Fairly summarized, the reports of Goose (1967) and Goose and Lee (1973) suggest that genetic factors perhaps are not quite as important as has been assumed generally, since their data "support the suggestion that a stronger environmental component is involved in immigrant populations" (Goose and Lee, 1973).

In summary, there is good reason to accept the consensus that some combination of intrinsic and extrinsic factors regulate sexual dental dimorphism. Of all the possible extrinsic factors, the effects of fluoridation appears to be the one about which the most abundant data exist, and this topic has the added interest of having been demonstrated to have some observable effect on amelogenesis.

EFFECT OF ENVIRONMENTAL FLUORIDES ON AMELOGENESIS

Quite aside from its well-known clinical effect of reducing the incidence of dental caries, fluoride ions seem in some way to intervene in odontogenesis. When administered systemically during odontogenic periods, changes in the size and/or shape of the teeth have been reported, but with seemingly conflicting results. Increase in human permanent tooth-crown diameters have been reported under these conditions (Møller, 1967; Wallenius, 1959). On the other hand, Cooper and Ludwig (1965), note a decrease in tooth size in the face of added fluoride ingestion. Seemingly additional fluoride does not alter the order of appearance of crown cusps (Cox et al., 1961).

In the rat, fluoride has been reported to cause either no significant dimensional change in molar teeth, or to cause smaller teeth (Kruger, 1966; Paynter and Grainger, 1956; Gray, 1973). However, these same reports clearly indicate that some interesting changes do occur in the enamel that significantly alter the shape (if not the overall size) of the tooth. Considering molar cuspal morphology, the depth of intercuspal fissures was decreased, while the angulation of the sides of these same occlusal fissures was increased (Paynter and Grainger, 1956, 1962). This would have the summative effect of producing observably "shorter" cusps, and such indeed has been reported (Kruger, 1966). Further, Gray (1973) notes that the absolute thickness of enamel in the base of the fissures is significantly greater than in non-fluoridated controls.

In a previously unpublished study in this laboratory, Dr Herbert P. Ostreicher studied the effects of 15 p.p.m. of fluoride added to drinking water of pregnant female rats (and offspring) on molar crown dimensions and occlusal cusp depths. No significant mesio-distal or bucco-lingual differences were noted. However, the depths of the grooves of the experimental teeth were significantly less than those of control teeth. Further, the amount of eruption of the third molars of the control animals was three times greater than that of rats ingesting 15 p.p.m. of fluoride, a finding supportive of earlier reports that fluoride in man could delay dental eruption (Short, 1944).

The possibility that environmental fluoride might act to produce a "flatter" occlusal morphology is supported explicitly by Kruger (1959) and by Simpson and Castaldi (1969). Consideration of the odontogenetic processes makes it clear that increased enamel deposition (more enamel in fissure depths), increased angulation between cusps, "shorter" cusps (measured vertically) and decreased intercuspal fissure depths can all be accounted for developmentally by increased amelogenesis, involving either increased rate or duration, or both. Interestingly this hypothesized explanation differs completely from that suggested for the hypodontia resulting from malnutrition, protein deficiency, or hypervitaminosis A (Tonge and McCance, 1973; Holloway et al., 1961; Holloway and Mellanby, 1961), where generalized odontogenic retardation is reportedly observed.

No review of the possible regulatory role of extrinsic factors in odontogenesis should omit the suggestive work of Tenczar and Boder (1966), who studied the dental effects of cross-fostering of mouse litters. The direction of the differences in molar dimensions between cross-fostered and normally fostered mice of the same litter was towards the dimensions phenotypic of the strain of the post-natal dam, and this with no detectable genetic variation within either strain of mouse.

Precise summarization of these data is difficult. There can be no question that dental dimorphism (of size as well as shape) may well reflect some sort of "interaction" between a variety of intrinsic and extrinsic factors, the nature of which are as yet rather unclear. But what does emerge from the materials cited above is a distinct possibility that the observed human canine dimensional sexual dimorphism could be the observed result of differential thickness of the enamel layer. Whatever the intrinsic and extrinsic factors may be that summate to produce this observable and measurable dimensional difference, they would then act upon the functioning ameloblasts—whether by affecting the rate and/or duration of amelogenesis is unclear. A further set of data relate to this hypothesis.

THE DENTINE LAYER

The data suggest that neither the size nor shape of either the pulpal outline or the dentine–enamel junction is related to sexual dental dimorphism. The internal outline of the coronal dentine (the pulp chamber outline) gives no indication of any sexual dimorphism (Carlsen and Anderson, 1966; Mjör and Hougen, 1974). Indeed, the relative independence of pulp chamber size, (and hence dentine layer thickness) and external coronal dimensions is obvious from a consideration of the essentially normal size of taurodont human teeth.

For the dentine–enamel junction, abundant data show, at least indirectly, that the outer dentine boundary is not the site of the dimensional canine dimorphism in man. Two principal techniques have been well used to study the morphology of this outer dentine surface in adult teeth: decalcification of enamel crowns (Dus, 1963; Knecht, 1965; Künzle, 1964; Nager, 1960) and selective destruction of coronal dentine, leaving the full thickness of the enamel cap intact (Korenhof, 1960, 1963). Other studies use alizarination of developing crowns (Kraus and Jordan, 1965). All of these studies converge in establishing that the morphology of the human dentine–enamel junction represents a generalized and simplified outline of the crown, one that is both ontogenetically and phylogenetically less well detailed and structurally differentiated than is the outer enamel surface (see also Adloff, 1937; Butler, 1956). In both sexes the further production of external coronal morphological detail and thickness is under control of the ameloblasts, derived from the inner enamel epithelium of the tooth germ (see Kraus and Oka, 1967, for a discussion of "wrinkling of the occlusal surface"). By this process of analytical reduction we are now left with the enamel layer itself as the possible site of dimorphic odontogenesis.

DIFFERENTIAL AMELOGENESIS

Consideration of the hypothesis that differential amelogenesis underlies human canine sexual dimorphism should, at some point, entail accurate determination of enamel layer thickness between appropriately paired teeth (cf. *above*). In this regard, it is critical to note that it would be inappropriate to simply measure enamel diameters in directions perpendicular (normal) to the dentine–enamel junction. The enamel prisms do not extend in a straight line from the dentine–enamel junction to the coronal surface; rather they are known to undulate (Osborn, 1967, 1973). Further, beyond this structural detail, the mean direction of the enamel prisms is not constant throughout the crown, most being occlusally directed, and others gingivally, while the mean angulation of all the prisms to the dentine–enamel junction is about 85°. All of these essentially geometric factors must be accounted for in more sophisticated measurements of enamel layer thickness in the future (Ramsey and Ripa, 1969).

Enamel Thickness

Despite the relatively large number of odontometric studies, relatively few have been devoted to the thickness of the several components of the dental crown. One group has reported on the total thickness of the crown wall (dentine plus enamel) (Kühl, 1969; Kühl and Schaaf, 1972), but such data are not useful presently. Recently, Fejerskov et al. (1973) studied the thickness of enamel in human maxillary premolars, finding that "the data conformed to a normal continuous distribution. . .", without kurtosis or skewness. While finding no correlation between the enamel depth in occlusal fissures and the angulation between adjacent cusp planes, they did find a high negative correlation between that angle and fissure depths.

Absolute thicknesses of the enamel layer in human incisor, premolar and molar teeth are reported, but, as in the papers mentioned above, without sexual segregation of the data (Gillings and Buoncore, 1961a, b). Similarly unsegregated are the data on human cuspids in the noteworthy work of Huszar (1971).

An exceptional paper by Shillingburg and Grace (1973) reports on enamel and dentine layer thickness of the complete human dentition (less the third molars) using 259 teeth. The thicknesses of both layers are recorded, in three dimensions, at each millimeter of the crown height. From their data we were able to compute the several coefficients of variation. Unfortunately, in this study their data were not sexually segregated. It is of considerable and possibly significant, interest to note that the coefficient of variation for canine enamel thickness ranges from 47–55% while canine dentine thickness is approximately 12%. Further, the coefficient of variation for enamel thickness found in all the other teeth ranged from $6\cdot7\%$–$16\cdot6\%$, with the corresponding statistic for dentine remaining about the same as that in the canines. When we compare these values with the coefficient of variation of total crown widths (cf. above) of between 5–11%, it is reasonable to suggest that the presence of two sexually dimorphic populations of enamel thickness account best for the exceptionally large variations of human canine enamel thickness observed.

Rate of Amelogenesis

Here again, little data are available. Two papers continue to serve this purpose in the absence of other substantial studies, and these suggest that deposition of human enamel occurs at rates ranging between 4 and 8 μm day $^{-1}$ (Schour and Massler, 1940; Massler and Schour, 1946). It should be noted that these rates vary from tooth to tooth (Massler and Schour, 1946), and from surface to surface on the same tooth (Yoshioka, 1970; Kraus, 1959, 1962). Further all of these rates were determined without consideration being given to the geometric problems, mentioned above, introduced by the undulations of enamel prism shape and the departure from true perpendicularity of their long axes; nevertheless they do serve as rough approximations.

Duration of Amelogenesis

At present we have no data suggesting a sexual difference in the rates of amelogenesis. However, substantial data support the hypothesis that the duration of amelogenesis is involved in the production of sexually dimorphic human canine crowns. Reporting on teeth other than canines, it has been noted that female teeth both erupt and complete their calcification earlier than male teeth (Garn et al., 1958), while both sexes show about equal variability in developmental sequences (Garn et al., 1959). The female teeth are developmentally more mature at comparable chronological ages by a mean factor of about $0\cdot32$ years (Lewis and Garn, 1960).

In the more precise terms of odontogenetic processes, males take 3–5% longer to pass between stages from the formation of the completed dental sac (dental follicle) to completion of crown formation, i.e. to completion of amelogenesis (Garn *et al.*, 1959). This figure is of interest when we remember that modern male canine teeth are about 3–5% larger than female teeth (cf. *above*).

Two papers of high significance for our present purpose are those of Fanning (1961) and of Moorrees *et al.* (1963). Reporting on a closely spaced longitudinal roentgenographic study of human permanent tooth formation, these papers report on five stages of crown formation (and seven stages of root formation), and this is done separately for each sex ($n = 48$ males, $n = 51$ females; Moorrees *et al.*, 1963); the data are presented graphically with mean values and two standard derivations shown. Utilizing these data, we were able to compare, within the limits of accuracy of the published figures, the temporal differences in duration of crown formation in permanent canine teeth. These derived data support the statements that, while "the earlier developmental stages of tooth formation in males coincided closely with those of females" (Fanning, 1961), crown completion was completed earlier in females.

Comparison of the male and female canine graphic data of Moorrees *et al.* (1963) for the stage of crown completion, suggests that the mean male time is about 0·2 years later than those of females, or about 73 days. Now when we multiply this time factor by 4 μm, 6 μm and 8 μm respectively, representing three presumed daily rates of amelogenesis, we obtain 0·29 mm, 0·44 mm and 0·58 mm of presumed additional enamel deposition during this time period.

The differences in enamel thickness of the several surfaces of teeth noted above, together with the reported differences in rate of formation of these same surfaces, make it reasonable to suggest further that the use of the several surface specific rates of amelogenesis presently employed may really reflect the normal biological state of affairs rather closely. Further, the geometric problems of non-linear and non-perpendicular prisms, noted above, persuade me to think that these several rates (and possibly others) must be used in such computations.

It is instructive to compare our theoretical results (above) with the actual size differences reported by Lunt (1969) for maxillary and mandibular canine teeth: maxillary canines, M-D = 0·28 mm, La-Li = 0·51 mm; mandibular canines, M-D = 0·45 mm, La-Li = 0·64 mm, with male values significantly exceeding the females.

I suggest that this close correspondence of theoretical and actual values strongly support the hypothesis that human canine sexual dimorphism is the result of a differential duration of active amelogenesis; a process occurring over a longer time interval in males than in females. This hypothesis is supported by a study of the first permanent mandibular molar in man in which "a slight linear increase in the precocity of female development was observed. The average span of active growth of this tooth in females is 96% of the male span, and the female tooth is also smaller by an equivalent amount in its linear dimensions" (Gleiser and Hunt, 1955).

GNOMONIC GROWTH

One problem inherent in the study of dental dimorphism cannot be resolved presently: the proposal that there is also a dimorphism of tooth shape, as well as of size, a point not yet definitely established. Some years ago we suggested that the growth of all vertebrate teeth could be analysed successfully by the use of the allometric, differential growth equation (Moss and Applebaum, 1957). Some years later we were able to demonstrate this again, and to refute the contrary statements of Kraus and Jordan (1965), using their own data (Moss and Chase, 1966). The correctness of our interpretation has been supported by the work reported in several other more recent publications by other workers. More recently, we have reapproached this theme again in another context, and have shown that, as is well known, any object whose dimensional growth can be described by the allometric equation, is also growing gnomonically, i.e. as it grows its size alters while its shape remains constant (Salentijn and Moss, 1971). It is of great interest, therefore, to note the earlier work of Herzberg and Massler (1940) in which the patterns of tooth formation are explicitly noted as gnomonic.

Returning to our problem, if it is true that the shape of male canine teeth differ from those of female canines, then it is reasonable to suggest that in both sexes, the shape of the developing enamel crowns also is always different. This could be accomplished by sexually differential rates of amelogenesis on comparable surfaces, or by differential geometries of these same surfaces. We do not now have the data to answer this question and its resolution must await further study.

CONCLUSIONS

This exercise in data analysis leads to the suggestion that the observed dimensional sexual dimorphism of human canine teeth is the result of a differential duration period of the amelogenesis, with male teeth forming enamel at the same rate as female teeth, but over a longer period of time. Although the developmental process related to the production of dimorphism has been identified, we come no closer to resolving the question of the relative influence of intrinsic and of extrinsic factors in the regulation of this same amelogenesis.

In view of the inability of skeletal geneticists to locate the primary site of genetic regulation within the osteoblasts or chondroblasts (Grüneberg, 1963; Grüneberg and Wickramaratne, 1974; Sawin and Hamlet, 1970; Sawin et al., 1970) and with the suggestion that a far greater precision must be employed by those who use the term "genetic" to designate a type of control mechanism (cf. Løvtrup, 1974), I would urge, at this time, that a rather vigorous re-examination of these concepts be undertaken by future workers in this field, to the end that greater clarity and closer approximations to biological correctness be achieved.

References

ADOLFF, P. (1937). Über die primitiven und die sogenannten "pithekoiden" Merkmale im Gebiss des rezenten und fossilen Menschen und ihre Bedeutung. *Z. Anat. EntwGesch.* **107**, 68–82.

ALMQUIST, A. (1974). Sexuai differences in the anterior dentition in African primates. *Am. J. phys. Anthrop.* **40**, 359–368.

ALVESALO, L. (1971). The influence of sex-chromosome genes on tooth size in man. *Suom. Hammaslääk. Toim.* **67**, 3–54.

ARYA, B. S., SAVARA, B. S., THOMAS, D. and CLARKSON, Q. (1974). Relation of sex and occlusion to mesiodistal tooth size. *Am. J. Orthod.* **66**, 479–486.

BUTLER, P. M. (1956). The ontogeny of molar pattern. *Biol. Rev.* **31**, 30–70.

CARLSEN, O. and ANDERSEN, J. (1966). Om pulpakammeret og rodkanaleme i mennekets temporaere taender. *Tandlaegebl.* **70**, 93–115, 181–198, 421–442, 529–561.

COOPER, W. K. and LUDWIG, T. G. (1965). Effects of fluoride and of soil trace elements on the morphology of the permanent molars in man. *N.Z. dent. J.* **61**, 33–40.

COX, G. J., FINN, S. B. and AST, D. B. (1961). Effect of fluoride ingestion on the size of the cusp of Carabelli during tooth formation. *J. dent. Res.* **40**, 393–395.

DUS, W. (1963). Vergleich des räumlichen Verhaltens von Dentinkronrelief und Schmelzrelief der Milchzähne. *Acta anat.* **54**, 101–136.

EBELING, C. F., INGERVALL, B., HEDEGÅRD, B. and LEWIN, T. (1973). Secular changes in tooth size in Swedish men. *Acta odont. scand.* **31**, 140–147.

FANNING, E. A. (1961). A longitudinal study of tooth formation and root absorption. *N.Z. dent. J.* **57**, 202–217.

FEJERSKOV, O., MELSEN, B. and KARRING, T. (1973). Morphometric analysis of occlusal fissures in human premolars. *Scand. J. dent. Res.* **81**, 505–510.

FRISCH, J. E. (1963). Sex-differences in the canines on the Gibbon (*Hylobates lar*). *Primates*, **4**, 1–10.

FURUHATA, T. and YAMAMOTO, K. (1967). "Forensic Odontology." C. C. Thomas, Springfield.

GARN, S. M., LEWIS, A. B., KOSKI, K. and POLACHECK, D. L. (1958). The sex difference in tooth calcification. *J. dent. Res.* **37**, 561–567.

GARN, S. M., LEWIS, A. B. and POLACHECK, D. L. (1959). Variability of tooth formation. *J. dent. Res.* **38**, 135–148.

GARN, S. M., LEWIS, A. B. and POLACHECK, D. L. (1960). Sibling similarities in dental development. *J. dent. Res.* **39**, 170–175.

GARN, S. M., LEWIS, A. B. and KEREWSKY, R. S. (1965). Size interrelationships of the mesial and distal teeth. *J. dent. Res.* **44**, 350–354.

GARN, S. M., KEREWSKY, R. S. and SWINDLER, D. R. (1966). Canine "field" in sexual dimorphism of tooth size. *Nature, Lond.* **212**, 1501–1502.

GARN, S. M., LEWIS, A. B. and KEREWSKY, R. S. (1967a). The relationship between sexual dimorphism in tooth size and body size as studied within families. *Archs oral Biol.* **12**, 299–301.

GARN, S. M., LEWIS, A. B. and KEREWSKY, R. S. (1967b). Sex difference in tooth shape. *J. dent. Res.* **46**, 1470.

GARN, S. M., LEWIS, A. B., SWINDLER, D. R. and KEREWSKY, R. S. (1967c). Genetic control of sexual dimorphism in tooth size. *J. dent. Res.* **46**, 963–972.

GARN, S. M., LEWIS, A. B. and KEREWSKY, R. S. (1968a). Relationship between buccolingual and mesiodistal tooth diameters. *J. dent. Res.* **47**, 495.

GARN, S. M., LEWIS, A. B. and WALENGA, A. (1968b). Evidence for a secular trend in tooth size over two generations. *J. dent. Res.* **47**, 503.

GARN, S. M., LEWIS, A. B. and KEREWSKY, R. S. (1971). Communalities in the size differences of teeth of brothers and sisters. *Archs oral Biol.* **12**, 575–581.

GILLINGS, B. and BUONCORE, M. (1961a). An investigation of enamel thickness in human lower incisor teeth. *J. dent. Res.* **40**, 105–118.

GILLINGS, B. and BUONCORE, M. (1961b). Thickness of enamel of the base of pits and fissures in human molars and bicuspids. *J. dent. Res.* **40**, 119–133.

GLEISER, I and HUNT, E. E., JR. (1955). The permanent mandibular first molar: Its calcification, eruption and decay. *Am. J. phys. Anthrop.* **13**, 253–281.

GOOSE, D. H. (1963). Dental measurement: an assessment of its value in anthropological studies. *In* "Dental Anthropology" (Brotherwell, D. R. ed.), pp. 125–148. Macmillan, New York.

GOOSE, D. H. (1967). Preliminary study of tooth size in families. *J. dent. Res.* **46**, 959–962.

GOOSE, D. H. and LEE, G. T. R. (1973). Inheritance of tooth size in immigrant populations. *J. dent. Res.* **52**, 175.

GRAY, H. S. (1973). A morphological study of the influence of fluoride on rat molar teeth. *Archs oral Biol.* **18**, 1451–1460.

GREENE, D. L. (1973). Gorilla dental sexual dimorphism and early hominid taxonomy. *Symp. IV Int. Cong. Primat.* **3**, 82–100.

GRÜNEBERG, H. (1963). "The Pathology of Skeletal Development." Wiley, New York.

GRÜNEBERG, H. (1965). Genes and genotypes affecting the teeth of the mouse. *J. Embryol. exp. Morph.* **14**, 137–159.

GRÜNEBERG, H. and WICKRAMARATNE, G. A. DE S. (1974). A reexamination of two skeletal mutants of the mouse, vestigial tail (*tv*) and congenital hydrocephalus (*ch*). *J. Embryol. exp. Morph.* **31**, 209–222.

GUSTAFSON, G. (1966). "Forensic Odontology." American Elsevir, New York.

HERZBERG, F. and MASSLER, M. (1940). The phylogenetic growth pattern of the conical forms of teeth. *J. dent. Res.* **19**, 511–520.

HOLLOWAY, P. J. and MELLANBY M. (1961). The effect of hyper-vitaminosis A on the development of rat tooth germs in tissue culture. *Archs oral Biol.* **5**, 190–194.

HOLLOWAY, P. J., SHAW, J. H. and SWEENEY, E. A. (1961). Effects of various sucrose: casein ratios in purified diets on the teeth and supporting structures of rats. *Archs oral Biol.* **3**, 185–200.

HOROWITZ, S. L., OSBORNE, R. H. and DE GEORGE, F. V. (1958). Hereditary factors in tooth dimensions, a study of the anterior teeth of twins. *Angle Orthod.* **28**, 87–93.

HUSZAR, G. (1971). Observations sur l'epaisseur de l'email. *Bull. Group. Int. Rech. Sc. Stomat.* **14**, 155–167.

KNECHT, H. (1965). Vergleich des räumlichen Verhaltens von Dentinkronrelief und Schmelzrelief in Rattengebiss. *Anat. Anz.* **116**, 59–72.

KORENHOF, C. A. W. (1960). Morphogenetical aspects of the human upper molar. A comparative study of its enamel and dentine surfaces and their relationship to the crown pattern of fossil and recent primates. *Acad. proefschrift, Utrecht. Uitg. mij. Neerl.* 368 pp.

KORENHOF, C. A. W. (1963). The enamel–dentine border: a new morphological factor in the study of the (human) molar pattern. *Ned. Tijdschr. Tandheelk.* Suppl. **70**, 30–57.

KRAUS, B. S. (1959). Differential calcification rates in the human primary dentition. *Archs oral Biol.* **1**, 133–144.

KRAUS, B. S. (1962). Areas of research in dental genetics. *In* "Genetics and Dental Health" (Witkop, C. J., Jr. ed.), pp. 57–69. McGraw-Hill, New York.

KRAUS, B. S. and JORDAN, R. E. (1965). "The Human Dentition Before Birth." Lea and Febiger, Philadelphia.

KRAUS, B. S. and OKA, S. W. (1967). Wrinkling of molar crowns: new evidence. *Science, N.Y.* **157**, 328–329.

KRUGER, B. J. (1959). Trace elements and dental morphology. *Pap. Dept. Dent. Univ. Qd.* **1**, 3–28.

KRUGER, B. J. (1966). Interaction of fluoride and molybdenum on dental morphology in the rat. *J. dent. Res.* **45**, 714–725.

KÜHL, W. (1969). Zur Eignung unterer Frontzähne für Kronenersatz. *Dt. Zahnärztl. Z.*, **24**, 707–711.

KÜHL, W. and SCHAAF, R. (1972). Untersuchungen über korrelatin Zusamussenhänge zurichen vestibulären und approxemalen Kronenwandstärken und Aussenmassen der Kronen untere Frontzähne und Prämolaren. *Dt. Zahnärztl. Z.* **27**, 706–708.

KÜNZLE, A. (1964). Vergleich des räumlichen Verhaltens von Schmelzrelief und Dentinkronrelief in Dauergebiss des Rindes. *Morph. J.* **106**, 500–540.

LEWIS, A. B. and GARN, S. M. (1960). The relationship between tooth formation and other maturational factors. *Angle Orthod.* **30**, 70–77.

LEWIS, D. W. and GRAINGER, R. M. (1967). Sex-linked inheritance of tooth size. A family study. *Archs oral Biol.* **12**, 539–544.

LØVTRUP, S. (1974). "Epigenetics." John Wiley and Sons, New York.

LUDWIG, F. J. (1957). The mandibular second premolars: morphologic variation and inheritance. *J. dent. Res.* **36**, 263–273.

LUNDSTRÖM, A. (1948). "Tooth Size and Occlusion in Twins," 2nd edition. S. Karger, Basle.

LUNDSTRÖM, A. (1949). An investigation of 202 pairs of twins regarding fundamental factors in the aetiology of malocclusion. *Dent. Rec.* **69**, 251–264.

LUNDSTRÖM, A. (1963). Tooth morphology as a basis for distinguishing monozygotic and dizygotic twins. *Am. J. hum. Genet.* **15**, 34–43.

LUNT, D. A. (1969). An odontometric study of mediaeval Danes. *Acta odont. scand.* **27**, Suppl. **55**, 1–173.

MASSLER, M. and SCHOUR, I. (1946). The oppositional life span of the enamel and dentin-forming cells. *J. dent. Res.* **25**, 145–150.

MEREDITH, H. V. and KNOTT, V. B. (1968). Coronal breadth of human primary anterior teeth. *Am. J. phys. Anthrop.* **28**, 49–64.

MJÖR, I. A. and HOUGEN, E. (1974). Pulp structure in bilateral and opposing pairs of teeth. *Scand. J. dent. Res.* **82**, 128–134.

MØLLER, I. J. (1967). Influence of microelements on the morphology of the teeth. *J. dent. Res.* **46**, Suppl., 933–937.

MOORREES, C. F. A. (1957). "The Aleut Dentition". Harvard University Press, Cambridge.

MOORREES, C. F. A. (1959). "The Dentition of the Growing Child." Harvard University Press, Cambridge.

MOORREES, C. F. A., FANNING, E. A. and HUNT, E. E., JR. (1963). Age variations of formation stages for ten permanent teeth. *J. dent. Res.* **42**, 1490–1502.

MOSS, M. L. and APPLEBAUM, E. (1957). Differential growth analysis of vertebrate teeth. *J. dent. Res.* **36**, 644–651.

MOSS, M. L. and CHASE, P. S. (1966). Morphology of Liberian Negro deciduous teeth. 1. Odontometry. *Am. J. phys. Anthrop.* **24**, 215–230.

NAGER, G. (1960). Der Vergleich zwischen dem räumlichen Verhaltens des Dentin-kronreliefs und dem Schmelzrelief der Zahnkrone. *Acta anat.* **42**, 226–250.

OSBORN, J. W. (1967). Three dimensional reconstruction of enamel prisms. *J. dent. Res.* **46**, 1412–1419.

OSBORN, J. W. (1973). Variations in structure and development of enamel. *Oral. Sci. Rev.* **3**, 3–83.

OSBORNE, R. H. (1962). Application of twin studies to dental research. *In* "Genetics and Dental Health" (Witkop, C. J., Jr., ed.), pp. 79–91. McGraw-Hill, New York.

OSBORNE, R. H., HOROWITZ, S. L. and DE GEORGE, F. V. (1958). Genetic variation in tooth dimensions. A twin study of the permanent anterior teeth. *Am. J. hum. Genet.* **10**, 350–356.

PAYNTER, K. J. and GRAINGER, R. M. (1956). The relation of nutrition to the morphology and size of rat molar teeth. *J. Can. dent. Assoc.* **22**, 591–531.

PAYNTER, K. J. and GRAINGER, R. M. (1962). Relationship of morphology and size of teeth to caries *Int. dent. J.*, **12**, 147–159.

RAMSAY, D. J. and RIPA, L. W. (1969). Enamel prism orientation and enamel-cementum relationship in the cervical region of premolar teeth. *Br. dent. J.* **126**, 165–167.

RIESENFELD, A. (1970). The effect of environmental factors on tooth development: an experimental study. *Acta anat.* **77**, 188–215.

SALENTIJN, L. and MOSS, M. L. (1971). Morphological attributes of the logarithmic growth of the human face: gnomonic growth. *Acta anat.* **78**, 185–199.

SAWIN, P. B. and HAMLET, M. (1970). Morphogenetic studies of the rabbit. XL. Growth gradient interaction and functions in morphology. *J. Morph.* **130**, 387–420.

SAWIN, P. B., FOX, R. R. and LATIMER, H. B. (1970). Morphogenetic studies of the rabbit. XLI. Gradients of correlation in the architecture of morphology. *Am. J. Anat.* **128**, 137–146.

SCHOUR, I. and MASSLER, M. (1940). Studies in tooth development: The growth pattern of human teeth. Part II. *J. Am. dent. Assoc.* **27**, 1918–1931.

SCHRANZE, D. (1964). Morphologische unterscheide männlicher und weiblicher Zähne. *Acta Morph.* **12**, 401–406.

SHILLINGBURG, H. T., JR and GRACE, C. S. (1973). Thickness of enamel and dentin. *J. S. Calif. dent. Assoc.* **41**, 33–52.

SHORT, E. M. (1944). The relation of fluoride domestic waters to permanent tooth eruption. *J. dent. Res.* **23**, 247–255.

SIMPSON, W. J. and CASTALDI, C. R. (1969). A study of crown morphology of newly-erupted first permanent molars in Wetaskiwin (optimum fluoride) and Camrose, Alberta (low fluoride). *Odont. Revy.* **20**, 1–14.

SIRIANNI, J. E. and SWINDLER, D. R. (1973). Inheritance of deciduous tooth size in *Macaca nemestrina*. *J. dent. Res.* **52**, 179.

SOFAER, J. A. (1973). A model relating developmental interaction and differential evolutionary reduction of tooth size. *Evolution* **27**, 427–434.

STÄHLE, H. (1959). The determination of mesiodistal crown width of unerupted permanent cuspids and bicuspids. *Helv. Odont. Acta.* **3**, 14–17.

TAYLOR, R. M. S. (1969a). Variation in form of human teeth: 1. Anthropologic and forensic study of maxillary incisors. *J. dent. Res.* **48**, 5–16.

TAYLOR, R. M. S. (1969b). Variation in form of human teeth: 2. An anthropological and forensic study of maxillary canines. *J. dent. Res.* **48**, 173–182.

TENCZAR, P. and BODER, R. S. (1966). Maternal effect in dental traits of the house mouse. *Science, N.Y.* **152**, 1398–1400.

TONGE, C. H. and MCCANCE, R. A. (1973). Normal development of the jaws and teeth in pigs, and the delay and malocclusion produced by calorie deficiencies. *J. Anat.* **115**, 1–22.

WALLENIUS, B. (1959). The mesiodistal width of the tooth in relation to the content of fluorine in drinking water. *Odont. Revy.* **10**, 76–83.

WOLPOFF, M. H. (1971). Metric Trends in Hominid Dental Evolution Studies in Anthrop. *Case Western Reserve Univ.* **2**, 1–244. The Press of Case Western University, Cleveland.

YOSHIOKA, M. (1970). Difference in time of crown completion among dental surfaces. *Okajimas Folia Anat. Jap.* **47**, 213–228.

ZINGESSER, M. (1968a). Sexual dimorphism in monkey canine teeth. *Proc. 8th Int. Cong. Anthrop. Ethnol. Sci.* **1**, 305–308.

ZINGESSER, M. R. (1968b). Functional and phylogenetic significance of integrated growth and form in occluding monkey canine teeth. *Am. J. phys. Anthrop.* **28**, 263–270.

12. Morphological and Histological Changes in the Developing Dentition of Aborted Human Foetuses with a Maternal History of Rubella

P. SMITH

Department of Anatomy, Hadassah Medical School and Laboratory of Dental Anthropology, Hebrew University, Israel

W. A. SOSKOLNE

Department of Oral Pathology, Hadassah School of Dental Medicine, Hebrew University, Israel

and

A. ORNOY

Department of Anatomy, Hadassah Medical School, Hebrew University, Israel

INTRODUCTION

Pathological changes in the primary dentition of individuals with a history of intra-uterine rubella infection have been described by Evans (1944, 1947) and Guggenheimer *et al.* (1971). The changes found by them included delayed eruption, enamel hypoplasia, malformed incisors and hypodontia. Over 50% of children examined were affected to some extent.

Following the recent epidemic of rubella in Israel, therapeutic abortions were carried out on a number of women who had contracted the disease in their first trimester of pregnancy. Diagnosis was based on a four-fold or higher rise in haemoglutination inhibition antibodies or complement fixation antibodies (Ornoy *et al.*, 1973). Interruption of pregnancy was carried out by currettage or intra-amniotic injection of hypertonic urea. Nineteen foetuses and placentae were examined both macroscopically and microscopically. Gross organ defects and growth retardation were found in eleven foetuses (Sekeles and Ornoy, 1975).

Specimens from this series were used in the present study to determine the effect of rubella infection on dental development.

MATERIALS AND METHODS

The specimens studied were divided into two groups: group 1 was made up of 13 foetuses with a maternal history of rubella, obtained following therapeutic abortion by intra-amniotic injection of hypertonic urea; group 2 contained 22 foetuses with no maternal history of infectious disease of which sixteen were obtained subsequent to therapeutic abortion carried out as above and six obtained after spontaneous abortion. In addition, one foetus with a maternal history of infectious mononucleosis was examined.

All foetuses were weighed, measured and examined for gross defects. They were fixed and stored in 10% neutral formalin for time periods up to one year. An incision was made from the angle of the lip to the lower border of the ear to separate the jaws. The tooth germs were dissected out from the right side and stained with alizarin red. They were then transferred to a 50% glycerine and water solution (Kraus and Jordan, 1965) and all intact specimens measured under the dissecting microscope. Findings for maximal mesio-distal diameter were recorded for all the teeth, and the correlation coefficient was calculated for the mesio-distal diameter and crown-heel length of all the maxillary tooth germs.

The left side of jaws from seven of the rubella group and eleven of the control group were decalcified, embedded in paraffin wax and serial sections 7 μm thick were cut. The sections were mounted on glass slides and every fifth section was stained with haemotoxylin and eosin.

FINDINGS

In the maxillary deciduous incisors, canine and first molar, tooth size increased linearly for crown-heel lengths from 19 to 40 cm in both rubella and control groups. No significant difference was found between the regression lines of these two groups for any tooth, or in the intercepts on the Y-axis. Correlation coefficients were lower in the rubella cases than in the control groups for all teeth except for the deciduous canine. This difference between the two groups was significant for the central incisors, $p < 0.05$, with control group $r = 0.91$ and rubella group $r = 0.52$. Because of the small crown-heel length variation in specimens with second deciduous molars, the t test was used to examine the significance of the difference in tooth size between rubella and control group molars. No significant difference was found. In six of the 12 rubella cases, a centripetal collapse of the molar cusp tips and infolding of the incisal tooth margins was found (Figs 1 and 2). This was accompanied by a splitting of the enamel organ from the underlying tooth germ. Some collapse of the molar cusp tips was also present in two of the 25

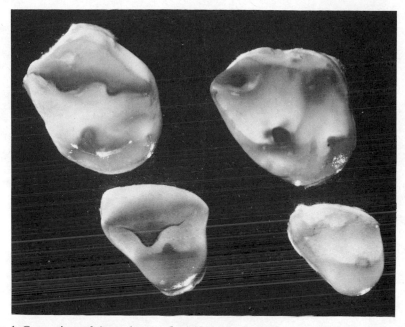

FIG. 1. Comparison of size and stage of calcification of tooth germs from foetuses of similar crown-heel length. Above are the Dm¹ and Dm² from a control foetus whilst those below are the Dm¹ and Dm² from a foetus of the rubella growth.

controls, but no splitting of the enamel organ from the underlying tooth germ was noted.

The most constant histological change seen in the rubella group was disarray of the tissues originating from the enamel organ. There was a disruption of the continuity of the ameloblast layer into smaller segments which had lost their relation to adjacent tissues in all seven rubella foetuses examined. This change was referred to as fractionation (Figs 3 and 4). There was an associated, but less frequent disruption of the stellate reticulum. This varied in degree from partial loss to complete absence of the stellate reticulum. The outer enamel epithelium was either partially or completely absent in all the rubella cases. The degree to which the outer enamel epithelium was absent seemed to depend on the extent of disruption of the stellate reticulum (Fig. 4).

The control group showed occasional disruption of the stellate reticulum and loss of outer enamel epithelium. Fractionation was seen in only three of these foetuses (Fig. 5). Perivascular infiltration of lymphocytes, polymorphonuclear leucocytes and plasma cells was seen in six of the seven rubella cases. This was particularly obvious around the thin-walled vessels between the tooth germs (Fig. 6). This perivascular infiltrate was also seen in the control group. It was present in three of the five induced and two of the six spontaneous abortions. Large swollen cells with eosinophilic cytoplasm and pyknotic

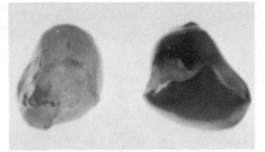

FIG. 2. Tooth germ dissected from a foetus with a maternal history of rubella. The Dm¹ shows more advanced calcification than the Dm². Centripetal collapse of the cusp tips of the Dm² is marked. Stained with alizarin red. × 10.

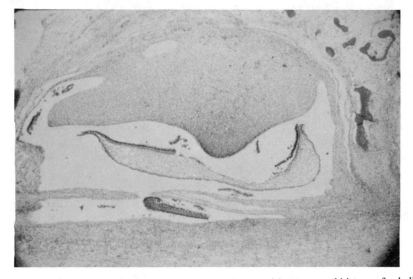

FIG. 3. Histological section of a tooth germ from a foetus with a maternal history of rubella showing fractionation of the internal enamel epithelium. Haematoxylin and eosin. × 30.

nuclei were seen in the rubella cases but were absent from the control group. They were especially frequent in the marrow spaces and loose mesenchymal tissue and often associated with the inflammatory cell infiltrate (Fig. 7). Large basophilic cells with pyknotic nuclei were found in the jaws of all foetuses aborted with urea (Sekeles and Ornoy, 1975).

In the case of infectious mononucleosis morphological and histological changes identical to those found in rubella were seen.

Discussion

Histologic studies of tooth germs in human foetuses with a maternal history of rubella have been carried out by Stocker (quoted by Grahnen, 1958) Bergman et al. (1958) and Töndury and Smith (1966). Stocker examined tooth germs of a stillborn infant with a gestational age of 8 months. He found that the permanent tooth germs were absent. He also found changes in the maxillary teeth of the primary dentition. He described invagination of the incisal region of the canines, malformation of the maxillary incisors and degenerative changes of the ameloblast layer.

Bergman et al. (1958) examined 23 foetuses. They found pathological changes to be present in only one of the 23 specimens examined, and even then the damage was limited to the maxillary central incisors, in which the greater part of the enamel organ was missing. Töndury and Smith (1966) found dental defects in four of the 67 foetuses that they examined. This series included the case described by Stocker. The only finding specifically described by them was necrosis of the ameloblasts.

The dental changes seen by us in human foetuses following intra-uterine rubella infection were severe and affected a far higher percentage of cases than was found in foetuses affected by the European rubella epidemic reported above. This is probably due to the highly teratogenic nature of the virus responsible for the epidemic in Israel (Ornoy et al., 1973). This would also account for the difference in the prevalence of dental abnormalities of the primary dentition in children with a history of maternal rubella described by Grahnen (1958), Evans (1944, 1947) and Guggenheimer et al. (1971).

The histological changes described in this work were localized in the developing enamel organ. The surrounding tissues including dental lamina, epithelial rests and salivary glands appeared normal. Although these changes were occasionally seen in the control group they were constantly present in the rubella group. The changes are undoubtedly degenerative in nature. This degeneration may be attributable to intra-uterine changes after foetal death but prior to abortion. However, the quantitative differences noted between the rubella and control groups suggests that the degenerative changes are, in part, related to the maternal rubella infection. The most constant finding in the rubella group, fractionation of the ameloblasts, was apparently due to degeneration of localized foci in the ameloblast layer, leaving isolated sheets of intact ameloblasts. This was associated with loss of the stellate reticulum leaving the ameloblasts unsupported. The centripetal collapse of the tooth cusps and infolding of the incisal enamel margins, noted in over 50% of the rubella tooth germs may be due to the loss of the stellate reticulum.

These features tend to support the hypothesis put forward by Driscoll (1969), and Guggenheimer et al. (1971), that some of the changes found in the rubella syndrome are due to cellular degeneration. The focal nature of the histological changes described above suggests that the damage is due to the direct local effect of the virus rather than a generalized vascular defect.

Tooth size in the rubella group was more variable in relation to crown-heel

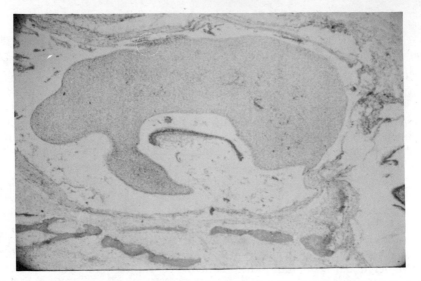

FIG. 4. Histological section of a tooth germ from a foetus with a maternal history of rubella. Fractionation of the enamel epithelium as well as degeneration of the stellate reticulum and the external enamel epithelium are evident. Haematoxylin and eosin. × 30.

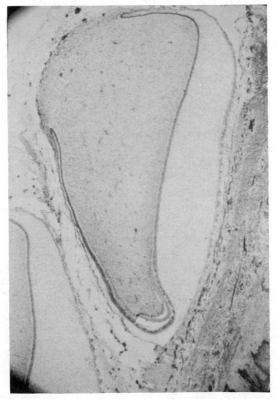

FIG. 5. Histological section of a tooth germ from a control foetus aborted by intra-amniotic injection of urea. Note the normal structure and relationship of the tissues of the enamel organ. Haematoxylin and eosin. × 30.

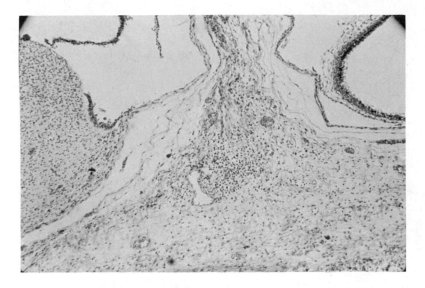

FIG. 6. Perivascular inflammatory cell infiltrate situated between two developing tooth germs. Haematoxylin and eosin. × 75.

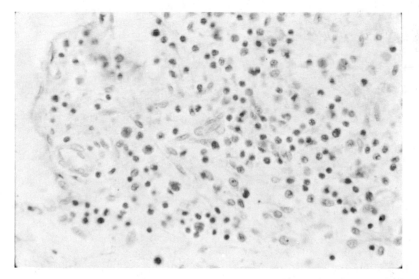

FIG. 7. Higher magnification of the perivascular infiltrate in a rubella foetus showing chronic inflammatory cells as well as large cells with eosinophilic cytoplasm and pyknotic nuclei. Haematoxylin and eosin. × 480.

length than in the control group. This difference was statistically significant only for the central incisor, the tooth which starts development earliest (Kraus and Jordan, 1965). This suggests that the rubella virus does affect tooth growth although we could detect no significant differences between growth rates and tooth size between the rubella and the control groups.

Naeye and Blanc (1965) found a general growth lag in rubella cases. Plotkin *et al.* (1969) attributed this to inhibition of mitotic activity. Since we used crown-heel length as an indicator of foetal age we may in fact have eliminated the possibility of observing a growth lag in tooth size as a result of the rubella virus.

Our results indicate that the virus may cause localized destruction of tissues as well as depression of mitotic activity. Neither of these changes may necessarily be specific to the rubella virus, since similar changes were found in the one foetus examined which was aborted following maternal infection with infectious mononucleosis.

ACKNOWLEDGEMENTS

This work was supported in part by grants from the Marcovitz Foundation (Jerusalem Mother and Child Development Center) and the Joint Research Fund of the Hebrew University-Hadassah Medical Organization and Alpha Omega Foundation.

REFERENCES

BERGMAN, G., LUNDSTROM, R. and LYSELL, L. (1958). Rubella during pregnancy. 2. Studies on the dental development in the foetus. *Acta path. scand.* **43**, 41–46.

DRISCOLL, S. G. (1969). Histopathology of gestational rubella. *Am. J. Dis. Child.* **118**, 49–53.

EVANS, M. W. (1944). Congenital dental defects in infants subsequent to maternal rubella during pregnancy. *Med. J. Aust.* **115**, 225–228.

EVANS, M. W. (1947). Further observations on dental defects in infants subsequent to maternal rubella during pregnancy. *Med. J. Aust.* **34**, 780–785.

GRAHNEN, H. (1958). Maternal rubella and dental defects. *Odont. Revy.* **9**, 181–192.

GUGGENHEIMER, J., NOWAK, A. J. and MICHAELS, R. H. (1971) Dental manifestations of the rubella syndrome. *Oral Surg.* **32**, 30–37.

KRAUS, B. S. and JORDAN, R. E. (1965). "The Human Dentition before Birth". Lea and Feabiger, Philadelphia.

NAEYE, R. L. and BLANC, W. (1965). Pathogenesis of congenital rubella. *J. Am. med. Ass.* **194**, 1277–1283.

ORNOY, A., SEGAL, S., NISHMI, M., SIMCHA, A. and POLISHUK, W. Z. (1973). Fetal and placental pathology in gestational rubella. *Am. J. Obstet. Gynec.* **116**, 949–956.

PLOTKIN, S. A., BOUE, A. and BOUE, J. G. (1965). The *in-vitro* growth of rubella virus in human embryo cells. *J. Epidem.* **81**, 71–85.

SEKELES, E. and ORNOY, A. (1975). Osseous manifestations of gestational rubella in young human foetuses. *Am. J. Obstet. Gynec.* **122**, 307–312.

TÖNDURY, G. and SMITH, D. W. (1966). Fetal rubella pathology. *J. Pediat.* **68**, 867–884.

13. Remnants of the Trigonid Crests in Medieval Molars of Man of Java

C. A. W. KORENHOF

Tandheelkundig Instituut, Rijksuniversiteit Utrecht, Utrecht, The Netherlands

INTRODUCTION

Between 1935 and 1940 von Koenigswald collected a large number of separate human teeth in the surroundings of Sangiran, Java. These teeth were found at the foot of the hills of a steep escarpment, formed by the main tuffaceous Trinil-beds about 15 km north of the town of Surakarta. Large parts of these are eroded every year by the tremendous rainfalls during the wet seasons. This leads to the destruction of many old graves, the remains of which can then be found regularly scattered over the ground.

The bones and skulls were badly disintegrated, and of the teeth not only the roots, but, in many instances, the dentine as well. In cases in which the dentine had not completely disappeared it was often so crumbled and loosened that it could be removed easily by hand instruments. In either case only the enamel crown was left, often beautifully preserved externally, but especially internally, giving the unique possibility to compare both the outer and inner enamel surfaces. This was done first by von Koenigswald (1940), whereas Kraus (1952) removed the enamel by acids, leaving more or less pure dentine crowns (Fig. 1).

From earlier studies (Korenhof, 1960, 1961, 1963) it appeared that the inner enamel surface not only showed a more complete and undamaged aspect, but also represented more conservative conditions than the outer surface, often displaying details which are unknown from the outer anatomy of man, but are known in earlier hominoid dentitions, especially in the Dryopithecinae. This could be expected on embryological grounds, because the inner enamel surface (of the Sangiran teeth) is identical to the original contact surface of ameloblasts and odontoblasts before both types of cell start producing the matrices of their specific tissues. Owing to the thickness

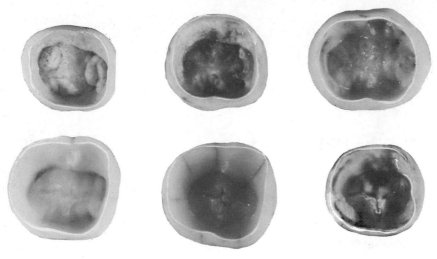

FIG. 1. Enamel caps from Sangiran, internal views.

of the enamel and its unequal distribution over the tooth, the external surface grows to a larger, rounder form reflecting the dentine surface only imperfectly. Factors which influence the development of the enamel thus secondarily modify the morphology of the tooth crown.

To facilitate comparison of the internal and external surfaces of the enamel caps, so-called "endocasts" were made using a hard dental stone-cement (Duroc). Because the upper molars are not the subject of this chapter (the result of the study of their anatomy has been previously published), only two anatomical examples will be given here to illustrate the remarkable differences in morphology between the outer and inner enamel surfaces:

(a) the presence of a complete or incomplete lingual cingulum round the protocone in the endocasts,

(b) the distinct visibility of both trigonal crests or their derivatives.

The Lingual Cingulum

It appeared that the endocasts show in many instances more original cingulum conditions than the outside enamel surfaces. This is the case in 20 % of upper molars with Carabelli cusps type *a*, in 23 % with type *b* and in 38 % with only type *c* fifth cusps on the outside. As is known a complete lingual cingulum never occurs in recent man on the outer anatomy, in contrast to the circumstances in *Gorilla* and *Pan* (see Figs 2 and 3). This finding, among others, brings the anatomy of the dentitions of man and the anthropoid apes into closer relation. In cases where no indication at all of remnants of the lingual cingulum or its derivatives existed on the outer surface, the endocasts show either a cingulum, indications of it or derivatives (pits of Carabelli, Carabelli cusps) in 307 out of 337 cases (i.e. 91 %).

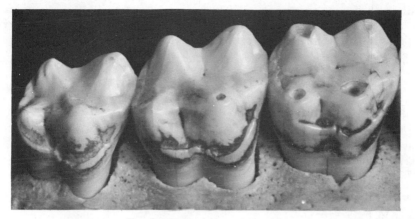

FIG. 2. Upper molars of *Gorilla*.

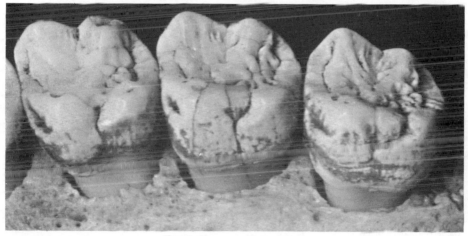

FIG. 3. Upper molars of *Pan*.

The Anterior Transverse Crest

From Tables 35 and 36 in Korenhof (1960) it appears that the crest occurs twice as frequently in the endocasts as in the outer configuration.

The Crista Obliqua

It also appears (Korenhof, 1960, Table 37, for example) that a type *a* crest, i.e. the most complete form (which runs uninterrupted by the longitudinal main groove from the tip of the protocone to the tip of the metacone) occurs in 64 % in the outer against 86 % on the inner enamel surfaces (endocasts).

These examples, which can be supplemented by many others, may demonstrate the importance of the Malayan dental material. For this reason the lower molar material was studied as well. The aim of this chapter is to give the results of a comparison of the outer and inner aspects of remnants of possible trigonid crests.

REMNANTS OF THE TRIGONID CRESTS

Material

The lower molars were classified according to the occlusal groove pattern and the cusp number as developed by Gregory (1916), Gregory and Hellman (1926) and Hellman (1928). The frequencies of the various types are given in Tables I and II (see also Fig. 4). Because of the circumstance that all molars

TABLE I. The types and frequencies of the lower molars from Sangiran.

	6	5	4	Total Number
Y	104	178	14	296
+	140	270	126	536
X	225	348	156	729
Total Number	469	796	296	1561

TABLE II. The types and frequencies of the lower molars from Sangiran from which endocasts could be made.

	6	5	4
Y	24	51	–
+	50	88	32
X	80	128	49

were found, or now are, separated from the jaws no attempt was made to place them according to their serial position in the dental arch (M1, M2, M3). In the following survey the types of molars from the left and right side have been counted together. The schematical drawings, however, always depict right-side teeth.

Types of Crest Pattern between Protoconid and Metaconid in the Endocasts

In many endocasts, distinct crests or remnants of them appear to run from

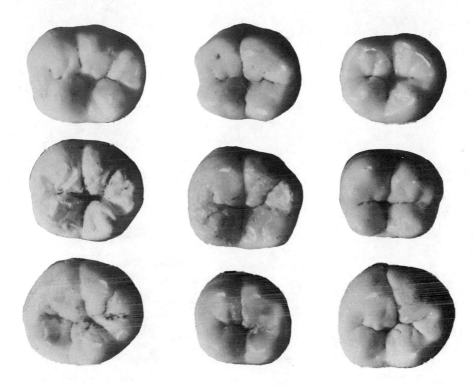

FIG. 4. Lower molar teeth from Java: top row, Y6, Y5 and Y4 patterns; middle row, +6, +5 and +4 patterns; and lower row, X6, X5 and X4 patterns.

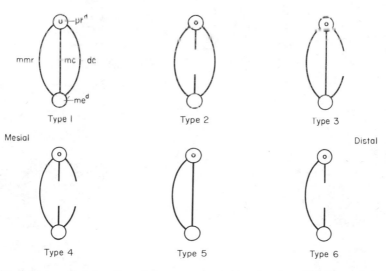

FIG. 5. Types of crest patterns between protoconid and metaconid in the endocasts.

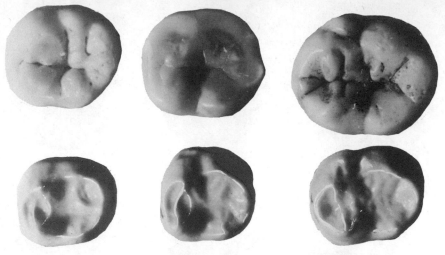

FIG. 6. Type 1 crest patterns. Lower row: endocasts.

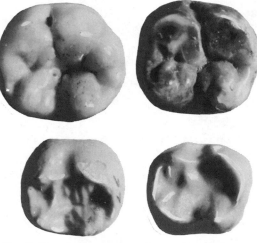

FIG. 7. Type 2 crest patterns. Lower row: endocasts.

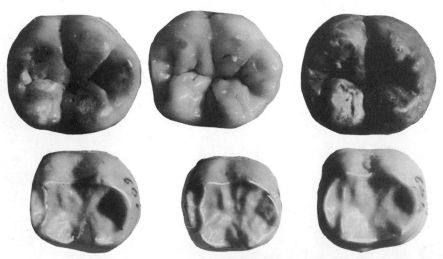

FIG. 8. Type 3 crest patterns. Lower row: endocasts.

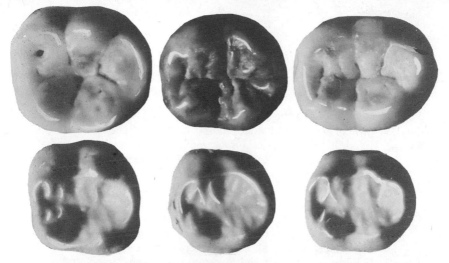

FIG. 9. Type 4 crest patterns. Lower row: endocasts.

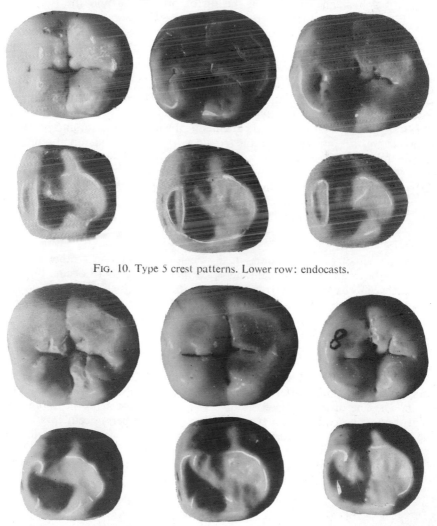

FIG. 10. Type 5 crest patterns. Lower row: endocasts.

FIG. 11. Type 6 crest patterns. Lower row: endocasts.

the tip of the protoconid (or its distal ridge) to (or near to) the tip of the metaconid (see Fig. 5). They may be distinguished into the following types:

Type 1: In addition to the mesial marginal ridge, two complete crests are present between protoconid and metaconid (Fig. 6).

Type 2: In addition to the mesial marginal ridge, two crests occur between protoconid and metaconid of which the mesial one is interrupted but the distal crest is complete (Fig. 7).

Type 3: In addition to the mesial marginal ridge, two crests occur of which the mesial one is complete but the distal crest is interrupted (Fig. 8).

Type 4: In addition to the mesial marginal ridge, two crests occur between the protoconid and metaconid, which are both interrupted or incomplete at a smaller or greater distance (Fig. 9).

Type 5: In addition to the mesial marginal ridge, one distinct and complete crest occurs between the tip of protoconid and the tip of the metaconid (Fig. 10).

Type 6: In addition to the mesial marginal ridge, one interrupted or incomplete crest is situated between the tip of the protoconid and the tip of the metaconid (Fig. 11).

Mesially from the crest(s) there is a fossa, often deep, which can be seen as a more intensive fovea anterior, or Hrdlička's (1924) precuspidal fossa, on the outer enamel aspect. If the hypothesis that the two crests running from the tips of protoconid and metaconid are identical with the anterior and posterior trigonid crests is accepted, then the sequence from type 1 to 6 might represent structural stages from a conservative towards an increasingly more progressive situation. In that case it would be expected that lower numbered crest-types occur in a high percentage in molars which on the outer enamel crown aspect show the more original pattern of grooves and cusp number (i.e. the upper left direction in Fig. 4).

Variations in Crest Patterns

In a number of cases variations in the position of the crests other than as defined above and schematically depicted in Figs 12 and 13 occur. In these instances the situation was translated into the type which they most closely resembled. When this was impossible or a deviation in structure was too arbitrarily added to one existing type, the molar in question was left out of the statistics. Figures 6–11 show some examples of variations in type.

Results

In Table III and Fig. 14, the frequency of occurrence of the six types of crests in each type of molar pattern, as defined by cusp number and fissure pattern, is shown. The distribution of the diverse types of crest gives the impression that more conservative crest types (i.e. low type numbers) occur in a higher percentage in the more original outer cusp patterns. In the Y6 and +6 pattern, for instance, type 1 and type 2 crests occur in 50 % and 20 % respectively of the total number of molars with endocasts of that type. In the Y5

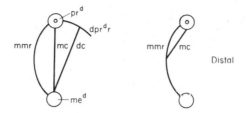

FIG. 12. Variations of type 1 crest patterns.

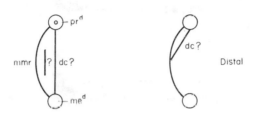

FIG. 13. Variations of type 5 crest patterns.

and +5 molar types these percentages are only about 6 and 16, respectively. On the other hand, the most progressive crest type 6 occurs in a much higher frequency in the Y5 and +5 types than in Y6 and +6 types (61 and 44 % against 21 and 32 %, respectively).

Because of the very low number of molars in several molar pattern groups and the consequently still much lower numbers of crest types it appeared impossible to compare these differences statistically. For that reason the crest type numbers of categories 1–3 and 4–6 were counted together. With the group "0", representing endocasts with no signs of crests at all, three new groups were formed (A, B and C) representing double crests, complete or partially complete (A = 1 + 2 + 3); single crests or remnants of double or single crests (B = 4 + 5 + 6); and no indications of crests at all (C = 0).

Going from A to C the sequence may be called progressive, just as holds true for the sequence 1 to 6 + 0 (see above). This progression appears to be weakly significant in relation to the progression in the cusp number pattern, going from six cusps (which equals Y6, +6 and X6 together), over five cusps (Y5, +5 and X5 together) to four cusps (+4 and X4 together). $\chi^2 = 11 \cdot 43$ (d.f. = 4, $p = 0 \cdot 05$; see Table IV and Fig. 15). However, this progression appears to be very strongly significant in relation to the progression in fissure pattern, i.e. going from Y (= Y6 and Y5 together) over + (+6, +5 and +4 together) to X (X6, X5 and X4 together). $\chi^2 = 48 \cdot 76$ (d.f. = 4, $p = 0 \cdot 01$; see Table V and Fig. 16).

CONCLUSIONS

If it is assumed that the sequences in crest type from 1 to 6 and 0 show a

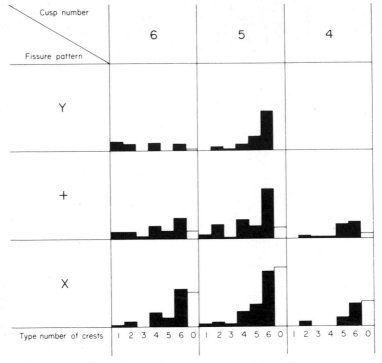

FIG. 14. Graphic representation of Table III.

TABLE III. Frequency of occurrence of the six types of crest patterns.

Fissure Pattern \ Cusp Number	6							5							4						
Y	7	5		6		5	1		3	1	5	11	31								
+	5	5	2	10	6	16	6	3	11	1	15	10	39	9		2	1	1	11	13	4
X	1	4		11	7	30	27	2	3	2	12	18	44	47		4			7	18	20
Type Number	1	2	3	4	5	6	0	1	2	3	4	5	6	0	1	2	3	4	5	6	0

progression (or reduction) in evolutionary development it may be stated that more conservative crest types occur in a higher percentage in more conservative molar types. This is much more significant with regard to the fissure pattern than with regard to the cusp number. Whatever the identity of the crests between protoconid and metaconid in relation to the original (or Gregory's secondary, 1922) trigonid crests may be, the occurrence of this feature has evolutionary significance and, in my opinion, the crests are not terminal products of changing anatomy. On the outer enamel anatomy only

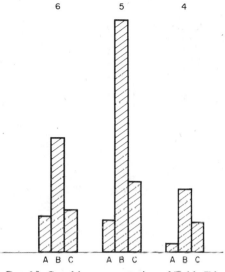
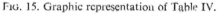

FIG. 15. Graphic representation of Table IV.

TABLE IV. Frequency of occurrence of three groups of crest patterns with regard to the cusp number.

		Progression in Cusp Pattern →			Total Number
		6	5	4	
Progression in Crest Type	A	29	26	7	62
	B	91	185	50	326
	C	34	56	24	114
Total Number		154	267	81	502

very weak indications of the crest may occur in man (Fig. 4), *Gorilla* (Fig. 17), *Pan* (Fig. 18) and *Pongo* (Fig. 19).

SUMMARY

Near Trinil, Java, a collection of medieval Malayan human teeth was found. Part of the teeth consisted of perfectly preserved enamel crowns (caps) because the cementum and dentine of the root and crown had disappeared.

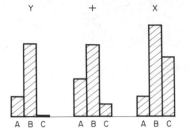

FIG. 16. Graphic representation of Table V.

TABLE V. Frequency of occurrence of three groups of crest patterns with regard to the groove pattern.

		Progression in Fissure Pattern			Total Number
		Y	+	X	
Progression in Crest Type	A	16	30	16	62
	B	58	57	73	188
	C	1	10	47	58
Total Number		75	97	136	308

Thus it became possible to study the anatomy of the enamel–dentine border surface. This was done by making duplicates of the (lost) dentine crowns by means of impression material.

The so-formed endocasts of 502 lower molars were divided into nine groups representing the original *Dryopithecus* pattern and their derivatives. As with the earlier investigation into the same aspect of the upper molar pattern, it appeared that the endocasts showed many additional anatomical details and/or more distinct details which represent earlier evolutionary stages than is the case with the outer enamel surface.

In the present investigation the crest (or crests) and their remnants occurring between the protoconid and metaconid were studied. Between both mesial cusps six different types of crests occur which from 1 to 6 seem to represent a sequence from conservative to progressive stages. The correlation was studied between the measure of evolution of the crest(s) and that of the outer enamel surface. There appeared to be a weakly significant relation between the evolutionary stage of the mesial crest(s) and the progression of

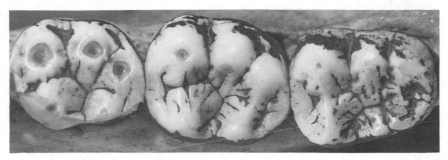

FIG. 17. Lower molars of *Gorilla*.

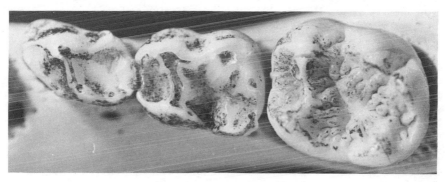

FIG. 18. Lower molars of *Pan*.

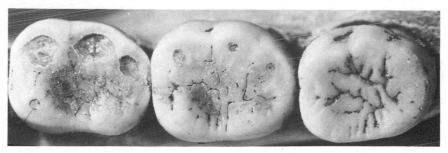

FIG. 19. Lower molars of *Pongo*.

cusp numbers (from 6 to 4). However, a highly significant relation exists between the evolutionary stage of the crest(s) and the progression of the fissure pattern (from Y to X). Thus more conservative molar patterns show a higher percentage of conservative crest patterns.

No attempt was made to suggest to what extent the crests were identical with the original mesial and/or distal trigonid crests as has been done by Remane (1921). However, the appearance of more complete and double crests in more conservative outer crown patterns suggests that at least one of these crests could be identical with the posterior trigonid crest.

REFERENCES

GREGORY, W. K. (1916). Studies on the Evolution of the Primates. *Bull. Am. Mus. Nat. Hist.* **35**, 239–355.
GREGORY, W. K. (1922). "The Origin and Evolution of the Human Dentition." Williams and Wilkins, Baltimore, U.S.A.
GREGORY, W. K. and HELLMAN, M. (1926). The Dentition of *Drypoithecus* and the Origin of Man. *Anthrop. Pap. Am. Mus. nat. Hist.*, *N.Y.* **28** (I), 1–123.
HELLMAN, M. (1928). Racial Characters in Human Dentition. I. A racial distribution of the *Dryopithecus* Pattern and its modifications in the lower molar teeth of man. *Proc. Am. Phil. Soc.* **67**, 157–174.
HRDLIČKA, A. (1924). New data on the teeth of early man and certain fossil European apes. *Am. J. phys. Anthrop.* **7**, 109–132.
KOENIGSWALD, VON, G. H. R. (1940). Neue Pithecanthropus-Funde 1936–1938. Ein Beitrag zur Kenntnis der Praehominiden. Dienst van den Mijnbouw in Ned.-Indië, *Wetensch. Mededelingen* **28**, 1–232.
KORENHOF, C. A. W. (1960). Morphogenetical aspects of the human upper molar. A comparative study of its enamel and dentine surfaces and their relationship to the crown pattern of fossil and recent primates. *Acad. proefschrift, Utrecht. Uitg. mij. Neerl.* 368 pp.
KORENHOF, C. A. W. (1961). The enamel–dentine border: a new morphological factor in the study of the (human) molar pattern. *Proc. K. ned. Akad. Wet. Ser. B* **64**, 639–664.
KORENHOF, C. A. W. (1963). The enamel–dentine border: a new morphological factor in the study of the (human) molar pattern. *Ned. Tijdschr. Tandheelk.* Suppl. **70**, 30–57.
KRAUS, B. S. (1952). Morphologic relationship between enamel and dentin surfaces of lower first molar teeth. *J. dent. Res.* **31**, 248–256.
REMANE, A. (1921). Beiträge zur Morphologie des Anthropoidengebisses. *Arch. Naturgesch.* **87**, 1–179.

14. Morphogenetic Gradients: Fields versus Clones

J. W. OSBORN

Anatomy Department, Guy's Hospital Medical School, London

INTRODUCTION

In 1934, Huxley and de Beer gave a detailed description of the way in which a concept of biological fields could be used to account for the ontogenetic differentiation of regions. Butler (1939) was the first to apply this concept to dentitions in an attempt to account for gradients in tooth shape. However, with regard to the development of patterns and gradients, the special province of field theories, Webster (1971) has stated that: "At present only formal explanations can be given and the concepts employed can only be defined operationally."

Edmund (1960) has described a *Zahnreihe* model in order to account for the development and evolution of the patterns of tooth replacement found in reptiles and mammals. This model is similar to field models (Osborn and Crompton 1973, Osborn 1974a) because it supposes that pattern formation is controlled by a source which is outside the developing dentition. Osborn (1970, 1971) studied the embryonic development of the above patterns and concluded that the data were not consistent with the *Zahnreihe* model. He has constructed a different type of model which is based on the view that the patterns are self-generated rather than "controlled" from outside (Osborn, 1973, 1974b, 1975a). In this chapter this model is extended to account for the development of gradients of tooth shape and is contrasted with the field model.

FIELD AND CLONE MODELS

In terms of biological fields the development of a gradient in structure is seen as the response to a gradient in environment: each quantum change in environment is matched by a quantum change in response. Several elegant models have recently been proposed in order to account for the development and maintenance of a gradient in the environment and to account for the different responses of cells to this environment (e.g. Wolpert 1969, Crick 1970, Goodwin and Cohen 1970, Webster 1971).

At its simplest, consider the development of five similar structures the shapes of which comprise a gradient (Fig. 1E). It is assumed that early in development a specialized region which I will call a field generator is different-iated (heavily stippled region in Fig. 1A). The field generator produces a field substance which diffuses through the growing region (light stipple in Fig. 1). The field substance is slowly destroyed by the tissues through which it

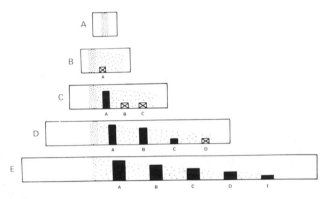

FIG. 1. An explanation in terms of fields for the development of five structures whose shapes are graded (A to E in E). A field generator (heavy stipple) is differentiated in (A) and produces a gradient of field substance (light stipple). All primordia (e.g. A in B, B and C in C and D in D) are identical. Each primordium develops into a shape determined by the concentration of field substance. This correspondence is indicated by matching the height of each structure (black rectangles) to the level of the field substance.

diffuses so that the further a region is from the field generator the lower is the concentration of the field substance (indicated by the gradient of light stipple in Fig. 1).

Due to some other control mechanism (for example a different field effect), primordia differentiate from the growing tissues. All the primordia are identical but each becomes surrounded by a different concentration of field substance. The final gradient in structure is the result of the different reactions of primordia to the different concentrations of field substance.

For the present model, the tissue equivalent to that in Fig. 1A contains three different regions (Fig. 2A), the middle of which (stippled) gives rise to our five structures together with all the tissues which surround them (stippled region in Fig. 2E). This middle region is referred to as a clone. The clone grows posteriorly. After a certain number of cell divisions the tissues become competent to initiate a primordium (Fig. 2B). New primordia are initiated as and when space becomes available within the posteriorly expanding clone. It

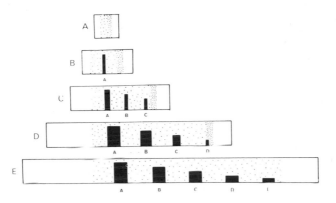

Fig. 2. An explanation in terms of a clone model for the development of the gradient of structures shown in Fig. 1E. All the structures develop from a clone of cells (stippled in A). The clone grows to the right (its growing edge is heavily stippled). New primordia are initiated when space becomes available inside the clone (light stipple). When a primordium differentiates out of the clone (A in B, B and C in C, D in D) its shape (represented by the height of the rectangle) is already determined.

is convenient to visualize around each newly developed primordium a zone of tissue in which the initiation of a new primordium is inhibited (Osborn, 1971). Clearly, successive primordia appear successively later and therefore the cells giving rise to a later primordium have divided more times than those giving rise to an earlier primordium. In other words there is a gradient in the cell ancestry of successive primordia. The gradient in the five fully developed structures is the result of the gradient in the cell ancestry of their related primordia.

Both the above descriptions are special examples of the way in which each model can be formulated. They have been simplified in order to focus attention on what might be termed axiomatic differences between the models:

(a) In a field model it is axiomatic that all primordia are equivalent: if they were different there would be no necessity for a field substance. In contrast, it is axiomatic in the clone model that all primordia are different. As soon as it has been initiated the final shape of a primordium has been largely determined.

(b) In a field model the shape into which a structure develops is controlled from outside. In a clone model it is self-generated from within. For field models, shape is induced; for the clone model, shape is intrinsic.

(c) In field models a primary gradient (of field substances) induces the development of a matching secondary gradient (of shapes). In the clone model gradients are the result of growth: until growth starts the gradient cannot exist and when growth stops the gradient ends. Growth "unfolds" the gradient.

TOOTH SHAPE

Studies of tooth primordia show that the soft-tissue interface between the ectodermally derived enamel organ and the mesodermal (ectomesenchymal) dental papilla folds in a three-dimensional pattern which closely approximates the shape of the later-to-be-developed tooth (Fig. 3). In 1956 Butler attempted

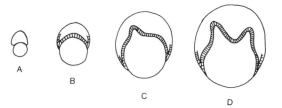

FIG. 3. A. A tooth primordium consists of a roughly spherical clump of ectomesenchymal cells (the dental papilla) surmounted by ectoderm (the enamel organ). B. At a later stage the inner cells of the enamel organ are arranged as a regular layer of columnar cells, the internal enamel epithelium (the IEE). The enamel organ becomes a cap on the papilla, the cap stage of development. C. The enamel organ continues to surround the papilla producing a bell shape, the bell stage of development. At this stage the IEE buckles in a region which later becomes the first cusp to develop. D. Subsequent growth leads to further folding of the IEE into a pattern which closely matches that of the fully developed crown of the tooth.

to analyse the mechanical aspects of this folding. The details of his analysis need not concern us here: suffice it to say that he reduced the problem to one in which each presumptive cusp in a tooth primordium becomes a site at which the soft tissues mature before their surroundings. My interpretation of his description is that prior to cusp development the soft tissue interface between the ectoderm and the mesoderm of a tooth primordium contains a set of discrete sites whose number and position correspond with the cusps of the presumptive tooth.

Measurements of molar teeth (e.g. Butler, 1939, 1952a, 1952b; van Valen, 1970) show that the height of a specific cusp, for example the paracone, is graded along the molar series, being highest at different teeth in different genera. Other features are maximally expressed in different molar teeth. In order to account for these observations Butler (1939), and later van Valen (1970), implied that all tooth primordia have the same set of hypothetical sites mentioned above (a statement of the "field axiom" that all primordia are equivalent). I will call these sites "targets." Towards the front of the jaw there is a field generator producing and maintaining a gradient of field substance. Different targets are sensitive to different concentrations of the field substance (Butler, 1952a). For example, if paracones are largest towards the front of a molar sequence and hypocones are largest towards the back, we can assume that paracone targets respond maximally to high concentrations and hypocone targets to low concentrations of field substance. It can be visualized that the model provides a formal explanation for gradients in any measurable characteristic shared by a row of molar teeth.

In a slightly different model, van Valen (1970) proposes the existence of several different field substances. Those parts of primordia which become either maximally or minimally expressed at the same tooth position in the molar series are assumed to have been sensitive (either activation or suppression) to the same field substance.

It should be noted that if all primordia are equivalent all must contain a full complement of incisor, canine and molar targets. A molariform tooth is one in which only the molar targets have been activated. Osborn (1975b) has described a model for the development of tooth shape which does not necessitate the existence of target sites. The model requires that the internal enamel epithelium (IEE) grows over the surface of the dental papilla (DP) at a constant rate in all directions. From an early spherical shape the DP grows at different (but constant) rates mesially, distally, lingually and buccally. A force equivalent to viscous drag restrains the IEE from sliding over the DP. An analysis of this mechanistic model shows that the shape into which the IEE folds (Fig. 3) could depend on the initial growth rates specified above. If this is true, in order to account for a gradient in tooth shapes we merely require a mechanism for providing a gradient in the initial growth rates of successive primordia.

It was earlier argued (Fig. 2A) that primordia "unfold" from the clone as it grows. Suppose that the clone itself grows progressively more slowly and that the initial growth rate of a primordium is the same as that of the segment of the clone from which it is initiated. There will be an equivalent reduction in the initial growth rates of successive primordia. Preliminary results from the mechanistic model referred to above suggest that the teeth developed from those primordia may not only be of different sizes but that they may also have surprisingly different, albeit graded, shapes.

In summary, the growth rate of the segment of clone from which a primordium is derived specifies the initial growth rates of the primordium which in turn prescribe the shape of the tooth. We can therefore conceive that successive generations of clone cells have different "shape potentials." The "shape potential" of cells is the shape of tooth that would be developed if they became incorporated into a primordium. The shape potential of successive cell generations changes as the clone unfolds. It should be noted that many clone cells do not become incorporated in primordia and therefore never express their shape potential.

The concept of changes in the shape potential of successive cell generations has something in common with changes in the competence of cells to interact during embryogenesis. The competence of cells to react to an inductive stimulus rises until it reaches a threshold at which the reaction can occur. Later the competence falls. For a given reaction it never falls and then rises again. In the same way the shape potential of cells in the growing margin of a clone, from which new primordia are initiated, cannot rise after it has fallen. This is an important addition to the clone model because, as will be argued later, it permits us to recognize clone borders in the fully developed dentition. For example, because the dentitions of most mammals contain three gradients of different tooth shapes (incisor, canine and molar regions) the embryonic jaws should contain at least three equivalent cell clones. The following experimental data seem to provide more support for a clone model than for a field model.

When isolated at a very early stage of development (cap stage) and cultured *in vitro* away from any possible field substances, a tooth rudiment continues to produce a normal cusp pattern (Glasstone, 1938, 1952; Fisher, 1971). In this laboratory Lumsden has isolated the developing rudiment (bud stage) of M1 from the jaws of 12-day embryo mice. This rudiment is cultured in the anterior chamber of the eye of homologous hosts, a region which can be presumed to lack any morphogenetic field substances associated with the normal developing dentition. After about 3 weeks the rudiment has generated perfectly shaped and mineralized crowns of the whole molar dentition: M1, M2 and M3 (Lumsden and Osborn, 1976). Glasstone (1952) has cultured a halved rudiment of a rabbit molar. This rudiment continued to develop the full cusp pattern. Therefore, at the cap stage of development a tooth germ possesses regulative rather than mosaic properties suggesting that all the cells in the dental papilla have the same potential (i.e. information) for becoming any target site. This is consistent with the clone model which proposes that the rates of cell division within a primordium determine the shape of tooth which is developed: removal of half a tooth germ does not change the initial growth rates and so the same shape is developed.

We might now question whether it is likely that a 2-month human embryo generates a complex pattern of targets in each deciduous incisor primordium at the front of the jaw which is identical to that generated by a 6-year-old child in its third molar primordium at the back of the jaw. It seems more probable that these gross differences in both time and space would lead to the production of different primordia. If this principle is accepted, equivalent differences in time and/or space can also account for differences between Dm4, M1 and M2, for example. Indeed, it seems unnecessary to propose a (field) model which is based on the premise that at an early stage in their development the related tooth primordia are identical, when all experiments in which tooth germs have been cultured show them to be different.

TOOTH NUMBER

Consider an ancestral eutherian mammal which possessed 11 tooth positions: 3 incisor, 1 canine and 7 molar positions (Fig. 4). The embryonic jaws contain a substrate in which 11 local variations ultimately lead to tooth development. How is the number 11 represented in the genome?

Neither Butler (1939, 1967) nor van Valen (1970), both of whom have measured the supposed field effect on dentitions, attempt to account for the number 11. However, there is little conceptual difference between a morphogenetic gradient which controls differences between the shapes of adjacent

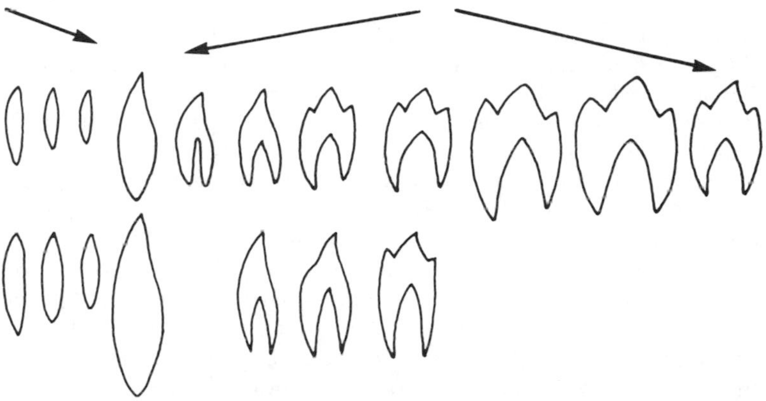

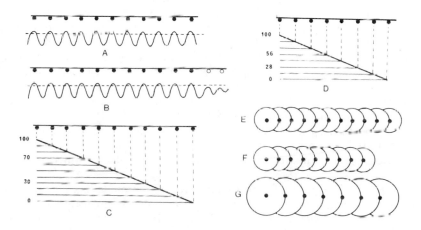

Fig. 4. A hypothetical dentition containing three incisors, a canine and seven molar teeth. Replacements for molars are called premolars. In each region of the jaw, teeth are graded in size. Arrows indicate the sequences in which the deciduous teeth and permanent molars develop.

Fig. 5. Methods for determining the number of teeth. A. Where oscillations in field strength rise above a threshold, indicated by the interrupted line, a tooth primordium (black circle) is initiated. The number of primordia would vary according to the length of tissue which contains the oscillating field. B. Similar to A, except that the number of potential primordia is determined in some other unspecified way and the field can vary this number by suppressing potential primordia (two open circles). C. A model based on positional information. A gradient of substance (the oblique line) extends along the jaw. Cells respond to concentrations of 100%, 90%, 80%, 70% and so on by producing primordia. D. Fewer teeth develop if cells are coded to respond to fewer critical concentrations. E. Tooth primordia are initiated in sequence from the front of the jaw (left). A newly initiated primordium is surrounded by a zone in which the initiation of primordia is inhibited. The number of primordia can be reduced either by shortening the jaws (F) or by increasing the sizes of the inhibitory zones (G).

teeth and a field whose strength peaks at 11 different places along the jaw (Fig. 5A). The field generator which controls tooth number may or may not be different from that which controls tooth shape.

Grüneberg (1951), working with M3 in mice, suggested that there is a critical size for tooth primordia; if a primordium is below this critical size, it fails to develop a tooth. In other words, reduction in the number of teeth seen in some mice (the loss of M3) is a discontinuous (threshold) step in a continuous variation in the size of the primordia for M3. The 11 tooth positions in our hypothetical dentition may have been derived from a larger number of tooth positions by suppressing the size of those primordia behind position 11 (Fig. 5B). This suppression could be brought about by the action of the same field which controls tooth shape. However, what determined the larger number of tooth positions in the ancestor to our mammal with 11 tooth positions?

Wolpert's (1969) variant of field theory is known as the "positional information" model. In the development of structures possessing an axial gradient in properties, the embryonic structure is permeated by a gradient of substance which has a concentration of 100 % (say) at one end falling to 0 % (say) at the other end. It can be appreciated if cells are coded to react in a specific way to a concentration 70 % (say) that, if the gradient is constant, this reaction will take place at a point $\frac{3}{10}$ from one end of the axis and $\frac{7}{10}$ from the other end. In other words, the cells might be considered to derive information about their position along the axis from the concentration of the substance. Cells are coded to react in the appropriate way to this "positional information." If the jaws contain a string of identical cells, all coded to react to concentrations of substance of 100 %, 90 %, 80 %, 70 % and so on by producing tooth buds, then 11 evenly spaced tooth buds will be initiated (Fig. 5C). Different numbers of teeth would require cells to react to different concentrations (Fig. 5D). It will be noted that tooth number is specifically represented within the genome by the number of different concentrations to which cells can react.

The above description of a positional information model is elementary for the sake of simplicity. Much more detailed and biologically acceptable descriptions have been provided by Wolpert (1969, 1971) and by Goodwin and Cohen (1970), who have constructed an ingenious variant based on the cyclic activity of cells.

Finally, suppose it is potentially possible to initiate tooth primordia anywhere within the lengthening clone but that once it has been initiated a primordium generates around it a zone which inhibits the initiation of further primordia (Osborn, 1971, 1974b). The number of primordia is now determined by the sizes of the inhibitory zones and the size to which the clone grows. The larger the inhibitory zones or the smaller the clone, the fewer the primordia (Fig. 5E, F and G). In contrast to a positional information model, the number 11 is the result of an expression of the potential of the genome rather than of a specific representation within the genome.

A consistent distinction between the two models persists in the different ways in which each accounts for tooth number. In field models the number is controlled from outside, in a clone model the number is self-generated. The latter model makes it easier to account for the anomalies in tooth number which are commonly described (e.g. Colyer, 1936).

Tooth Class

There are obvious gradients of tooth shape in nearly all mammalian dentitions (Fig. 4). From the way in which the clone model has been formulated it is evident that any set of teeth whose shapes are graded have probably developed from the same clone. In the upper jaw the gradients are generally interrupted immediately in front of and behind the most anterior tooth on the maxilla. The isolated tooth (the canine) therefore belongs to a different clone from anterior (incisor) and posterior (molar) clones. It can be concluded that the jaws of most mammals contain three clones, each generating a different tooth class (incisor, canine and molar). The number of teeth within a class depends on the size to which its clone grows (see section on tooth number).

The above simple and natural method of recognizing tooth classes has not been adopted by comparative anatomists. They favour the following system which is based on the premaxillary/maxillary suture:

(a) there can only be one canine in a jaw quadrant,
(b) the upper canine is the tooth posteriorly adjacent to the premaxillary/ maxillary suture (unless there is a large diastema), and
(c) the lower canine is the tooth which articulates immediately in front of the upper canine.

This system automatically defines an incisor class (all teeth in front of the canines) and a molar class (all teeth behind the canines)

The tooth classes recognized by the clone model do not always correspond with those defined by the "maxillary suture" system. For example, in artiodactyls the tooth defined by the latter system as a lower canine looks like an incisor and is therefore recognized as such in the clone model. The validity of the distinction between the three tooth classes recognized by the clone model is universally accepted; it is a subject for elaboration of a theory of morphogenetic fields. Butler (1939) proposed that the dentitions of mammals contain three morphogenetic fields equivalent to incisor, canine, and molar classes and that their influence may spread into an adjacent class. For example, in artiodactyls the incisor morphogenetic field extends beyond the incisor class primordia into the canine class primordium, sensitizing the incisor targets of the canine primordium and thereby inducing it to become incisiform.

Both field and clone models seek to understand the evolution and development of dentitions in terms of embryology, the only certain basis for establishing homologies. I visualize that an anterior limb bud might contain three clones: "humerus", "radius and ulna" and "hand" clones. In the same way the jaws contain incisor, canine and molar clones. The three clones of an anterior limb and of a jaw quadrant are conceptually equivalent. The individual bones of a hand are equivalent to the individual teeth of an incisor clone. The shape potential of each unfolds with the growing clone.

It is possible that the "maxillary suture" system of classifying teeth takes a similar view of its three tooth classes (but see later). A canine primordium, the middle class of the dentition, may be embryologically specified in much the same way as a radius and ulna, the middle "class" of the upper limb. But the radius and ulna class of the upper limb is recognized by its shape and by reference to its adjacent "classes," humerus and hand. In contrast, the upper canine is neither recognized by its shape nor by reference to its adjacent classes, incisor and molar; it is recognized by an outside reference point, the premaxillary/maxillary suture (cf. the recognition of the parietal bone by reference to an outside structure; Parrington, 1967). This prompts the question, if all primordia are identical, what can be embryologically unique to the upper canine primordium which ensures that it always captures the position posteriorly adjacent to this suture? And if it is unique it is not identical to all other primordia. The lower canine primordium which invariably captures the region anteriorly adjacent to the upper canine is even more of an enigma.

THE SEQUENCE OF TOOTH INITIATION

In nearly all eutherian mammals, the incisors develop in sequence from front to back, the deciduous molars from back to front and the permanent molars from front to back (Fig. 4; Osborn, 1970). The only exception is that in some mammals (e.g. man) Dm3 develops before Dm4.

For the clone model teeth are initiated where sufficient new tissue has been generated by the growing clone. This is supported by some data for reptiles (Osborn, 1971) and mammals (Osborn, 1973). Space becomes available at the margins of the clone produced by successive cell generations, and cell ancestry determines the shape potential of primordia. Therefore gradients of tooth shape should match the sequences in which teeth are initiated. This prediction matches data for all dentitions in which sequences of tooth initiation have been studied (remembering that within a clone these gradients can fall, or rise and fall, but cannot fall and rise again).

For a field model, because all primordia are equivalent, some outside influence must control the sequences in which they are initiated. Leche (1895) suggested that, apart from molars, the primordia of smaller teeth are initiated later. We can visualize that primordia influenced by a "weakening" field become late developers and poor growers. But there are too many exceptions. For example, I3 in Carnivora, Pm2 in lemurs and Dm1 in the European mole are all the largest in a sequence and develop last. If Leche's "rule" (Butler, 1963) reveals a basic principle underlying the ontogeny of dentitions, there seems no logical reason for the exclusion of molars, except that the last developed molar, M3, is often the largest. No doubt an *ad hoc* explanation can be proposed to account for this anomaly, but explanations of this type must weaken confidence in a rule. It might also be argued that the sequences have evolved in response to the requirements of the animal, but, of course, this suggests a selective advantage for a sequence, not a mechanism for its control.

THE TIMING OF TOOTH INITIATION

The field generator responsible for inducing the initiation of molar primordia must appear before the first primordium is initiated. In man the first deciduous molar (the so-called Dm3 in man) appears at about the end of the second month *in utero*; the primordium for M3 appears in a 6-year-old child. It is scarcely credible that the field generator continues to act as a generator for nearly 7 years. However, even if it does continue producing field substances for 7 years it can only be possible to initiate a primordium when the jaws have grown sufficiently to accommodate (or to develop) the tissues which will later generate the primordium for M3. In other words the most significant control for timing the initiation of M3 is unlikely to be a rate of diffusion of field substances but is almost certainly the growth of tissues capable of differentiating into a primordium of M3 (as in the clone model). If this is true for the initiation of M3 and, almost equally certainly, for the initiation of M2 in man, it seems probable that the same would be true for the remaining tooth primordia. In which case field generators and substances are not necessary to account for either the timing or sequence in which tooth primordia appear.

TOOTH LOSS DURING EVOLUTION

It was suggested above for the clone model that the number of teeth is a self-generated expression by the clone of its genetic potential. New primordia are generated when space becomes available in the growing clone. However, if the shape potential of the clone cells falls below a threshold before the clone has finished growing, primordia might be generated but fail to grow thereby leaving tooth-free regions. Remembering that shape potential cannot rise after it has fallen, the model predicts that teeth can only be lost in sequence from the margins of the classes generated by the clones. The margins of classes can be recognized by observing changes in gradients of tooth shape and/or the sequences in which primordia are initiated. Provided that tooth classes are recognized by a clone analysis, the above prediction accurately accounts for the sequences in which teeth have been lost by all mammals. In every case the relevant tooth has been lost from the margin of its class.

Field models account for the loss of teeth by a weakening of the field effect. The positional information variety of model would conclude that there had been a change in the response to positional information. In both cases the field, or its equivalent, is like an ace of trumps which can be played to account for any card of variation. I suggest that in their application to dentitions, i.e. the number of teeth, their shapes, gradients of shape, sequences of initiation and evolutionary loss, field models can usually do little more than disguise the statement of an observation as an explanation. Nothing can be predicted because fields seem to be infinitely variable.

THE UNITS OF DENTITIONS

Thus far little has been concluded for the clone model which might be objected to by comparative anatomists as opposed to embryologists. Before describing some areas of contention which result from the interpretation of dentitions in terms of clones, it is as well to give a brief account of the development of a dentition and to introduce replacement teeth into the discussion.

Dentitions contain three types of unit: individual teeth, tooth families and tooth classes, the tooth class being the largest unit (Fig. 6) and the product of a dental clone.

A tooth class consists of a set of tooth families. The first tooth to be initiated in a tooth family is the family progenitor; the remaining teeth are replacements. The first family to be initiated in a tooth class is the stem family. Starting from the stem family, new tooth families may be initiated

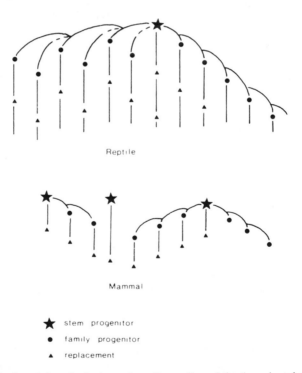

FIG. 6. The single dental clone in the lower jaw of a reptile and the three dental clones in the lower jaw of a mammal are represented. Time runs vertically, from which it can be seen that the stem progenitors (stars) of each clone are the first teeth to be initiated. Curved lines connect the members of a tooth class. In the reptile, progenitors of anterior (left) branch families are initiated in alternation; posterior (right) branch families are initiated in sequence.

anteriorly or posteriorly either in sequence or in alternation; they are referred to as anterior or posterior branch families of the class (Fig. 6).

A tooth class is one of the products of a dental clone. Each lower jaw quadrant of a mammal is partly developed from anterior, middle and posterior dental clones. In addition to contributing other connective tissue elements of the anterior part of the jaw, the anterior dental clone is also involved in producing incisor class teeth. Similarly, the posterior dental clone contributes much of the jaw tissue behind the canine together with the molar class teeth; the middle dental clone contributes the canine and associated tissues. The upper jaws are also developed from anterior, middle and posterior dental clones.

The lower jaw of a recent reptile contains a single tooth class (Fig. 6) but the upper jaw probably contains two tooth classes (see later). In front of the lower-jaw stem progenitor, family progenitors are initiated in alternation; behind the stem progenitor they are initiated in sequence (Osborn, 1971, 1974a).

The jaws of an embryo mammal contain three dental clones (Figs 6 and 7A). The origin of these three clones is as obscure as the origin of three equivalent clones (upper arm, middle arm and hand) in an anterior limb bud. In eutherian mammals, the anterior (incisor) clone grows posteriorly; the canine clone generally accommodates a single tooth family; the molar clone grows anteriorly to generate deciduous molar primordia and posteriorly to generate permanent molar primordia (Fig. 7B to D).

In order to account for the fact that within a molar clone the progenitors of anterior branch families (deciduous molars) have different shapes from those of posterior branch families (permanent molars) we must conclude that the shape potential of cells at the anterior margin of a clone is different from the shape potential of those at the posterior margin. But it is already clear that anterior clone cells must differ from posterior clone cells otherwise we could not have some clones growing only posteriorly (e.g. incisor clones of eutheria) while others grow both anteriorly and posteriorly (molar clones).

If we accept that the shape potential of cells at the anterior margin of a clone differs from that of cells at the posterior margin it can readily be conceived that the shape potential of cells at the growing inferior margin of a clone is different from both. This can account for the different shapes of premolar (replacement) teeth, a difference for which Patterson (1956) found it necessary to postulate the existence of a premolar morphogenetic field.

SHAPE, SIZE AND EMBRYONIC COMPETENCE

The results of Kollar and Baird (1969, 1970) suggest that shape determination, and therefore probably shape potential, is a property of the ectomesenchymal cells which colonize the embryonic jaws. The shape potential of these cells may be closely related to the embryonic competence of these same cells to initiate a tooth primordium and later to produce dentine.

Osborn (1971) deduced for the lizard, *Lacerta vivipara*, that the earliest

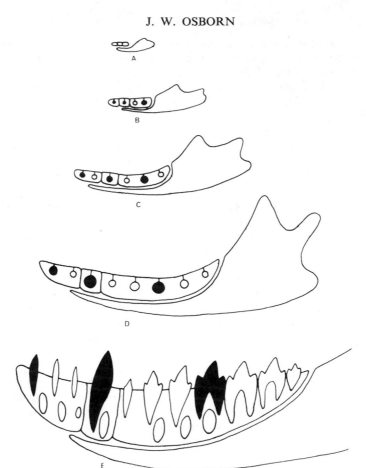

FIG. 7. The lower jaw of an embryo mammal contains three clones (A) which generate the three tooth classes (E). Stem progenitors are black. The incisor clone grows posteriorly, the molar clone grows both anteriorly and posteriorly. The ovals represent replacement teeth. In this diagram it is suggested that the teeth and alveolar bone (clone derivatives) have a different origin from the basal bone of the jaws. This suggestion accords with the view of orthodontists who conceive that many irregularities in the human dentition are due to an incorrect relationship between alveolar bone and the basal bone of the jaws.

initiated tooth primordia cannot yet produce dentine, and the primordia (rudimentary buds) rapidly degenerate. Those primordia initiated a little later develop small knobs of dentine (rudimentary teeth) which are either resorbed or shed into the oral cavity before hatching. Later and all subsequent primordia produce functional teeth. These data indicate that embryonic competence rapidly increases during early embryonic life to achieve the thresholds at which all tooth tissues can be formed. It is possible that embryonic competence could fall to zero in old reptiles because Bellairs and

Miles (1961) have described a very large (old) toothless monitor lizard in which there is no evidence of tooth replacement.

Until cells have achieved the embryonic competence to produce all the tooth tissues, we cannot know their shape potential because teeth cannot yet be formed. The teeth of *L. vivipara* hatchlings possess small anterior and posterior accessory cusps which are gradually lost in successive replacement teeth (Cooper, 1963). Therefore as the hatchling grows, shape potential decreases to reach a certain minimal level represented by simple conical teeth. However, although shape potential decreases early in life, successive replacement teeth seem to be successively larger (Osborn, 1974b). The above data for embryonic competence, shape potential and tooth size are represented in Fig. 8.

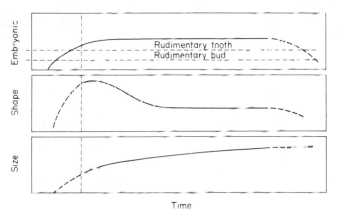

Time

FIG. 8. Curves in which the embryonic competence of jaw tissue, the shape complexity and the size of teeth in *L. vivipara* are plotted against time. Interrupted parts of the curves indicate that data are absent or unobtainable.

Sexual dimorphism in dentitions probably indicates that both shape potential and size can be influenced by hormonal controls. An interesting example is the salamander, *Desmognathus fuscus*. The premaxillary teeth in males are long and monocuspid while those in females are short and bicuspid. Castrated males produce the short bicuspid premaxillary teeth which are typical of females (Noble and Pope, 1929).

Embryonic competence may also be affected by hormones. Male salamanders (*Eurycea bislineata bislineata*) collected at the end of the breeding season are partially edentulous (Stewart, 1958); however, this loss may have been due to trauma provoked by female reluctance rather than due to a temporary loss of embryonic competence which had caused a delay in tooth replacement. Many of the replacements for the lost monocuspid teeth are small and bicuspid. Later, these are replaced by the more usual monocuspid teeth.

The above data indicate a relationship between tooth shape and tooth size in salamanders which is similar to that in lizards, small teeth having more complex shapes. A progressive decrease in shape potential within each tooth family, similar to that in *L. vivipara*, has been demonstrated for *Thrinaxodon* (Osborn and Crompton, 1973), a Triassic cynodont which is generally presumed to have been close to the line of mammal evolution. Each postcanine tooth family appears to have been capable of producing at least three, and probably four, teeth whose complexity successively decreased, the last being a very small conical tooth. However, unlike *L. vivipara*, successive teeth generally decreased in size, although the decrease may only be obvious in the last tooth in the four tooth sequence.

Diademodon, a gomphodont cynodont from the Triassic, produced six teeth in each postcanine tooth family, the largest and most complex being the fifth tooth in the sequence (Fourie, 1963). In this animal, size and shape complexity are closely matched (Fig. 9). Although each tooth family in mammals contains at most two teeth, the relationship between size and shape in postcanine families is similar to that in *Thrinaxodon* (Fig. 9). However, in

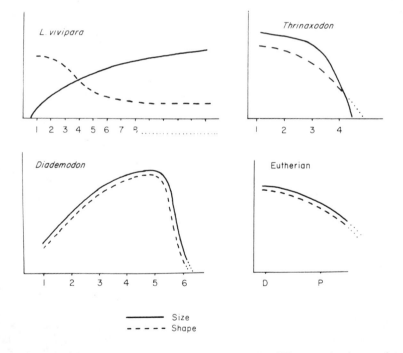

FIG. 9. Curves in which size and complexity of shape for different animals are plotted against the number of each replacement tooth.

canine and incisor families, the permanent teeth are larger than, but of similar shape to, the deciduous predecessors.

Numerous mammals seem to produce vestigial deciduous teeth or tooth primordia which do not develop into functional teeth: the insectivores, *Suncus orangiae* (Kindahl, 1959a), *Erinaceus europaeus* (Kindahl, 1959b) and *Sorex araneus* (Kindahl 1959a); the bat, *Hipposideros caffer* (Gaunt, 1967); the albino ferret, *Mustela putorius* (Berkowitz and Thompson, 1973); and strains of laboratory mice (Fitzgerald, 1973). They have also been observed in three metatherians (Berkowitz 1966, 1968, 1972). Thus, the phylogenetic loss of deciduous teeth seems to be related to a change in shape potential and/or embryonic competence rather than the loss of genetic coding for specific primordia. This change could take place in two ways: either by initiating primordia before the embryonic competence and/or shape potential have risen sufficiently to generate a viable tooth, or by changing the time at which these competencies develop (Fig. 10).

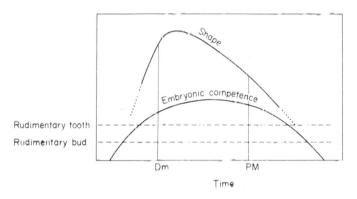

FIG. 10. The embryonic competence and shape potential of the jaw tissues responsible for producing a molar tooth family are plotted against time. Dm and PM are the times at which the deciduous and replacement teeth are initiated. Below a threshold level the tissues have only sufficient embryonic competence to produce a rudimentary tooth. Below a further threshold they are not competent to form a tooth bud (primordium).

By increasing the above changes it becomes possible to repress not only deciduous but also permanent teeth. Even some edentulous mammals such as *Ornithorhynchus* (Green, 1937), the pangolin, *Manis* (Röse, 1892) and whalebone whales, the Mysticeti (Julin, 1880) still produce vestigial teeth or primordia.

I conclude that the genetic coding for dental clones *per se* is phylogenetically very stable. Phylogenetic change, not only in the shape of teeth but also in the number of tooth families, and the number of replacement teeth, are all related to variations in competence at the clone rather than at the tooth level.

EVOLUTION OF MAMMALIAN FROM REPTILIAN CLONES

A single dental clone fills each lower jaw quadrant in *L. vivipara*, the stem progenitor being at position 11 (Osborn, 1971). For the upper jaw, the break in tooth replacement waves and the separation of the dental lamina at the premaxillary/maxillary suture (Edmund, 1960; Cooper, 1963) suggest that the premaxillary teeth may belong to a different clone from the maxillary teeth. A median premaxillary tooth family, whose replacements are identical to the remaining premaxillary teeth, has the egg tooth as its progenitor (Cooper, 1963). It is possible that the egg tooth is the stem progenitor of a clone which includes both left and right premaxillary teeth; in other words, all premaxillary teeth belong to a single premaxillary clone which colonizes both left and right sides of the jaw.

The clone model can readily account for the evolution of the dentitions found in many Cotylosaurs, the stem reptiles of the Permian, if their ancestors possessed dentitions like that suggested above for *L. vivipara*. In these animals two or three very large premaxillary teeth are followed by a sequence of smaller teeth which gradually increase in size, reaching their largest somewhere towards the middle of the maxilla (Fig. 11). It will be recalled

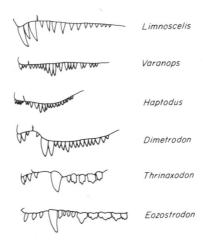

Limnoscelis

Varanops

Haptodus

Dimetrodon

Thrinaxodon

Eozostrodon

FIG. 11. Upper dentitions of a Cotylosaur (*Limnoscelis*) and three Pelycosaurs (after Romer, 1966), *Thrinaxodon* (after Crompton, 1963) and *Eozostrodon* (after Parrington, 1971). Not to scale. A tooth in the middle of the maxilla of *Varanops* is small because it is erupting.

that the clone model requires, starting from the stem family, that a sequence of anterior or posterior members of a clone does not decrease in size and then increase in size. If the stem family of maxillary teeth in the Cotylosaurs were in the middle of the maxilla, the premaxillary teeth would belong to a different clone because of the increase in the size of these teeth when compared with those posteriorly adjacent. Thus, the large anterior teeth must belong to a different clone from the remaining teeth. The evidence of *L. vivipara* suggests that the egg tooth may have been the stem progenitor of the premaxillary clone in Cotylosaurs (there may have been two egg teeth, left and right).

While in the upper jaws of Cotylosaurs differences had evolved between the teeth in anterior and posterior clones, many of the descendant Pelycosaurs, judged from the sizes of their teeth (Fig. 11), seem to have evolved three clones, the condition found in mammals. In *Dimetrodon*, behind the pre-maxillary teeth, two anterior maxillary teeth dwarf the small posteriorly adjacent maxillary tooth and from here size increases, reaching a peak somewhere in the middle of the maxilla (Fig. 11). The clone model predicts that the maxilla contained two tooth clones. In the ancestral Cotylosaurs, the stem families of the anterior and posterior clones were widely separated, the former containing the egg tooth (or left and right egg teeth) and the latter being in the middle of the maxilla. Early in the embryogenesis of later Pelycosaurs the space between the stem families of the anterior and posterior clones became colonized by a middle clone which generated the large teeth at the anterior end of the maxilla.

An alternative method of deriving three clones in the lower jaw (and, by implication, the upper jaw) has been given by Osborn (1973). He suggested that the enlarged "canine" evolved from the stem family of the clone which had occupied the whole jaw of an ancestral homodont reptile. Later, anterior (precanine) and posterior (postcanine) clones evolved, leaving the canine as the sole representative of the ancestral clone which, at one time, had occupied the whole jaw. The view presented here is that the anterior clone evolved from the egg tooth and the canine clone was the last to evolve. The choice between these alternatives awaits a more detailed study of the Cotylosaurs and Pelycosaurs.

Fossil data seem to indicate that the evolution of two, and then three, clones in the lower jaw lagged behind that of the upper jaw. For example, judged from gradients in tooth size, the Cotylosaurs seem to have a single lower clone while the Pelycosaurs have only two lower clones. The lower anterior clone in Pelycosaurs may have evolved in the same way as the upper anterior clone in Cotylosaurs. In support of this view, I have noticed (unpublished observations) a small median knot of cells situated at the front of the jaw within the lower dental lamina of an early embryo of *L. vivipara* (this was in embryo A; Osborn, 1971). This knot of cells, like similar but more obvious early proliferations in the dental lamina of the lower jaw (Osborn, 1971), does not produce a recognizable tooth bud. However, its position suggests that it corresponds with the egg tooth in the upper jaw. A similar knot of cells in the early Pelycosaurs could have been ancestral to a stem progenitor for the lower anterior clone of teeth in later Pelycosaurs. The subsequent evolution of a lower canine clone would have followed a similar sequence to the evolution of the upper canine clone.

The mammal-like reptiles retained the three tooth clones of the Pelycosaurs and evolved intra-family heterodonty; that is, families in which successive replacement teeth developed different shapes. This grade of evolution, which has been discussed by Osborn (1973) is demonstrated by the post-canines of *Thrinaxodon* (Osborn and Crompton, 1973) and *Diademodon* (Osborn, 1974a). Dentitions were polyphyodont but the post canine families developed a limited number of replacement teeth: three or four in the case of *Thrinaxodon* and six in the case of *Diademodon*. Just as in earlier grades of dental evolution, the postcanine clone appears to have continued to generate new tooth families at the back of the growing jaw throughout life.

By the time the earliest known mammal, *Eozostrodon*, was evolved tooth families had been reduced to a progenitor, the deciduous tooth, and a single replacement, the permanent tooth (discussed by Osborn, 1975a). Furthermore the jaws no longer increased in length throughout life with the result that during subadult or early adult life, no more posterior branch families were budded out of the molar clone. Finally, in these posterior branch families replacement teeth were not developed, thus introducing permanent (unreplaced) molar teeth.

Since the upper Triassic the dental evolution of mammals has, with few exceptions such as the Cetacea, been characterized by a further reduction in the growth of dental clones.

HOMOLOGIES BETWEEN TOOTH CLASSES

Although it is a subject for the exercise of philosophy and logic, the conventional concept of homology implies development from the same embryological primordium. The position or shape of structures in adults may indicate a probable homology but, because of the way in which it is conceived, homology can be most firmly established by studies of comparative embryology. Conversely, where two different structures are thought to be homologous, we conclude that their differences have been brought about by a change in the developmental controls operating on the same primordium.

For the clone model, a clone is a primordium and it generates a tooth class. Changes in the number and shapes of teeth within a class are brought about by changes in the developmental controls operating at the primordium level, the clone. A tooth primordium is a "secondary" primordium in the sense that it develops out of a "primary" primordium, the clone.

For field models a tooth primordium is a "primary" primordium: the separation of teeth into classes is an artificial but helpful means of describing dentitions. For example, an ancestral eutherian mammal possessed 11 identical primordia in each jaw quadrant (ignoring replacement teeth) which could be labelled 1 to 11 without any loss of precision in terminology; there is no more difference between 1 and 3 than between say 3 and 11. Primordia 1 to 3 (incisors) are grouped together, not because they are different from the remainder, but because they are usually subjected to similar developmental controls (the incisor morphogenetic field). In contrast, primordia 1 to 3 are an embryological group for the clone model; they are the members of the incisor clone.

In the following examples clone and field models recognize different tooth homologies. Each model bases its recognition on the identification of its "primary" primordia. The clone model first identifies tooth classes, by the boundaries between gradients of shape, and then individual teeth. The field model identifies "individual" teeth, ignoring shape. Identification automatically places a tooth in its class.

Some Early Mammals

In several Mesozoic mammals the so-called second premolar is smaller than the tooth posteriorly adjacent to the canine (the so-called PM1). This is true for the upper jaw of *Eozostrodon* (Parrington 1971), the upper and possibly lower jaw of *Megazostrodon* (Crompton, 1974) and the upper jaw of *Erythrotherium* (Crompton, 1974), which constitute the most completely known mammalian dentitions from the Triassic/Jurassic boundary. It is also true for the lower jaw of *Docodon* (Simpson, 1929; see Fig. 12). I suggest that in each case the so-called PM1 may be a second canine.

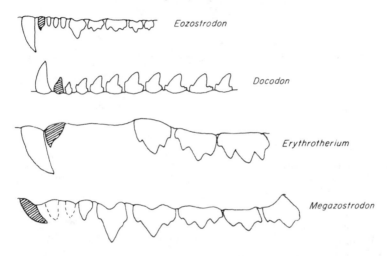

Eozostrodon

Docodon

Erythrotherium

Megazostrodon

FIG. 12. Dentitions of some early mammals in which the so-called PM1 is larger than PM2. It is suggested that PM1 (shaded in the diagram) may be a member of the canine clone. For *Erythrotherium*, the roots of the teeth contained in the gap indicate that the most anterior lost tooth was smaller than the retained adjacent tooth. *Eozostrodon* is after Parrington (1971); *Erythrotherium* and *Megazostrodon* are after Crompton (1974); and *Docodon* is after Simpson (1929). Not to scale.

Recent Insectivores

In the lower dentition of the European mole, *Talpa europaea*, the supposed lower canine is shaped like a fourth incisor and PM1 is a large caniniform tooth which articulates behind the upper canine (Fig. 13). Clearly, from the way in which the clone model has been formulated (see above), this large caniniform tooth does not belong to the molar clone; therefore it is a canine. And the shape of the supposed canine suggests that it is a fourth incisor. The lower jaw of *T. europaea* would have the dental formula $I_4 C_1 PM_3 M_3$.

To those who are disturbed by the suggestion that a eutherian mammal might possess four incisors in a jaw quadrant it is worth mentioning that Berkovitz and Thompson (1973) have demonstrated that a high percentage of albino ferrets (*Mustela putorius*) develop four upper deciduous incisors (by the standard definition) in each jaw quadrant. This "inconsistency" is similar

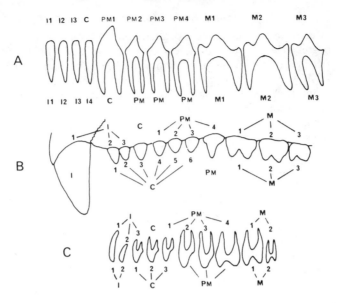

Fig. 13. Dentitions of *Talpa europaea* (A), *Desmana* (B) and *Elephantulus* (C). The generally accepted interpretation is given above, and the present interpretation is given below each dentition. Not to scale.

to the possession of four permanent molars by the eutherian carnivore, *Otocyon*, and the possession of five permanent lower molars by the metatherian insectivore, *Myrmecobius*.

Many of the Talpidae have a large upper central incisor followed by five or six similarly shaped conical teeth; for example, *Desmana* (Fig. 13). It seems possible that these conical teeth are canines, giving *Desmana* the dental formula I^1, C^6, PM^1, M^3. Additionally, in the two skulls I have examined, the so-called upper second and third incisors appear to be sited on the maxilla in *Desmana*, in which case they are not incisors even by currently accepted definitions.

The shapes of teeth in *Elephantulus*, a Macroscelid, indicate that the third and fourth teeth from the front of the upper jaw, and probably the fifth, are members of the canine clone (Fig. 13). The same is true of the other Macroscelididae I have examined. The sequence of tooth development in *Elephantulus* (Kindahl, 1957a) does not conflict with the view that its upper dentition might have the formula I^2 C^3 PM^3 M^2.

An analysis based on gradients of tooth shape suggests that in the upper dentition of *Sorex araneus*, the anterior clone contains a single specialized incisor (Fig. 14C), the middle clone contains five almost identically shaped teeth (the second being the largest and the fifth being the smallest) and the posterior clone contains four teeth. In other words the upper dentition has the formula I^1, C^5, PM^1, M^3. Fortunately Kindahl (1959a) has studied

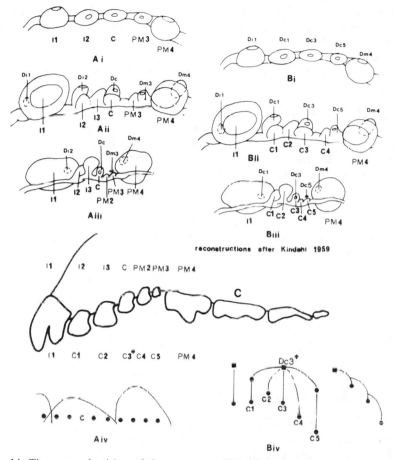

FIG. 14. The upper dentition of *Sorex araneus* (C). Kindahl's interpretation of her re-construction A (i–iii) and the present interpretation B(i–iii). Also indicated in C are the conflicting interpretations of the tooth classes. A (iv) shows the dentition in terms of fields, the canine field spreading to affect morphogenesis of five primordia. B (iv) shows the dentition in terms of the clone model. A (iii) is not to scale with A (i) and A (ii).

dental development of *S. araneus* so that it is possible to analyse this un-orthodox interpretation.

Kindahl (1959a) reached the conclusion that the permanent teeth were initiated before their deciduous predecessors (Fig. 14A), the latter being resorbed before they erupted. It can be seen (Fig. 14A) that Kindahl's data are difficult to interpret. I suggest that the five buds in the smallest embryo are the incisor (Di^1), canine (Dc^3) and molar (Dm^3) stem progenitors together with Dc^1 and Dc^5 (Fig. 14Bi). Subsequently the canine clone spreads apart enabling two more canines (C^2) and C^4) to develop in the interspaces between Dc^1, Dc^3 and Dc^5 (Fig. 14Bii). The three deciduous canines develop permanent successors. It will be noted that teeth in the canine clone are initiated in alternation and that the gradient in shape matches the sequence of development (Fig. 14B iv).

It should be pointed out that in all the above animals the upper and lower anterior cheek teeth have imprecise occlusal relationships. There has been no strong selection pressure for evolving the precise relationships that are seen between the upper and lower cusps of the posterior cheek teeth. The absence of necessity for precise occlusal relationships in the anterior cheek region allows it to be colonized by either molar or canine clones, and one may colonize one jaw while the other colonizes the other jaw.

The above descriptions suggest that a new approach to dental formulae might improve our understanding of the relationships between different groups of insectivores.

Prosimians

The dentitions of several prosimians together with the probable extent of the canine clones are shown in Fig. 15.

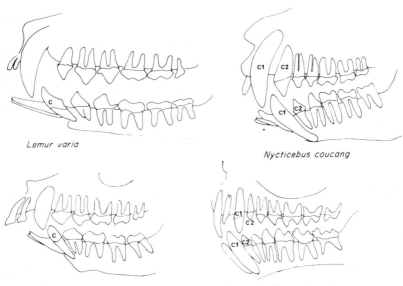

Lemur varia

Nycticebus coucang

Indri brevicaudata

Tarsier spectrum

FIG. 15. The present interpretation of some prosimian dentitions.

Pecora

It seems likely that in Pecora the so-called lower canine might in fact be a fourth member of the incisor clone and that the canine clone has been lost. Fossil data reviewed by Romer (1966) are consistent with this interpretation. *Homacodon*, an archaic artiodactyl (Fig. 16), clearly had a lower dentition:

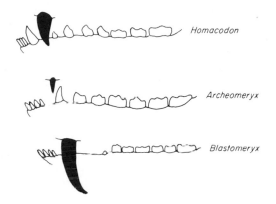

FIG. 16. Stages in the evolution of recent pecoran dentitions. The upper canine is indicated in black (after Romer, 1966). Not to scale.

I_3, C, PM_4, M_3. The Eocene and Oligocene hypertragulids (e.g. *Archeomeryx*), which were close to the stem of the pecorans, have a large isolated tooth occupying a space between the cheek teeth behind and four incisiform teeth in front (Fig. 16). Within a sequence of teeth budded from a clone it is not possible for size drastically to increase after it has decreased suggesting that the large isolated tooth does not belong to the molar clone. Therefore it is the canine, and the four incisiform teeth belong to the incisor clone. This tooth was later lost in the Old World traguloids (e.g. *Blastomeryx*), a stock from which the higher pecorans appear to have descended. It is, therefore, possible that the pecorans have a dental formula I_4, C_0 . . . , rather than I_3, C_1 . . . . Against this interpretation it should be noted that in some pecorans the fourth incisor (or canine) has a shape which is slightly different from the remaining incisors.

TOOTH HOMOLOGIES

In the current premaxillary/maxillary system of tooth recognition (which is the starting point for the elaboration of a field analysis of dentitions) the molar class is subdivided into deciduous and permanent molars. The most posteriorly replaced molar is considered to be homologous in all dentitions and is called Dm4 (the fourth deciduous molar). In front of it lie the remaining deciduous molars and behind it lie the permanent molars. Any replacement for a molar is called a premolar (PM) although there is some doubt as to whether un-replaced molars anterior to Dm4 are retained deciduous molars or are premolars whose deciduous predecessors have been suppressed during evolution.

Comparative anatomists clearly consider that the first permanent molar (M1) is homologous in all eutherian and metatherian dentitions. This implies that PM4 has never been lost without the loss of Dm4: if such a PM4 had been lost the ancestral (now unreplaced) Dm4 would be the most anterior permanent molar in the descendant dentition. Because this tooth is always designated M1, Dm4 can never be unreplaced.

There is no embryological reason for believing that a replacement for Dm4 cannot be lost; fields seem to be infinitely variable. We can only assume that it has never been lost because such loss would constitute too severe a selective disadvantage. However, there is an undoubted example of a dentition where a replacement for Dm4 is lost and an embryological argument which suggests that it may have commonly been lost during evolution.

Man's is the most intensively studied of all dentitions and it is well recognized that his second premolar (supposedly homologous with PM4) is commonly absent. The most frequently absent tooth is M3 (an incidence which can be as great as 25% in some populations) but 11% of individuals lacking an M3 also lack a PM4 (Garn and Lewis, 1962). If there were some selective advantage for shortening the dentition of man there is little doubt that PM4 and M3 would be suppressed. It is interesting that where M3 is lost, the development of the premolars and remaining molars is delayed (Garn *et al.*, 1961). This suggests the possibility that man's dentition would be shortened by delaying the times at which teeth were initiated beyond the time at which embryonic competence had dropped below a threshold (cf. Fig. 10). In conclusion PM4 can be lost while Dm4 is retained and in such a dentition Dm4 apparently becomes M1, the most anterior of the permanent molars.

Although the clone model can be used to recognize homologies between tooth classes, it can be argued that the teeth within a class are, like hairs or leaves, serially homologous structures and that it would be equally meaningless to look for (historical) homologies (Simpson, 1961). However, every clone must have a stem progenitor and it seems reasonable to suggest that the stem progenitors of all molar classes, for example, are homologous teeth. At least this would establish an embryological foundation for homologies. Comparative anatomists might be expected to treat embryological arguments with caution: faced with the closely similar problem of cusp homologies, embryologists suggested that the paracone, the first initiated cusp on the mammalian upper molar, and not the protocone, was homologous with the single cusp of a conical reptilian tooth. Palaeontological data finally proved the embryologists to have been correct.

In most mammals Dm4 is the molar stem progenitor, but it is Dm3 in man, the tree shrew, *Tupaia javanica* (Kindahl, 1957b), the bat, *Hipposideros caffer* (Gaunt, 1967), the cat (Gaunt, 1959) and possibly the ferret (Berkowitz and Thompson, 1973). Eruption times (Kremenak *et al.*, 1969) indicate that the dog may be included in this list. These embryological data suggest that the Dm3 in these animals, and possibly many other primates, Cheiroptera and Carnivora, is homologous with the Dm4 of other mammals. In which case the following definition which is currently applied to the molars of mammals is based on analogy; any member of an uninterrupted sequence of unreplaced teeth at the back of the maxilla is a permanent molar and the most anterior of these is M^1. Stated in this way it seems clearly possible, and even probable, that M¹ is currently recognized by analogy rather than by homology. However, even if this is true there seems as little point in changing the present useful and workable system of tooth designation as, in a closely similar situation, there would be in renaming the cusps of upper molar teeth. Nevertheless, it is worth drawing attention to the sequences of dental evolution which the above homologies seem to imply.

It is currently accepted that any eutherian mammal with a molar formula 3 PM, 3 M has been derived from an ancestral formula 4 PM, 3 M by the loss of the most anterior molar family which consists of Dm1 and PM1. In some dentitions (e.g. *Tupaia*, see above) the stem progenitor must have shifted from Dm4 to Dm3 (dentitions (i) and (ii), Fig. 17). While recognizing the recapitulationist nature of the argument, I suggest that this is as unlikely as the equivalent suggestion that the first developed cusp in a eutherian upper molar could be either the paracone or the protocone, and by extension, could even be the metacone or hypocone. If the ancestral eutherian mammal possessed dentition (i) (Fig. 17) we can more reasonably account for the new position of the stem progenitor by a loss of the two anterior families and the addition of a new premolar and molar (dentition (iii), Fig. 17). But this seems too complex and I suggest that the solution shown in Fig. 18 is more probable.

The mammals ancestral to both Eutheria and Metatheria possessed a molar

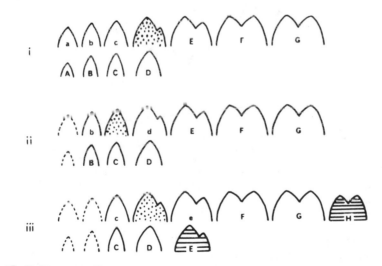

FIG. 17. (i) The generally accepted molar dentition of an ancestral eutherian mammal. Deciduous teeth are lettered in lower case, permanent teeth in capitals. The stem progenitor (d = Dm4) is stippled. (ii) Here, the generally accepted homologies between (i) and a dentition containing three premolars are illustrated, even when Dm3 (= c) is the stem progenitor. It is argued that if (i) is the true dentition of an ancestral eutherian mammal, the evolution of a dentition containing three premolars where the stem progenitor is the penultimate deciduous molar, can more reasonably be explained by the loss of aA and bB, and the addition of a new premolar (E) and permanent molar (H), as shown in (iii).

formula 5 PM, 3 M with Dm4 being the stem progenitor (dentition (i), Fig. 18). The generally accepted eutherian ancestor evolved by shortening the molar dentition from behind (dentition (ii), Fig. 18); other Eutheria shortened the molar dentition from in front (dentition (iii), Fig. 18). Only in the latter group has the stem progenitor remained the penultimate deciduous molar. The dentitions of Metatheria evolved by the loss of aABC and E (dentition (iv), Fig. 18).

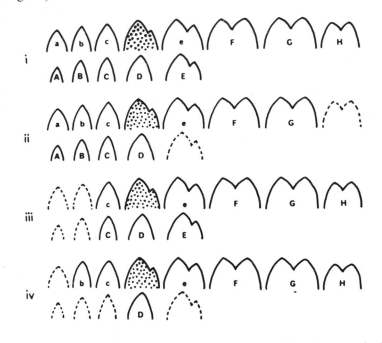

FIG. 18. A new interpretation of the evolution of molar dentitions in mammals. (i) The mammals ancestral to Eutheria and Metatheria had a molar dental formula 5 PM, 3 M with Dm4 (= d), the penultimate deciduous molar, as the stem progenitor. When the dentition has initially been shortened from behind in (ii) the most posterior deciduous molar has become the stem progenitor. When the dentition has been initially shortened from in front as in (iii), the stem progenitor has remained as the penultimate deciduous molar. A metatherian dentition (iv) is achieved by losing a, A, B, C and E.

It is convenient to mention here that in the Muridae, which have no deciduous molars or premolars, M1 is the stem progenitor. Presumably such a dentition consists of d, e and F from dentition (i) (Fig. 18).

The embryological data quoted above indicate that Dm3 is the stem progenitor in some primates, Cheiroptera and Carnivora. I doubt whether this is taxonomically important at the ordinal level. An apparent forward shift of the stem progenitor from Dm4 to Dm3 merely represents a shortening of the dentition from behind and this could probably take place within a species (e.g. man, see above).

Finally, the clone model might be of importance in anthropological studies. For example, it provides a different interpretation of gradients in the sizes of molar teeth. The tooth Dm4 is smaller than M1. If PM4 and M3 are lost (see above) the small Dm4 becomes the most anterior of three permanent molars with the result that the largest molar is now found in a different position.

Interestingly enough, the M1 of Old World Monkeys is so small that it could be an example of a tooth which at one time was the last deciduous molar of an ancestral dentition. If the penultimate deciduous molar was the stem progenitor in an ancestral Old World Monkey (having three premolars), the most posterior deciduous molar would be the stem progenitor in recent Old World Monkeys (having two premolars) (cf. Simons, 1972, his Fig. 78). However, there are too few observations of recent primates, let alone data for fossil primates, to determine whether there is any foundation for the above speculations, but they do suggest possible avenues for research.

REFERENCES

BELLAIRS, A. D'A. and MILES, A. E. W. (1961). Apparent failure of tooth replacement in monitor lizards. Br. J. Herpet. 3, (1), 14–15.

BERKOWITZ, B. K. B. (1966). The homology of the premolar teeth in *Setonix brachyurus* (Macropodidae: Marsupialia). *Archs oral Biol.* **11**, 1371–1384.

BERKOWITZ, B. K. B. (1968). Some stages in the early development of the post-incisor dentition of *Trichosurus vulpecula* (Phalangeroidea: Marsupiala). *J. Zool., Lond.* **15**, 403–414.

BERKOWITZ, B. K. B. (1972). Tooth development in *Protemnodon eugenii*. *J. dent. Res.* **51**, 1462–1473.

BERKOWITZ, B. K. B. and THOMPSON, P. (1973). Observations on the aetiology of supernumerary upper incisors in the albino ferret (*Mustela putorius*). *Archs oral Biol.* **18**, 457–463.

BUTLER, P. M. (1939). Studies of the mammalian dentition. Differentiation of the postcanine dentition. *Proc. zool. Soc. Lond.* **109**, 1–36.

BUTLER, P. M. (1952a). The milk-molars of Perissodactyla, with remarks on molar occlusion. *Proc. zool. Soc. Lond.* **121**, 777–817.

BUTLER, P. M. (1952b). Molarization of the premolars in the perissodactyla. *Proc. zool. Soc. Lond.* **121**, 819–843.

BUTLER, P. M. (1956). The ontogeny of molar pattern. *Biol. Rev.* **31**, 30–70.

BUTLER, P. M. (1963). Tooth morphology and primate evolution. In "Dental Anthropology" (Brothwell, D. R., ed.), pp. 1–13. Pergamon, London.

BUTLER, P. M. (1967). Dental merism and tooth development. *J. dent. Res.* **46**, 845–850.

COLYER, F. (1936). "Variations and Diseases of the Teeth of Animals." John Bale, Sons and Danielsson, London.

COOPER, J. S. (1963). The dental anatomy of the genus *Lacerta*. Ph.D. thesis, Bristol, England.

CRICK, F. (1970). Diffusion in embryogenesis. *Nature, Lond.* **225**, 420–422.

CROMPTON, A. W. (1963). Tooth replacement in the cynodont *Thrinaxodon liorhinus* Seeley. *Ann. S. Afr. Mus. Cape Town* **46**, 479–521.

CROMPTON, A. W. (1974). The dentitions and relationships of the Southern African Triassic mammals, *Erythrotherium parringtoni* and *Megazostrodon rudnerae*. *Bull. Br. Mus. nat. Hist. (Geol)* **24**, No. 7.

EDMUND, A. G. (1960). Tooth replacement phenomena in the Lower Vertebrates. *Contr. Life Sci. Div. R. Ont. Mus.* **52**, 1–90.

FISHER, A. R. (1971). Morphological development in vitro of the whole and halved lower molar tooth germ of the mouse. *Archs oral Biol.* **16**, 1481–1496.

FITZGERALD, L. R. (1973). Deciduous incisor teeth of the mouse (*Mus musculus*) *Archs oral Biol.* **18**, 381–389.

FOURIE, S. (1963). Tooth replacement in the gomphodont cynodont, *Diademodon*. *S. Afr. J. Sci.* **59**, 211–213.

GARN, S. M. and LEWIS, A. B. (1962). The relationship between third molar agenesis and reduction in tooth number. *Angle Orthod.* **33**, 14–18.

GARN, S. M., LEWIS, A. B. and BONNE, B. (1961). *Nature, Lond.* **192**, 989.

GAUNT, A. W. (1959). The development of the deciduous cheek teeth of the cat. *Acta anat.* **38**, 187–212.

GAUNT, A. W. (1967). Observations on the developing dentition of *Hipposideros caffer* (Microchiroptera) *Acta anat.* **68**, 9–25.

GLASSTONE, S. (1938). A comparative study of the development in vivo and in vitro of rat and rabbit molars. *Proc. R. Soc. B.* **126**, 315–330.

GLASSTONE, S. (1952). The development of halved tooth germs. A study in experimental embryology. *J. Anat.* **86**, 12–15.

GOODWIN, B. C. and COHEN, M. H. (1970). A phase-shift model for the spatial and temporal organisation of developing systems. *J. theor. Biol.* **25**, 49–107.

GREEN, H. L. H. H. (1937). The development and morphology of the teeth of *Ornithorhyncus*. *Phil. Trans. R. Soc. Lond.* (B) **228**, 367–420.

GRÜNEBERG, H. (1951). The genetics of a tooth defect in the mouse. *Proc. R. Soc. B.* **138**, 437–451.

HAY, M. F. (1961). The development in vivo and in vitro of the lower incisor and molars of the mouse. *Archs oral Biol.* **3**, 86–109.

HUXLEY, J. S. and DE BEER, G. R. (1934). "The Elements of Experimental Embryology." Cambridge University Press, Cambridge, England.

JULIN, C. (1880). Recherches sur l'ossification du maxillarie inférieur et sur la constitution du système dentaire chez le foetus de la Balaenoptera. *Arch. Biblogie Gand,* **1**, 75–136.

KINDAHL, M. (1957a). Some observations on the development of the tooth in *Elephantulus myurus* Jamesoni. *Ark. Zool.* **11**, Nr 2, 21–29.

KINDAHL, M. (1957b). On the development of the tooth in *Tupaia javanica*. *Ark. Zool.* **10**, Nr 11, 463–479.

KINDAHL, M. (1959a). Some aspects of the tooth development in Soricidae. *Acta odont. scand.* **17**, 203–237.

KINDAHL, M. (1959b). The tooth development in *Erinaceus europaeus*. *Acta odont. scand.* **17**, 467–489.

KOLLAR, E. J. and BAIRD, G. R. (1969). The influence of the dental papilla on the development of tooth shape in embryonic mouse tooth germs. *J. Embryol. exp. Morph.* **21**, 131–148.

KOLLAR, E. J. and BAIRD, G. R. (1970). Tissue interaction in embryonic mouse tooth germs. II. The inductive role of the dental papilla. *J. Embryol. exp. Morph.* **24**, 131–148.

KREMENAK, C. R., RUSSELL, L. S. and CHRISTENSEN, R. D. (1969). Tooth eruption ages in suckling dogs as affected by local heating. *J. dent. Res.* **48**, 427–430.

Leche, W. (1895). Zur Entwicklungsgeschichte des Zahnsystems der Saugethiere, Zugleich ein Beitrag zur Stammesgeschichte dieser Thiergruppe. 1. Ontogenic. *Zoologica, Stuttgart* **6**, Heft. 17, 1.

Noble, G. K. and Pope, S. H. (1929). The modification of the cloaca and teeth of the adult salamander, *Desmognathus*, by testicular transplants and by castration. *Br. J. exp. Biol.* **6**, 399–411.

Osborn, J. W. (1970). New approach to Zahnreihen. *Nature, Lond.* **225**, 343–346.

Osborn, J. W. (1971). The ontogeny of tooth succession in *Lacerta vivipara* Jacquin (1787). *Proc. R. Soc. Lond. B.* **179**, 261–289.

Osborn, J. W. (1973). The evolution of dentitions. *Am. Scient.* **61**, 548–559.

Osborn, J. W. (1974a). On tooth succession in *Diademodon*. *Evolution*, **28** 141–157.

Osborn, J. W. (1974b). On the control of tooth replacement in reptiles and its relationship to growth. *J. theor. Biol.* **46**, 509–527.

Osborn, J. W. (1975a). Tooth replacement: efficiency, patterns and evolution. *Evolution* **29**, 180–186.

Osborn, J. W. (1975b). The control of tooth shape. *J. dent. Res. IADR Abst. L.* 57.

Osborn, J. W. and Crompton, A. W. (1973). The evolution of mammalian from reptilian dentitions. *Breviora* **399**, 1–18.

Parrington, F. R. (1967). The identification of the dermal bones of the head. *J. Linn. Soc. (Zool.)* **47**, 231–239.

Parrington, F. R. (1971). On the Upper Triassic mammals. *Phil. Trans. R. Soc. Lond. B.* **261**, 231–272.

Patterson, B. (1956). Early cretaceous mammals and the evolution of mammalian molar teeth. *Fieldiana Geol.* **13**, 1–105.

Romer, A. S. (1966). "Vertebrate Paleontology," 3rd edition. University of Chicago Press, Chicago, U.S.A.

Röse, C. (1892). Über rudimentaire Zahnlagen der Gattung *Manis*. *Anat. Anz.* **7**, 495–512.

Simons, E. L. (1972). "Primate Evolution." Macmillan, New York.

Simpson, G. G. (1929). American Mesozoic Mammalia. *Mem. Peabody Mus. nat. Hist.* **3**, 1–235.

Simpson, G. G. (1961). "Principles of Animal Taxonomy." Oxford University Press, London.

Stewart, M. M. (1958). Seasonal variation in the teeth of the two-lined salamander. *Copeia* **3**, 190–196.

van Valen, L. (1970). An analysis of developmental fields. *Devl. Biol.* **23**, 456–477.

Webster, G. (1971). Morphogenesis and pattern formation in Hydroids. *Biol. Rev.* **46**, 1–46.

Wolpert, L. (1969). Positional information and the spatial pattern of cellular differentiation. *J. theor. Biol.* **25**, 1–47.

Wolpert, L. (1971). Positional information and pattern formation. *Curr. Top. devl. Biol.* **6**, 183–224.

15. A Factor Analysis of Morphogenetic Fields in the Human Dentition

A. VINCENT LOMBARDI

University of Pittsburgh, Pennsylvania, U.S.A.

INTRODUCTION

The concept of morphogenetic dental fields derives from Butler's (1939) analysis of the morphodifferentiation of teeth in fossil Cenozoic mammals. He postulated that the mammalian dentition could be differentiated along an anterior–posterior axis into three morphogenetic fields corresponding to the incisor, canine and molar tooth groups. Each tooth group by virtue of its position was subject to a distinct genetic field which governed the size and form of the teeth within the group. Moreover, the intensity of morphogenetic control varied within each field so that particular teeth within each group were the most stable in size and form.

Dahlberg (1945) subsequently applied Butler's field concept to the human dentition. Identifying each of the regional tooth groups, incisor, canine, premolar and molar, with a morphogenetic field, he then determined within each group the tooth which was least variable in size, form and the occurrence of certain morphologic traits. The tooth with the lowest coefficients of variation was believed to be nearest the centre of morphogenetic influence, whereas more variable teeth were believed to approach the extremities of the field. The most stable tooth was thought to be the polar tooth for the morphogenetic field. In the human dentition, $I^1_2 \, C^1_1 \, PM^1_1 \, M^1_1$ were proposed as the polar teeth.

In a study of the dentition of the Liberian chimpanzee, Schuman and Brace (1954) found the relative variation of crown dimensions to be largely consistent with Dahlberg's findings in man and generally supportive of his field model. There have been other investigations of non-human populations, but most have been concerned with the patterns of morphologic integration within the postcanine teeth rather than the evaluation of tooth fields *per se* (Olson and Miller, 1958; van Valen, 1962; Wallace and Bader, 1967; Wallace,

1968; Gould and Garwood, 1969; Leutenegger, 1971; Fleagle, 1972). Although the investigations differed in methodology and the mammalian species studied, common to most was the finding that crown width (bucco-lingual diameter) is an important axis of dental morphologic integration.

Potter *et al.* (1968) used principal components analysis to reveal the associations among crown length and crown width measurements taken from dental casts of Pima Indians. They extracted and identified three components, none of which could be strictly identified with tooth groups. The first had high loadings for length and width dimensions of the posterior teeth and appeared to represent overall posterior tooth size. The second component had high correlations with the crown widths of the anterior teeth, and the third was identified by its strong loadings for the crown lengths of the anterior teeth. Size in the dentition was seemingly controlled by three factors: one controlling posterior crown size and two identified with the anterior teeth influencing, respectively, crown width and crown length.

In the present study, the multivariate statistical technique of factor analysis was used to evaluate the morphogenetic fields attributed to the human dentition, the goal being to reduce a correlation matrix of dental dimensions to a smaller number of determining "factors" which would account for most of the common variance in the matrix. By disclosing the patterns of correlations among the individual teeth, the morphogenetic fields that account for most of the covariation in dental dimensions would hopefully be identified or, at least, suggested.

Material and Methods

A series of 66 Mexico City skulls housed at the University of the Pacific was used in the study. While the provenience of the skulls is minimal, they are apparently representative of a modern Mexican Indian population. Most importantly, the skulls had unworn and relatively complete dentitions. No attempt was made to analyse the sexes separately because of the small sample and the lack of supporting material to confirm sex assignments. Combining the sexes in a single group will tend to increase the value of the correlation coefficients because of sexual dimorphism in size, but as found by Potter *et al.* (1968), it does not affect the factor solution significantly. Crown length and crown width measurements were made on the individual teeth with a Helios dial caliper, and crown indices, a rough approximation of crown shape, were computed following the formula:

$$\text{crown index} = \frac{\text{crown width} \times 100}{\text{crown length}}.$$

Third molar measurements were excluded from the analysis because of the high frequency of third molar agenesis in the skulls. The principal factors analysis routine (BMDO 3M) of the Biomedical Computer Programs statistical package (Dixon, 1970) was used for reduction of the correlation matrix and the Varimax rotation was used to transform the initial factor solution to the terminal solution. Factor analysis was applied to crown length, crown width and crown index dimensions separately and to combined crown length–crown width dimensions.

RESULTS

Crown Length and Crown Width

Factor analysis of crown length and crown width separately generated four factors which could be identified with tooth groups and which accounted for 69% and 75%, respectively, of the total variance (Tables I and II).

TABLE I Rotated factor matrix of crown length.

Variable	I	II	III	IV	Communalities[a]
M^2	0·75	0·16	0·36	0·20	0·75
M^1	0·80	0·30	0·14	0·13	0·76
PM^2	0·49	0·19	0·62	0·15	0·68
PM^1	0·25	0·32	0·69	0·33	0·74
C	0·29	0·36	0·24	0·70	0·76
I^2	0·25	0·46	0·26	0·08	0·34
I^1	0·31	0·74	0·17	0·20	0·70
M_2	0·71	0·15	0·36	0·32	0·75
M_1	0·67	0·29	0·24	0·32	0·69
PM_2	0·59	0·28	0·60	0·05	0·79
PM_1	0·25	0·28	0·69	0·23	0·66
C	0·33	0·40	0·31	0·66	0·80
I_2	0·13	0·75	0·23	0·24	0·68
I_1	0·13	0·71	0·15	0·18	0·57
Trace	3·25	2·63	2·36	1·51	9·75
Common variance (%)	33·4	27·0	24·2	15·5	

[a] Communalities are for four factors.

Molar size (I). The first rotated factor in the crown-length and crown-width analyses had its highest correlations with molar dimensions in both jaws. The maxillary and mandibular second premolars loaded strongly on the factor, especially in the crown-length analysis. The canines also were correlated with this factor, but their highest loadings were in the crown width analysis.

Incisor size (II). The second rotated factor in both analyses had strong loadings for the upper and lower incisors. In the crown length analysis, the maxillary lateral incisor correlated less highly than the other incisors. Also,

TABLE II. Rotated factor matrix of crown width.

Variable	I	II	III	IV	Communalities[a]
M^2	0·71	0·27	0·47	0·18	0·82
M^1	0·69	0·46	0·42	0·10	0·87
PM^2	0·31	0·19	0·78	0·13	0·76
PM^1	0·22	0·28	0·76	0·06	0·71
C	0·39	0·50	0·44	0·48	0·82
I^2	0·19	0·61	0·21	0·03	0·45
I^1	0·26	0·73	0·36	0·01	0·72
M_2	0·69	0·27	0·45	0·23	0·80
M_1	0·72	0·41	0·35	0·19	0·84
PM_2	0·45	0·19	0·76	0·17	0·84
PM_1	0·29	0·28	0·55	0·20	0·50
C	0·38	0·51	0·32	0·58	0·83
I_2	0·23	0·79	0·08	0·37	0·82
I_1	0·25	0·72	0·23	0·26	0·70
Trace	2·92	3·31	3·32	0·99	10·54
Common variance (%)	27·7	31·4	31·5	9·4	

[a] Communalities are for four factors.

the canines were associated with this factor, but in the crown width analysis, tooth size integration was greater, with both canines and first molars loading strongly.

Premolar size (III). This factor had its highest loadings for the premolars in both the crown-length and crown-width analyses. In the crown-length analysis, the second molars had moderate correlations. Both first and second molars loaded on this factor in the crown-width analysis, but the second molars had somewhat higher values.

Canine size (IV). The last rotated factor in both analyses, which accounted for less covariance than the preceding factors, had its highest correlations with the upper and lower canines. In the crown-length analysis, the maxillary first premolar and the mandibular molars had moderate loadings. The mandibular lateral incisor loaded in the crown-width analysis.

Crown Index

When the crown index was factored, six factors emerged which corresponded in a general but not exclusive way with the tooth groups (Table III). This analysis accounted for only 51 % of the total variance, less than the other analyses, which suggests that unique variance is high among the crown indices of the teeth.

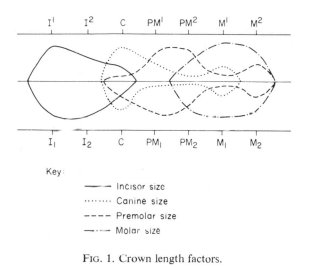

FIG. 1. Crown length factors.

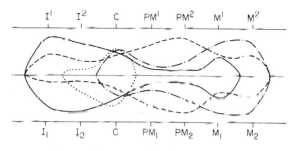

FIG. 2. Crown width factors (Key as Fig. 1).

TABLE III. Rotated factor matrix of crown index.

Variable	I	II	III	IV	V	VI	Communalities[a]
M^2	0·22	0·06	0·09	0·20	0·14	0·06	0·65
M^1	0·09	0·20	0·07	0·21	0·79	0·17	0·75
PM^2	0·05	0·69	0·26	0·21	0·17	0·01	0·61
PM^1	0·15	0·60	0·09	0·08	0·06	0·10	0·40
C	0·62	0·10	0·01	0·08	0·33	0·39	0·66
I^2	0·10	0·03	0·34	0·18	0·16	0·40	0·34
I^1	0·06	0·09	−0·03	0·13	0·13	0·71	0·55
M_2	0·06	0·11	0·10	0·54	0·12	−0·09	0·33
M_1	0·03	0·12	0·02	0·57	0·17	0·14	0·39
PM_2	−0·05	0·35	0·52	0·25	0·11	0·01	0·47
PM_1	0·12	0·19	0·59	−0·01	0·02	0·26	0·46
C	0·59	0·23	0·15	0·11	0·16	0·33	0·56
I_2	0·18	0·03	0·29	−0·13	−0·01	0·66	0·57
I_1	0·22	0·03	0·10	−0·03	0·05	0·54	0·35
Trace	0·93	1·14	0·95	0·90	1·44	1·79	7·15
Common variance (%)	13·0	15·9	13·3	12·6	20·1	25·0	

[a] Communalities are for six factors.

Canine index (I). On the first crown-index factor extracted, only the maxillary and mandibular canines loaded strongly.

Maxillary premolar index (II). The maxillary premolars correlated the highest with this factor; the mandibular second premolar had a lower but significant loading.

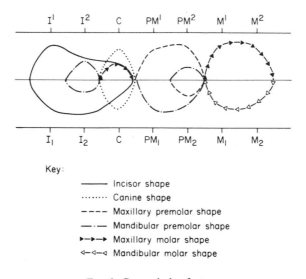

Key:

———— Incisor shape

········ Canine shape

– – – – Maxillary premolar shape

—·— Mandibular premolar shape

▸—▸—▸ Maxillary molar shape

◃—◃—◃ Mandibular molar shape

FIG. 3. Crown index factors.

Mandibular premolar index (III). On this factor the mandibular premolars correlated the strongest. Interestingly, the maxillary lateral incisor had a moderate loading. Fleagle (1972) found a size association between the maxillary lateral incisor and the heteromorphic anterior premolar in the gibbon, which he suggested might indicate functional integration related to sharpening of the opposing projecting canines.

Mandibular molar index (IV). Only the mandibular molars loaded strongly on this factor.

Maxillary molar index (V). This factor had its highest correlations with the maxillary molars; however, the maxillary canine loaded also.

Incisor index (VI). The factor which accounted for the most covariance in crown index had its strongest correlations with the maxillary and mandibular incisors, of which the maxillary lateral incisor loaded the least. The maxillary and mandibular canines had moderate loadings.

Combined Crown Length and Crown Width

Factor analysis of combined crown length and crown width dimensions generated five factors, not always identifiable with tooth groups, accounting for 73% of the total variance in the matrix (Table IV).

Molar size (I). The first factor had high loadings for maxillary and mandibular molar crown length and crown width, but somewhat higher correlations with length. Maxillary second premolar length also loaded on this factor.

TABLE IV. Rotated factor matrix of crown length and crown width.

Variable	I	II	III	IV	V	Communalities[a]
Crown length						
M^2	0·77	0·20	0·12	0·34	0·10	0·77
M^1	0·82	0·25	0·15	0·11	0·21	0·81
PM^2	0·56	0·29	0·05	0·55	−0·00	0·70
PM^1	0·25	0·43	0·17	0·66	0·17	0·73
C	0·22	0·57	0·42	0·34	−0·05	0·67
I^2	0·21	0·39	0·02	0·16	0·66	0·65
I^1	0·28	0·72	0·17	0·14	0·27	0·72
M_2	0·67	0·18	0·41	0·33	0·07	0·76
M_1	0·62	0·33	0·39	0·19	0·13	0·70
PM_2	0·58	0·24	0·11	0·55	0·26	0·78
PM_1	0·28	0·35	0·15	0·63	0·16	0·64
C	0·30	0·57	0·49	0·29	0·06	0·74
I_2	0·15	0·78	0·17	0·12	0·11	0·68
I_1	0·14	0·67	0·14	0·11	0·15	0·52
Crown width						
M^2	0·50	0·13	0·42	0·56	0·09	0·77
M^1	0·43	0·22	0·33	0·49	0·19	0·78
PM^2	0·22	0·17	0·19	0·82	0·09	0·80
PM^1	0·09	0·21	0·22	0·77	0·18	0·73
C	0·18	0·27	0·74	0·47	0·05	0·87
I^2	0·09	0·10	0·44	0·19	0·65	0·66
I^1	0·22	0·17	0·46	0·36	0·47	0·64
M_2	0·57	0·08	0·42	0·53	0·09	0·79
M_1	0·58	0·23	0·49	0·41	0·12	0·81
PM_2	0·36	0·07	0·30	0·77	0·07	0·82
PM_1	0·19	−0·09	0·39	0·60	0·17	0·59
C	0·21	0·27	0·79	0·33	0·03	0·85
I_2	0·24	0·20	0·74	0·07	0·35	0·77
I_1	0·19	0·31	0·61	0·20	0·38	0·68
Trace	4·74	3·50	4·61	5·74	1·80	20·39
Common variance (%)	23·2	17·2	22·6	28·1	8·8	

[a] Communalities are for five factors

Anterior crown length (II). Maxillary and mandibular anterior crown lengths correlated with this factor. The maxillary median incisor and the mandibular lateral incisor had the highest loadings. The maxillary lateral incisor correlated less, having a smaller loading than the maxillary first premolar. Most of the common variance of the maxillary lateral incisor loaded on another factor described subsequently.

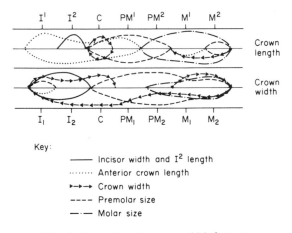

FIG. 4. Crown length–crown width factors.

Crown width (III). This factor had high loadings for the crown widths of all the teeth except for the maxillary premolars, but the loadings were the highest for the widths of the mandibular anterior teeth, with the mandibular canine having the strongest correlation. The maxillary canine also had a high loading, suggesting that the canines are the polar teeth for this factor. Although this appears to be a general crown-width factor, the crown lengths of several maxillary teeth loaded on it. The strongest correlations in the tooth groups resided with the assumed polar teeth, with the exception of mandibular molar length, where the second molar had a slightly higher loading than the first molar.

Premolar size (IV). The highest loadings on this factor were for the maxillary premolar crown widths, followed closely by the widths of the mandibular premolars and premolar crown lengths. The crown widths of the lower molars but not the upper molars also correlated with this factor.

Incisor crown width and maxillary lateral incisor crown length (V). This factor, which accounted for relatively little of the total variance in the matrix, associated crown width of the maxillary incisors to the crown length of the maxillary lateral incisor, and, to a lesser extent, to the crown widths of the mandibular incisors. The length of the maxillary central incisor loaded weakly.

Discussion

The factors extracted in the crown-length and crown-width analyses are consistent with Dahlberg's morphogenetic field model for the human dentition. Each factor comprises a functional occlusal grouping, encompassing teeth in both dental arches that correspond with the tooth fields: molar, incisor, canine and premolar. In general, the strength of the loadings for the individual teeth in each field corresponds with Dahlberg's evaluation of the relative stability of the teeth. Other teeth loaded to a lesser degree in a seeming but not invariable pattern, teeth immediately adjacent to the group and the polar teeth in other tooth groups correlating most strongly. In crown width, the factors were less distinct; although tooth groups dominated each factor, non-group teeth were often strongly correlated.

The factors extracted in the crown-index analysis also appear to support Dahlberg's model. Factors were easily identified with tooth groups, although in the premolar and molar groups functional antagonists were not joined on the same factor. This may indicate that molar and premolar form is functionally specific for each dental arch, whereas the incisors and canines are of more general form. It could also mean that there are morphogenetic fields operating on the dentition that do not necessarily coincide with the tooth groups. Consideration of the combined crown length–crown width analysis gives support to the latter possibility.

When crown length and crown width were combined, a different pattern of factors emerged. Factors were identified as molar size, anterior crown length, crown width, premolar size, incisor crown width and maxillary lateral incisor crown length. Whereas the molar and premolar tooth groups were segregated by factors, the other factors did not correspond with the traditional fields. The five factors appear similar to the three components found by Potter et al. (1968), the difference possibly being attributable to the different level of variance described. Potter's factors accounted for 52% of the total variance, whereas 73% of the variance was determined by the factors identified here. Potter's factor of posterior tooth size may have been further resolved here into two factors, one centring on the molars and dominated by crown lengths and the other centring on the premolars, with somewhat higher loadings for crown widths. Anterior crown length emerges as a separate factor in both investigations. What appears as a single factor of anterior crown width in Potter's analysis may be present as two factors here: overall crown width, which had its highest correlations for the mandibular anterior teeth, and incisor crown width.

The factor analyses of dental dimensions revealed that factors can be identified exclusively with tooth groups in certain circumstances only, i.e. when dimensions such as crown length, crown width and crown index are considered separately and as independent variables. Treating the dimensions as independent variables, however, provides more information about the dimensions than the teeth, which are obviously multidimensional. It would appear that the univariate statistical approach is not adequate for identifying morphogenetic fields in the human dentition. While the traditional fields describe the way individual traits behave within the dentition, the tooth group associations may, in some instances, only reflect longstanding dental homologies and not morphogenetic fields. It is apparent that some morphogenetic fields extend beyond the tooth groups and are multidimensional in effect. They are best discerned by considering the teeth as multidimensional units where the correlation among dimensions is accounted for. For this reason, it is likely that only the combined crown length–crown width factors have morphogenetic significance. The crown length–crown width analysis revealed that crown width is an important organizing influence in the human dentition; it is perhaps related to the transverse grinding motions that characterize the masticatory patterns of many mammals. Other factors encompassed non-group teeth and different dimensions but their functional correlates are not readily apparent; perhaps the inclusion of more variables in factor analysis would clarify their significance. Crown height, crown volume, occlusal area and morphologic traits such as cusp and wear patterns would be relevant variables to include if they could be quantified satisfactorily.

SUMMARY

The traditional morphogenetic fields of the human dentition were evaluated by means of factor analysis of dental dimensions taken from a series of human crania. When crown length, crown width and crown index were considered separately, factors emerged which were readily identified with the traditional tooth-group fields. But a combined crown length–crown width analysis generated factors which extended beyond the regional tooth groups. Crown width itself was revealed to be an important axis of morphologic integration. It was concluded that univariate statistical methods are not adequate for identifying morphogenetic fields; the teeth must be treated as multidimensional units where the correlation among dimensions is accounted for.

ACKNOWLEDGEMENTS

I am grateful to Dr W. W. Howells, Dr J. S. Friedlaender, Dr J. H. Shaw, Dr C. F. A. Moorrees and the late Dr A. Damon for advice and assistance given during the conduct of this investigation.

REFERENCES

BUTLER, P. M. (1939). Studies of the mammalian dentition. Differentiation of the post-canine dentition. *Proc. zool. Soc. Lond.* **109**, 1–36.

DAHLBERG, A. A. (1945). The changing dentition of man. *J. Am. dent. Ass.*, **32**, 676–690.

DAHLBERG, A. A. (1949). The dentition of the American Indian. *In* "The Physical Anthropology of the American Indian" (Laughlin, W. S., ed.) pp. 138–176. Viking Fund, New York.

DIXON, W. J. (ed.) (1970). "Biomedical Computer Programs." University of California Press, Los Angeles, U.S.A.

FLEAGLE, J. (1972). Patterns of variability and organization in the dentition of the white-handed gibbon, *Hylobates lar*. Unpublished paper, Harvard University.

GOULD, S. J. and GARWOOD, R. A. (1969). Levels of integration in mammalian dentitions: an analysis of correlations in *Nesophontes micrus* (insectivora) and *Oryzomys couesi* (rodentia). *Evolution*, **23**, 276–300.

LEUTENEGGER, W. (1971). Metric variability of the postcanine dentition in Colobus monkeys. *Am. J. phys. Anthrop* **35**, 91–100.

OLSON, E. C. and MILLER, R. L. (1958). "Morphological Integration". The University of Chicago Press, Chicago, U.S.A.

POTTER, R. H. Y., YU, P.-L., DAHLBERG, A. A., MERRITT, A. D. and CONNEALLY, P. M. (1968). Genetic studies of tooth size factors in Pima Indian families. *Am. J. hum. Genet.* **20**, 89–100.

SCHUMAN, E. L. and BRACE, C. L. (1954). Metric and morphologic variations in the dentition of the Liberian chimpanzee: comparisons with anthropoid and human dentitions. *Hum. Biol.*, **26**, 239–268.

VAN VALEN, L. (1962). Growth fields in the dentition of *Peromyscus*. *Evolution*, **19**, 272–277.

WALLACE, J. T. (1968). Analysis of dental variation in wild-caught California house mice. *Am. Midl. Nat.*, **80**, 360–380.

WALLACE, J. T. and BADER, R. S. (1967). Factor analysis of morphometric traits in the house mouse. *Syst. Zool.*, **16**, 144–148.

16. Morphogenetic Influences and Patterns of Developmental Stability in the Mouse Vertebral Column

J. A. SOFAER

School of Dental Surgery and Department of Human Genetics, University of Edinburgh, Scotland

INTRODUCTION

Developmental stability can be assessed through a study of the variation shown by adult populations. Two aspects of this variation are: firstly, the asymmetry of bilaterally represented structures within individuals; and secondly, in experimental situations, differences between members of a genetically homogeneous population. Asymmetry provides information about the ability of the individual to produce the same developmental result on two occasions, and is perhaps the most controlled indication of instability of development, since, under normal circumstances, the genotype and general external environment are the same for both sides of the body. Between-individual variation in a genetically homogeneous population expresses the lack of ability of a given genotype to produce the same developmental result on several occasions, though it must be assumed that all individuals are in fact genetically identical and that the general environment is constant. If different organs or regions of the body are studied with respect to asymmetry and between-individual differences, the resulting patterns of variation can be regarded as patterns of relative developmental instability, and can, perhaps, throw some light on the distribution of morphogenetic influences that may be operating during development. A further dimension can be added to such an investigation by examining the response of these patterns to a standard environmental disturbance imposed at different stages of development.

A Suitable System

In a series of homologous structures divided into morphologically distinct segments, such as the teeth of most mammals, differences within and between segments with respect to asymmetry or the response to an imposed environmental disturbance can provide patterns of instability that may suggest how these morphologically distinct regions are established during development. However, the dentition of the most convenient experimental mammal, the mouse, is far from ideal for such a study. There are only two morphological classes of teeth, incisors and molars, represented by only one and three teeth respectively in each quadrant. A series of homologous structures more suitable for the study of patterns of developmental stability is found in the mouse vertebral column. Anterior to the sacrum there are three morphological segments: cervical, thoracic and lumbar, normally composed of 7, 13 and 5 or 6 vertebrae respectively. The potential for disclosing patterns of morphogenetic influence is much greater among these 25 or 26 presacral vertebrae than among the smaller number of teeth, since the effect of any such influence can, as it were, be "sampled" at a greater number of positions.

The vertebrae, of course, are not bilaterally represented structures, so asymmetry cannot be studied in the same way as for teeth; but each vertebra has a right and a left half that can be measured and compared. It was therefore decided to investigate vertebral asymmetry, and the response of vertebral size and asymmetry to an environmental disturbance, in an inbred strain of mice; the aim being to assess the value of the mouse vertebral column for studying the way in which morphological segments in a series of homologous structures arise during development.

Embryological Background

Before proceeding to the experiment itself, it is relevant to consider briefly the early embryology of vertebral development.

Figure 1 is a summary of early mouse development. If the day on which fertilization occurs is regarded as day 0, then implantation occurs between days 4 and 5, mesoderm starts to appear between days 6 and 7, and somite development starts on day 8. The first five somites contribute to the occipital region of the skull, and the vertebrae are derived from subsequent somites. Each vertebra is formed from the neighbouring caudal and cranial halves of two adjacent somites, so there is a one-to-one somite–vertebra correspondence, though the sequence of vertebrae is displaced by half a unit relative to that of the somites. The somites from which the presacral vertebrae are formed have all appeared by the end of day 10 (Grüneberg, 1963; Snell and Stevens, 1966; Theiler, 1972). It is during the time when their somites are forming that the vertebrae have been found to be most sensitive to teratogenic treatments. Variations in both vertebral number and form have been produced by a variety of such treatments, including fasting, hypoxia, X-radiation and a number of different chemical agents (Dagg, 1966).

MATERIAL AND METHODS

The material consisted of a control group and six groups of mice that were day: 0   fertilization

        1

        2

        3

        4
               implantation
        5

        6
               mesoderm appears
        7

vertebrae ⎧   8   somites: 0
sensitive to ⎪   5 occipital
teratogenic ⎨   9   13 cervical
treatments ⎪   21 upper and middle thoracic
          ⎩   10   30 lower thoracic and lumbar

        11

        12   segmentation complete

FIG. 1. A summary of early mouse development.

the progeny of females starved for 24 h on one of six different days of pregnancy. All mice were from the highly inbred strain CBA/Cam, so for practical purposes they could be considered genetically identical.

Females were caged with males (three females to one male per cage) and were examined for vaginal plugs on the following morning. Plugged females were then caged individually with *ad libitum* supplies of food and water. The day on which a plug was found was regarded as day 0. Females for starvation were transferred to individual clean cages without food, but with water as before, at 16·00 h on day $n-1$ and returned to their original cages supplied with food and water at 16·00 h on day n, where n was one of the following: 5, 6, 7, 8, 10 or 12. Litters from starved and control mothers, if larger than six, were reduced to six as soon as possible after birth. All offspring were weaned at 4 weeks, stored six to a cage, and sacrificed at 6 weeks after birth. The numbers of mice used and the numbers of litters from which they came are shown in Table I. Within each group there were approximately equal numbers of the two sexes.

After sacrifice, each vertebral column down to the sacrum was dissected out with its immediately adjacent tissues, and a hard stainless steel wire (0·25 mm diameter) was threaded down the neural canal and twisted at each end. The column was then subjected to papain digestion, normally formed and unbroken vertebrae remaining in the correct order on the wire. A search

TABLE I. The numbers of mice used and the numbers of
litters from which they came.

Starvation day	Individuals	Litters
5	50	12
6	35	6
7	25	7
8	29	6
10	50	12
12	50	10
Control	39	8

was made following papain digestion for any abnormally formed or broken vertebrae that may have fallen from the wire.

Measurement Technique

Vertebrae from each column were attached, cranial surface uppermost, onto a $3 \cdot 25$ inch square lantern slide glass by means of double-sided transparent self-adhesive tape, and silhouettes of each complete set of presacral vertebrae, plus the first sacral vertebra, were projected onto a screen at a convenient standard magnification ($\times 17 \cdot 5$). Figure 2 illustrates the kind of picture that was produced. Vertebra no. 1 is the first cervical, and vertebra no. 26 is the first sacral. The first sacral vertebra was included because, as it articulates with the pelvis, it was thought likely to be a relatively stable structure with which the presacral vertebrae could be compared. Even though the vertebrae vary considerably, each one, except the first, has a dorsal mid-line spinous process, and all have lateral transverse processes; though in some vertebrae they are poorly developed. The first cervical vertebra has a mid-line ventral tubercle.

Two measurements were taken from each of these vertebral silhouettes by placing a grid of millimetre squared graph paper against the screen and adjusting its position until the transverse processes of each silhouette came to lie along one axis. The two measurements taken were the distances along this axis from the end of each transverse process to a perpendicular line passing through the spinous process, or, in the case of the first cervical vertebra, the centre of the ventral tubercle. This is illustrated in Fig. 3.

In the few cases where the complement of presacral vertebrae differed from 25, adjustments in numbering were made so that the first sacral vertebra always occupied position 26 in the series. When there was an additional vertebra, one was removed from the series, and when there was one less than the normal 25, a space was left in the appropriate position in the series. This was done so that sets of measurements in such cases would be comparable with those of the majority of individuals with the normal vertebral number.

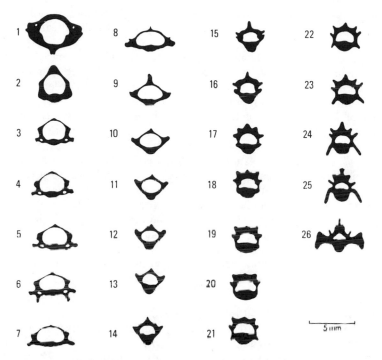

FIG. 2. Silhouettes from a control vertebral column.

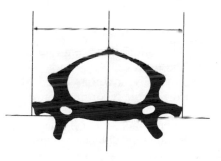

FIG. 3. Silhouette of vertebra no. 6 showing the measurements that were made.

Measures of Developmental Instability

Asymmetry was expressed by V_a, the variance of $(R - L)/(R + L)$, where R and L are corresponding measurements on the right and left sides of each vertebra. This measure of asymmetry is therefore adjusted for the size of the particular vertebra being considered. The response to starvation was expressed firstly by relative asymmetry, the ratio of the experimental asymmetry variance to the control asymmetry variance for each vertebra and for each starvation group; and secondly by the percentage change of full vertebral width (the sum of right and left side measurements) associated with starvation at each stage.

Since the anatomical landmarks used to provide reference points for measurement are not equally well defined in all vertebrae, different degrees of measurement error could arise for different vertebrae. In order to minimize the possibility of such differences masking or distorting any underlying pattern of instability, the control group of vertebrae was measured on a second occasion. A repeatability variance, V_r, for each vertebra, comparable with the asymmetry variance, could then be calculated as the variance of *(1st — 2nd)/(1st + 2nd)* measurements, for the right and left sides separately. Right and left side repeatability variances were combined to give a single overall estimate of the repeatability variance for each vertebra, and two asymmetry variances, one calculated from the first and the other from the second set of measurements, were similarly combined to give a single overall estimate of the asymmetry variance for each vertebra. The "instability variance", V_i, of the control group was considered to be the difference between the asymmetry and repeatability variances for each vertebra. Thus, for each vertebra,

$$V_i = V_a - V_r.$$

Patterns of developmental instability were expressed graphically, with the measure of instability (control instability variance, relative asymmetry or % change of width) plotted against vertebral position number. Positions 1–7 refer to the cervical segment, 8–10 the thoracic segment, 21–25 the lumbar segment and 26 the first sacral vertebra. All measures of instability were based on vertebral measurements expressed in mm.

Results

The numbers of presacral vertebrae that were found in the different groups are shown in Table II. The halves arise because sometimes there is asymmetrical articulation with the pelvis (McLaren and Michie, 1954). However, for the purpose of standardizing the recording of measurements, cases falling

Table II. The numbers of presacral vertebrae found in the different groups.

Starvation	Vertebrae				
day	24	$24\frac{1}{2}$	25	$25\frac{1}{2}$	26
5	–	–	50	–	–
6	–	–	35	–	–
7	–	–	25	–	–
8	2	–	23	3	1
10	–	–	49	1	–
12	–	–	50	–	–
Control	–	–	39	–	–

into the $25\frac{1}{2}$ category were regarded as having 26 presacral vertebrae, so in these cases one complete lumbar vertebra was removed from the series. Exceptions to the normal presacral number of 25 in this strain occurred only in the groups starved on days 8 and 10.

Figure 4 shows the pattern of instability variances in the control group for

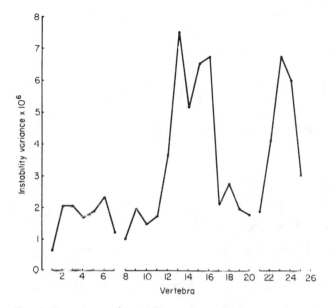

FIG. 4. The pattern of instability variances in the control group.

the 26 vertebrae that were measured. The most striking feature is that vertebrae towards the extremes of each segment were the least unstable, and those towards the centre of each segment were the most unstable. However, at the very centre of the cervical and thoracic segments there was evidence of a small localized decrease of instability.

The relative asymmetry for the different groups, that is, the variance ratio of the experimental asymmetry variance to the control asymmetry variance, is shown in Fig. 5. There was little by way of a consistent response to starvation on days 5, 6 and 7, though, at least in the cervical segment, vertebrae towards the centre tended to be more affected by starvation than those at the extremes. However, there was a definite response to starvation on day 8 in the thoracic segment. Vertebrae at the extremes of the segment tended to be least affected by starvation, whereas those towards the centre showed a marked increase of asymmetry, with a localized decrease of the starvation effect a little anterior to the very centre of the segment. Starvation on days 10 and 12 tended to increase asymmetry on the whole, though there was no very definite pattern of response.

The response of the full width of each vertebra to starvation is shown in

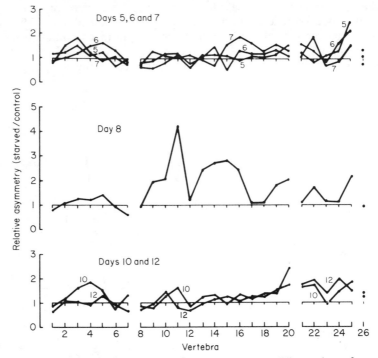

FIG. 5. Patterns of relative asymmetry following starvation on different days of pregnancy.

Fig. 6. Surprisingly, the general effect of starvation on days 5 and 6 was to increase vertebral width. However, by day 8 the effect of starvation was definitely to reduce vertebral width, and this applied also to starvation on days 10 and 12. For days 5 and 6 the cervical and thoracic segments again tended to show least response at their extremes and most response towards their centres, with some suggestion of localized resistance to the starvation effect at the very centre of each segment. By day 8 the pattern became one of relative stability at the anterior end and instability at the posterior end of each segment, particularly of the thoracic segment. A similar pattern in the thoracic segment was found for day 10, with some relaxation of the effect by day 12.

DISCUSSION

Theoretical Considerations

Three different patterns of developmental instability that might result from different kinds of morphogenetic control are illustrated in Fig. 7. In the first scheme, against (a), the morphogenetic influence for each segment, cervical (C), thoracic (T) and lumbar (L), has its origin at the anterior end of each segment and spreads posteriorly. Against (b) is the associated pattern of instability that might be expected. Vertebrae at the anterior end of each

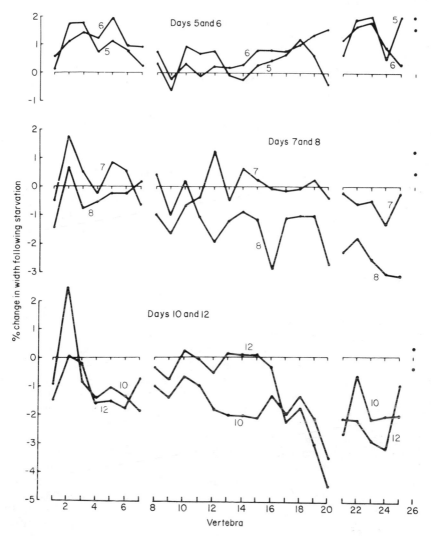

FIG. 6. Patterns of percentage change in width following starvation on different days of pregnancy.

segment, closest to the source of morphogenetic influence, show least instability, whereas those at the posterior end, furthest away from the morphogenetic source, are most unstable. In the second scheme, the morphogenetic influence has its origin at the centre of each segment and spreads outwards. The corresponding pattern of instability shows least instability at the centre of each segment and greatest instability at their extremes. The third scheme shows the sources of morphogenetic influence defining the

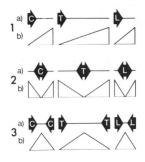

FIG. 7. Possible alternative schemes of morphogenetic control.

limits of each segment and spreading towards their centres. The corresponding pattern of instability is characterized by least instability at the ends and greatest instability at the centre of each segment.

Observed Patterns of Instability

The most common pattern of instability observed within segments was one of least instability towards the extremes and greatest instability towards the centre, corresponding to morphogenetic scheme no. 3 in Fig. 7. This pattern was found in all three segments for the control instability variance, in the cervical and thoracic segments of some of the starvation groups for relative asymmetry, and in the cervical segment for percentage change in full width. Superimposed on this pattern was some evidence of morphogenetic scheme no. 2, that is, a localized tendency towards a low level of instability at or near the very centre of a segment. This appeared in the cervical and thoracic segments for the control instability variance, in the thoracic segment for relative asymmetry on day 8, and also possibly in the lumbar segment for relative asymmetry. There was also some suggestion of morphogenetic scheme no. 1, particularly in the thoracic segment for percentage change in full vertebral width after starvation on days 8, 10 and 12. The first sacral vertebra was relatively stable in almost all situations.

The apparent increase in vertebral size following starvation on days 5 and 6 could perhaps have been due to physiological over-compensation by the pregnant female on her return to a cage supplied with food. Such over-compensation would have coincided with the time when the developing vertebrae were most sensitive to environmental effects. Even though this response was in the opposite direction to that produced by starvation at later stages, the pattern of low instability (resistance to size increase) towards the ends, and high instability (maximum size increase) towards the centre of the cervical segment, with a localized tendency towards less instability at the very centre, still applied.

Components of Asymmetry

The expression of asymmetry used here was the total observed asymmetry, without regard to details of its underlying basis. However, the observed differences between sides can be thought of as having three components: fluctuating asymmetry, directional asymmetry and antisymmetry (van Valen, 1961). Fluctuating asymmetry is due to inability to buffer against minor developmental accidents and non-specific local environmental differences between sides, the distribution of $R - L$ being normal and having a mean of 0. Directional asymmetry is due to a consistently greater degree of development of the organ on one particular side of the body, presumably due to a consistent and "normal" difference in the local environment of the developing organ between sides. Here the distribution of $R - L$ is probably approximately normal, but the mean is different from 0. Antisymmetry occurs when a difference between sides is regularly induced by negative, presumably competitive, interaction between sides, $R - L$ having a mean of 0, but not being normally distributed, since individuals with a near-zero difference between sides are relatively rare. All three components arise through a lack of rigid intrinsic control by the organ over its own development, so an overall expression of asymmetry is a reasonable indication of developmental instability in its broadest sense. However, a difficulty arises if the directional and antisymmetry components take up more than a small proportion of the total observed asymmetry, for the observed distribution of $R - L$ would then deviate from normality. In this event, the variance of the difference between sides would not be a strictly valid measure. However, the general consistency of the patterns of instability obtained from the different measures in the different segments of the vertebral column suggests that this difficulty has not given rise to undue error in the present case. Nevertheless, it would perhaps be informative to look more deeply into the developmental basis of vertebral asymmetry and vertebral size variation as a whole, particularly with regard to possible interactions between sides within vertebrae, and interactions between adjacent vertebrae.

Implications of the Results

The results therefore suggest that the predominant morphogenetic influence in the establishment of the segments in the vertebral column is one in which a prominent feature is the defining of the limits of each segment. There is evidence that superimposed on this is an influence originating at the centre of the cervical and thoracic segments; and there is also evidence for an effect that originates at the anterior end of the thoracic segment, spreading posteriorly. All effects related to starvation showed a maximum with starvation on day 8, which is consistent with previous teratological experiments. The segmental response of asymmetry and vertebral width to starvation indicates that division of the vertebral column into prospective morphological segments is already established at the stage of somite development. The thoracic segment, the longest segment, showed the greatest range of effect for all measures of instability, which tends to support the concept of morphogenetic influences spreading outwards from well defined sources, their effects weakening with distance.

An analysis of truly morphological, rather than size, variation over the length of the vertebral column could perhaps serve to confirm these findings and be more specific about the way in which vertebral development is controlled. The value of a detailed morphological analysis of the vertebral column, in terms of underlying morphogenetic gradients, has already been suggested (van Valen, 1970). The possibility of investigating vertebral development through direct experimental manipulation in embryos of oviparous amniotes has also been suggested (van Valen, 1970), and, more recently, manipulations of this type have been performed on chick embryos with a view to investigating regional determination in the vertebral column (Kieny et al., 1972). In these experiments, segmented or even unsegmented somitic or presomite mesoderm from the cervical region of a donor embryo was transferred to the thoracic region of a host embryo from which a corresponding piece of mesoderm had been removed. A similar transfer of segmented or unsegmented thoracic mesoderm was made to the cervical region. In both types of transfer the transplanted mesoderm developed according to its origin, resulting either in a rib-free region within the thoracic segment, or supernumerary ribs in the cervical segment. The fact that unsegmented mesoderm behaved in this way indicates that, in the chick, the somitic mesoderm has acquired regional determination before segmentation occurs.

SUMMARY

Patterns of developmental instability in the mouse vertebral column have been studied with a view to drawing general conclusions about influences that divide a series of homologous structures into morphologically distinct segments. It is suggested that the results indicate patterns of morphogenetic control that might be less easily disclosed in dentitions, where the number of elements in each segment is smaller. In addition, the possibilities for more detailed investigation discussed, particularly direct experimental interference at an early embryonic stage in the chick, make the vertebral column a useful system for studying the way in which morphological segments in a series of homologous structures arise during development.

ACKNOWLEDGEMENTS

The material was collected at the University of Cambridge, Department of Genetics, and for this thanks are due to Professor J. M. Thoday for laboratory facilities, the Nuffield Foundation for a Dental Research Fellowship and the Medical Research Council for a Research Project Grant. Edith Redpath made the measurements in Edinburgh.

REFERENCES

DAGG, C. P. (1966). Teratogenesis. In "Biology of the Laboratory Mouse" (Green, E. L., ed.), Ch. 14. McGraw-Hill, New York, Toronto, Sydney and London.

GRÜNEBERG, H. (1963). "The Pathology of Development". Blackwell, Oxford.

KIENY, M., MAUGER, A. and SENGEL, P. (1972). Early regionalisation of the somitic mesoderm as studied by the development of the axial skeleton of the chick embryo. *Devl Biol.* **28**, 142–161.

McLAREN, A. and MICHIE, D. (1954). Factors affecting vertebral variation in mice. I. Variation within an inbred strain. *J. Embryol. exp. Morph.* **2**, 149–160.

SNELL, G. D. and STEVENS, L. C. (1966). Early embryology. *In* "Biology of the Laboratory Mouse" (Green, F L., ed.), Ch. 12. McGraw-Hill, New York, Toronto, Sydney and London.

THEILER, K. (1972). "The House Mouse. Development and normal stages from fertilisation to 4 weeks of age." Springer-Verlag, Berlin, Heidelberg and New York.

VAN VALEN, L. (1961). A study of fluctuating asymmetry. *Evolution* **16**, 125–142.

VAN VALEN, L. (1970). An analysis of developmental fields. *Devl Biol.* **23**, 456–477.

17. Metric Analysis of Primate Tooth Form

C. L. B. LAVELLE*

Department of Oral Pathology, University of Birmingham, England

INTRODUCTION

Odontological investigation of extant primates provides a background for the assessment of fossil teeth. Yet the principal method for studying tooth form has relied upon the experienced eye and the creative mind behind the eye. Hence the taxonomic classification of teeth has tended to rely upon the reputation of the worker making the classification. Additional information has been provided by the use of the bucco-lingual and mesio-distal crown measurements together with univariate and bivariate analyses of the data. Moreover, combinations of such measurements, as exemplified by the use of indices, have served to provide elementary definitions of tooth shape. Tooth dimensions assessed in this way, however, rarely do more than confirm the results already obtained by visual techniques. Indeed, as shown in Fig. 1A and B, variation in the mesio-distal and bucco-lingual crown diameters between different populations is often so marked that it is difficult to discriminate between the teeth of one population sample compared with another.

There remains, amongst others, a deficiency in such studies that is shared by both observation and simple measurement. Tooth form is complex, often exhibiting different modes of variation and varying kinds of multiple correlation in its many dimensions. In order to obtain an accurate metrical definition of a tooth, therefore, many dimensions are required. Furthermore such multidimensional data require multivariate statistical analysis in order to compare tooth form between one population and another. Multivariate statistical analysis of multidimensional data is capable of allowing for perturbations of data, whereas these are difficult to evaluate visually and impossible to reveal by simple analysis of the mesio-distal and bucco-lingual crown dimensions. Primarily, therefore, the multivariate approach based upon many dimensions per tooth facilitates better descriptions of

* Present address: Department of Oral Boilogy, University of Manitoba, Canada

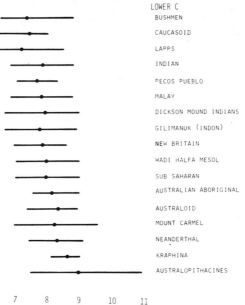

LOWER C

BUSHMEN
CAUCASOID
LAPPS
INDIAN
PECOS PUEBLO
MALAY
DICKSON MOUND INDIANS
GILIMANUK (INDON)
NEW BRITAIN
WADI HALFA MESOL
SUB SAHARAN
AUSTRALIAN ABORIGINAL
AUSTRALOID
MOUNT CARMEL
NEANDERTHAL
KRAPHINA
AUSTRALOPITHACINES

```
5     6     7     8     9     10    11
```
M.D. (MEAN + RANGE)

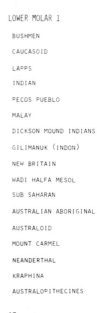
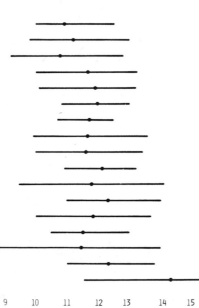

LOWER MOLAR 1

BUSHMEN
CAUCASOID
LAPPS
INDIAN
PECOS PUEBLO
MALAY
DICKSON MOUND INDIANS
GILIMANUK (INDON)
NEW BRITAIN
WADI HALFA MESOL
SUB SAHARAN
AUSTRALIAN ABORIGINAL
AUSTRALOID
MOUNT CARMEL
NEANDERTHAL
KRAPHINA
AUSTRALOPITHECINES

```
8   9   10   11   12   13   14   15   16   17
```
M.D. (MEAN + RANGE)

overall morphological patterns and frequently provides information that is unsuspected from visual inspection alone.

METHODS OF STATISTICAL ANALYSIS

Physical anthropology became a science early in the nineteenth century, although it fell into disrepute in the first few decades of this century when it was realized that comparison of phenotypes as such were of little significance. The evolution of techniques ostensibly suited for the analysis of anthropometric measurements subsequently progressed rapidly and physical anthropology has once more gained its self respect. It is now commonplace for physical anthropologists to employ sophisticated methods of multivariate analysis in an attempt to gain insight into morphology, heritability, classification and discrimination. The advantages of such sophisticated techniques are beginning to be exploited in odontometry (Ashton et al., 1957; Lavelle, 1972). Hence it is high time to examine the virtues and vices of such statistical procedures before they are uniformly adopted in odontometry.

The main problem of multivariate statistics revolves around the need to keep measures of distances between populations or population samples under analysis as simple and communicable as possible. Sokal (1961) recommended the use of Pythagorean distances in a variety of taxonomic problems. Blackith (1965) however noted that this choice is not valid when the parameters studied exhibit little intragroup variation. This is precisely the situation where the discriminative or classification procedures might be expected to be most sensitive, e.g. discriminating between ape and human teeth. The only solution, therefore, is to compute more sophisticated measures of distance.

The meaning of distance or measure of separation between population or sample groups may be obscure. Dempster (1969) presented a case for more than a single distance measure to be computed, i.e. the same body of data must be subjected to a battery of tests before any conclusions can be ascertained with confidence. This may be overstating the problem, although at present there is little experience as to how discrimination behaves when different tests are applied to the same odontometric data. Corruccini (1973) compared pongid and hominid tooth dimensions by a variety of quantitative measures of distance and similarity. Only size differences were detected by the Coefficient of Racial Likeness, Penrose's size distance, D^2 and canonical variates. As a result, these statistical tests failed to produce an accurate taxonomic classification. Penrose's shape distance and Q-mode correlation coefficients produced better results due to their discrimination of similarity on the basis of more important shape and morphological differences. The D^2 and canonical variate methods were converted to shape methods through Q-mode standardization of the raw data, whereupon they also produced more meaning-

---

FIG. 1. Means and ranges of mesio-distal crown diameters of lower permanent teeth:
A. first molar,
B. canine.

ful results. There is a great need however for further research on the effect of different statistical methods of analysis on odontometric data.

Marked differences are apparent when the same statistical test is applied to different bodies of data from the same biological source. For instance, varying degrees of discrimination become apparent when canonical analysis is applied to the same tooth samples, but based upon different dimensions (Fig. 2).

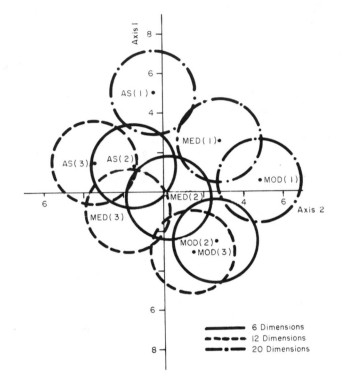

Fig. 2. First two canonical axes based on analysis of three Anglo-Saxon (AS), three Medieval (MED) and three modern (MOD) population samples. Three analyses are superimposed upon one another, based upon 6, 12 and 20 dimensions of the lower three permanent molars. The figure shows centroids (means) and 90% confidence limits.

It is not uncommon in practice to find significant differences at a given level of significance by applying the Student's t-test on each individual measurement, whereas the squared generalized distance statistic (D^2) utilizing all the measurements simultaneously fails to indicate significance at the same level. This may result from univariate comparisons exhibiting varying patterns of contrast between the various parameters. Also the chance of finding significant differences by multivariate statistics may be reduced when variables which do not contain information about group differences are included in the analysis.

Nevertheless the selection of tooth dimensions to be compared has yet to be subjected to scrutiny.

Ultimately there must be some choice as to which parameters should be compared. In the pectoral girdle, for instance, the parameters related to certain muscle groups can be readily identified (Ashton and Oxnard, 1964), but the selection of odontometric parameters presents a much more difficult selection. The mesio-distal and bucco-lingual crown diameters merely provide a sketchy metrical profile of a tooth.

Yet even when the same dimensions of permanent molars measured by

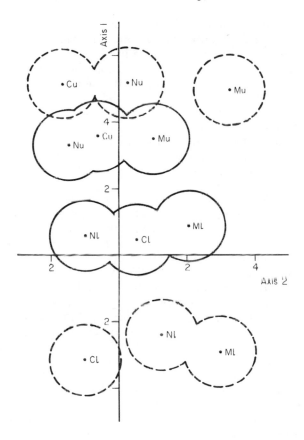

Fig. 3. First two canonical axes based on analysis of Caucasoid (C), Negroid (N) and Mongoloid (M) upper (u) and lower (l) teeth. In this analysis, six dimensions were measured for each upper and lower molar tooth, and the dimensions were combined together in the same analysis. Furthermore, the same dimensions were measured on the same samples by another experienced observer (Observer 1 represented by whole circles; Observer 2 by intermittent circles). The two analyses are superimposed to illustrate the contrast in the degree of separation between the samples by the two observers. The figure shows centroids and 90% confidence limits.

two experienced observers are contrasted by canonical analysis, different patterns of discrimination between different ethnic groups emerge (Fig. 3). This problem is compounded by the limited knowledge as to the sensitivity of multivariate tests. Many workers have conjectured that the robustness and power of the univariate t-test would carry over to the multivariate test, but the available evidence tends to indicate that this anticipation is unfounded (Holloway and Dunn, 1967). Nevertheless, whether such an assumption is applicable to odontometric data has yet to be examined.

Maintaining equal sample sizes tends to maintain the actual level of significance close to the nomimal level, but does not help in maintaining the power of the test. In addition, it is difficult to attempt to obtain equal sample sizes when the covariance matrices are unequal, for increasing the number of variables causes a direct increase in the level of significance. The use of separate univariate t-tests confuses the composite level of significance, but unless the covariance matrices are equal, the same sort of phenomenon affects the multivariate test and the greater the number of variables, the greater the distortion of the nominal significance level. Thus multivariate analysis exhibits some disadvantages which are often not appreciated in odontometric studies. Multivariate statistical analysis, however, holds great promise, but more information about their operating characteristics must be elucidated before they can tell us much about the informational content of our data.

Fisher (1938) defined the discriminant function as the linear combination of the elements of the response vector which maximizes the ratio of the variance between two groups to that within the groups. Rao (1952) subsequently generalized this concept to the case of several groups. These procedures depend on the assumption of equal covariance matrices and multivariate normality of the response vector. When the covariance matrices are unequal, a quadratic discriminant function may be appropriate (Smith, 1947), although non-linear discriminant functions have received scant attention. Yet estimation of the probabilities of miscalculation may be considerably biased if the linear function is used when the covariance matrices are unequal (Gilbert, 1969). Perhaps odontometric data could be exploited in examining the behaviour of non-linear discriminant functions.

In addition to the selection of distance measures between populations or samples, the determination of the dimensionality of the space within which to define the groups, and the number of groups one is to have, provide two problems in the development of any discriminatory procedure. In discriminant analysis, the number of groups into which a sample is to be partitioned is assumed to be known. Thus the discriminant function serves to allocate the new individual into one or other of the specified groups. The rationale of forcing each new individual into one or other of the existing groups may be questioned, and Kendall (1957) makes out a case for some intermediate category where some isolated samples could be allocated. For instance, an isolated tooth might not belong to a known fossil group but to an unknown fossil taxon, yet multivariate statistical techniques might not recognize this phenomenon. Thus the taxonomic identification of an isolated tooth may be inaccurate when exploiting multivariate statistical techniques.

When applying the discriminant function to odontometric data, the variables included in the discriminant function often have a marked dependency on attrition (Fig. 4). The question, therefore, is what is the proper

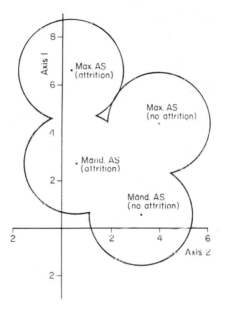

FIG. 4. First two canonical axes based on analysis of the upper (max) and lower (mand) permanent molar dimensions of an Anglo-Saxon (AS) population sample, contrasting the discrimination between teeth with or without attrition. The figure shows centroids and 90% confidence limits.

definition of the best linear discriminator of a sample in the presence of covariates. Although tooth size is important, tooth shape variables need to be defined which are independent of size. This would enable large and small teeth from the same population to be classified into the same group. Alternatively it is possible that two groups may contrast in some aspect of tooth shape yet conventional multivariate tests along the discriminant function may fail to indicate a significant difference (Blackith, 1965). When measurements alone are used as descriptive data, there is general concurrence that "shape" coefficients of affinity are superior to "size" (distance) coefficients (Giles, 1956; Kowalski, 1972). Tooth size and shape are however intimately interrelated, so that it is difficult to identify shape variables which are theoretically or practically independent of size (Mosimann, 1970). Some form of covariance adjustment is required, although how this can be achieved without loss of data accuracy and how tooth shape varies with tooth size requires urgent study.

The basic strategy behind a canonical analysis of discriminance is to describe the variation of N points in a p-dimensional space by introducing a new set of orthogonal linear coordinates in such a way that the sample variances of the given points with respect to these new coordinates are in decreasing order of magnitude. Thus the first principal component is such that the projections of the points onto it have maximum variance among all possible linear coordinates; the second principal component has maximum variance subject to being orthogonal to the first, and so on. This analysis, therefore, commences with measurements and a search is made for the components which may be able to reduce the dimensions of variation and assign them with some biological significance. This rationale appears eminently reasonable and would seem to be useful in the study of odontometry, since odontologists are typically interested in the determination of what measurements or combination of measurements show considerable variation. The main problem is that the solution depends upon the units of measurement. For instance, in the analysis of crown form, both linear (e.g. cusp heights) and angular (e.g. cusp slopes) measurements may be used yet, in the interpretation of the distances between different population samples, how can these be interpreted in biological terms if both angles and linear measurements are combined together (Anderson, 1958)? Indeed, unless measurements are all in the same units, univariate statistical techniques may be preferable.

Another problem is that odontometric data may be too sparse to permit exploitation of sophisticated statistical techniques. For instance, there is a limit as to the number of parameters that can be measured for a single tooth, and even these may exhibit diminished biological significance due to attrition. Thus simple univariate statistical techniques may be relevant to some biological data and produce meaningful results. In the case of isolated fossil tooth fragments, subjective visual inspection may be the only means of taxonomic identification.

No complex statistical analysis will have relevance, unless it is based on sound data. Measurements provide information only relating to the points from which measurements are made. Data from positions between datum points are ignored, i.e. the mesio-distal and bucco-lingual crown diameters provide no data as to intercusp distances or cusp heights. Increasing the number of datum points helps to avoid this, but there are practical limits, although scanning methods have been evolved to make mensuration and recording easier and more accurate so that it becomes possible to characterize patterns and shape almost *in toto*.

Errors of the observer may also be significant, and may arise either from the incorrect use of calipers or copying the data. Inappropriate definition or location of datum points may also contribute to the error. In addition, there are random errors which are unpredictable and are always present to a certain extent in any physical data, e.g. from differential environmental influences on tooth size and shape or from errors of sampling populations (this latter error may present problems when categorizing fossils). There may also be contrasts when comparing the data from different workers. For instance, Tobias (1964) compared his measurements of South African Australopithecines with those of the same specimens measured by Robinson (1956) and noted differences of 0·1–0·3 mm, whereas a comparison of Robinson's measurements with those of Leakey (1961) reveal a difference of 1·4 mm. Hunter and Priest (1960) report a mean difference of 0·153 ± 0·026 mm between observers, whereas Bailit et al. (1968) cite an average error between observers of 0·052 ± 0·032 mm for 105 casts of the Nasioi dentitions. For this reason, comparison between the data of other workers may negate any conclusions.

Mensurational data also frequently depend upon the particular orientation of specimens along standard lines or planes. Yet truly homologous lines or planes in different teeth need not be straight or flat, although there are practical problems in taking this into account. More recently, attempts to allow for the possible curvature of homologous lines or planes include coordinate measurements together with such techniques for their examination as trend-surface analysis (Sneath, 1967). But apart from the study of Hine et al. (1971), such techniques have yet to be exploited in odontometry. Other techniques in dealing with three-dimensional aspects of form are also available, e.g. stereoscopic image analysis (Rohlf, 1968) and Moire fringe methods with coherent light (Chmielowski and Varner, 1969). It is because teeth are small and readily available that they make ideal biological objects for the exploitation of such techniques.

Evolutionary Trends

An evolutionary trend can be defined as a "sustained prevailing tendency in a phylogenetic progression" (Simpson, 1953). Such trends are of interest since they provide a fundamental insight into the adaptive orientating factors in hominid evolution. Due to their sustained trend, adaptively important and so taxonomically relevant characteristics are constructed by evolutionary trends. Tooth size has adaptive significance, since in addition to mastication, teeth are used for grasping, holding and other manipulative functions (Campbell, 1925; Brace, 1962). Indeed tooth size seems to be one of the major adaptive mechanisms with which hominids meet their environment. Traditionally a general trend for a reduction in tooth size is recognized in hominid evolution (Robinson, 1956). Other workers, by contrast, find no taxonomic chasm between Homo sapiens and H. erectus in tooth size (Garn, 1964) and no systematic reduction in tooth size in modern man (Garn et al., 1969).

Using the odontometric data provided by Wolpoff (1971), however, different evolutionary trends can be computed from hominoid odontometry, depending upon the dimensions actually included in the analysis. For instance, as shown in Fig. 5A and B, the evolutionary trend differed when all the mesio-distal crown dimensions were combined together compared with analysis of all the upper mesio-distal crown dimensions combined together. It is possible, however, that each tooth follows a different evolutionary

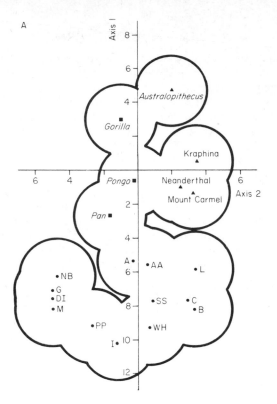

FIG. 5 (A and B). First two canonical axes based on hominoid mesio-distal tooth dimensions combined together, the data being derived from Wolpoff (1971). Populations represented by letters refer to various *Homo sapiens* samples.

A. Analysis of all the upper and lower mesio-distal tooth dimensions combined together.

B. See facing page.

trend, although little work has been undertaken relating to the metric changes in the dentition as a whole. Different evolutionary trends can also be obtained depending upon the taxonomic groupings. As shown in Fig. 6A and B analysis of all the mesio-distal crown dimensions combined together contrasts when *H. sapiens* is regarded as a single group, rather than a number of population samples as shown in Fig. 5A and B. This is particularly important, since the taxonomic identification of fossil specimens often changes as more evidence becomes available, and this may result in considerable confusion regarding the computation of evolutionary trends. This therefore indicates that much more research is required before odontometric evolutionary trends can be elucidated with confidence. Moreover, the factors affecting crown form must also be investigated before the significance of such odontometric trends can be discussed.

Tooth size has long been considered to be relatively independent of the environment,· and so provides a useful genetic marker between populations

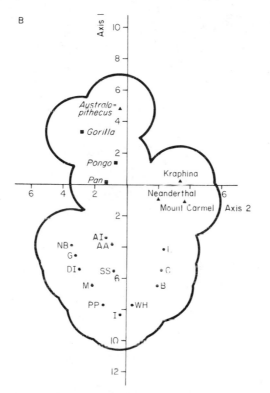

FIG. 5. B. Analysis of all the upper mesio-distal tooth dimensions combined together, The figure shows centroids and 90% confidence limits.

(Garn *et al.*, 1969). Using correlations to measure similarity, however, Goose (1967) has reported that the correlation coefficients in a family study are smaller than should be expected if genetic factors were the principal factors concerned. Twin studies show a low nutritional and maturational component, but high genetic components of tooth size variation (Garn *et al.*, 1965) and Garn *et al.* (1967) have shown that sexual dimorphism in tooth size is under genetic control. Nevertheless, when a number of dimensions are recorded from surgically extracted unerupted human lower third molar teeth, an increase in size is noted between 17 and 25 years of age (Fig. 7). It must be emphasized that such changes cannot be recognized from analysis of merely the mesio-distal and bucco-lingual crown dimensions and possibly a complex change is indicated in overall tooth form, although the mechanisms of such a process remain obscure. One possibility is that such a change merely reflects a peculiar sample of teeth, although in this instance, all the teeth were from male Caucasoids. Furthermore, a similar trend is beginning to emerge from analysis of unerupted, but surgically removed, upper canine teeth. Tooth size also differs between subjects derived from fluoridated compared

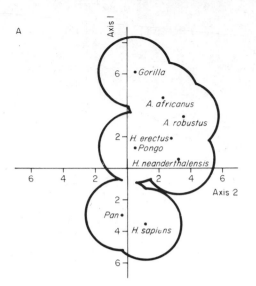

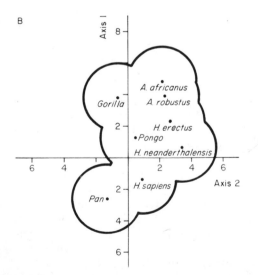

Fig. 6. First two canonical axes based on the same tooth dimensions as listed above, but with regrouping of the population samples.
A. analysis of all the upper and lower mesio-distal tooth dimensions combined together;
B. analysis of all the lower mesio-distal tooth dimensions combined together.
The figure shows centroids and 90% confidence limits.

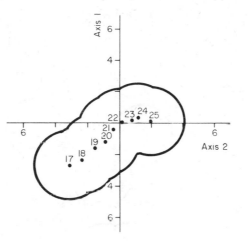

FIG. 7. First two canonical axes based on analysis of 12 dimensions of surgically removed unerupted lower third mandibular molar crowns. The figure shows centroids (listed according to the age of the individual) and their 90% confidence limits.

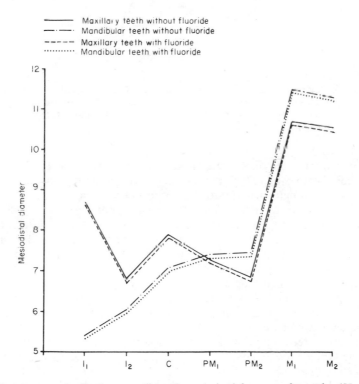

FIG. 8. The mean mesio-distal crown dimensions derived from equal samples (50 males) derived from fluoridated and non-fluoridated regions of the United Kingdom.

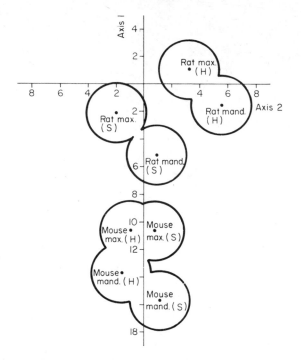

FIG. 9. First two canonical axes based on analysis of the mesio-distal and bucco-lingual crown dimensions of the upper (max) and lower (mand) teeth combined together from rats (Birmingham inbred strain) and mice (C57) fed on hard (H) and soft (S) diets. The figure shows centroids and their 90% confidence limits.

with non-fluoridated areas (Fig. 8). In addition, the molar tooth dimensions have been shown to differ between laboratory animals fed upon hard and soft diets, although such variation may reflect variation in the loss of tooth substance due to attrition (Fig. 9). Secular trends can also be detected in tooth size (Fig. 10), and these changes appear to vary in different regions (Fig 11). Finally it is possible to discriminate between the dimensions of teeth derived from subjects living in different parts of England (Fig. 12). These features, therefore, appear to throw open the whole question as to how reliable is odontometric data, i.e. how closely does the phenotype of a tooth reflect the genotype? How representative of a population is a tooth sample, i.e. how large should a sample of teeth be before any meaningful odontometric data can be obtained?

Permanent teeth could well be influenced by dietary factors (Hunt, 1960), and the type of food (oats, barley or wheat) has a selective effect on mouse tooth size (van Valen, 1963). Nevertheless, Swindler *et al.* (1963) report closely related species of *Macaca* exhibiting significant differences in tooth size yet sharing apparently identical diets. It is possible, however, that

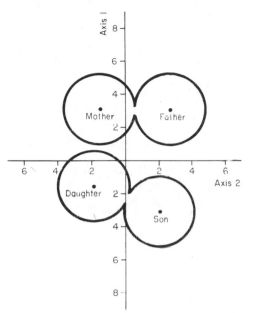

FIG. 10. First two canonical axes based on analysis of the mesio-distal and bucco-lingual crown dimensions of all the upper and lower teeth combined together of parents and offspring. The figure shows centroids and their 90% confidence limits.

different diets may have differential effects on different taxonomic hominoid groups.

Finally, there may be problems when measuring casts of fossil teeth. For instance, Lundstrom (1943) obtained 1–2% higher values from measuring casts compared with measurement of teeth actually from the mouth, a feature which was subsequently confirmed by Hunter and Priest (1960). Also, as illustrated in Fig. 13A and B, variation in tooth dimensions may be recorded between casts derived from different impression materials and between teeth measured using different measurement techniques, i.e. calipers or dividers.

CONCLUSIONS

Teeth provide the primary biological structures for morphological investigation in evolutionary studies, due to their preferential fossilization compared with the remainder of the skeleton. Nevertheless, more research is required into how representative a tooth sample must be before any conclusions can be accurately derived. Also more information is required about the importance of various odontometric dimensions to the metrical profile of a tooth and the performance of multivariate statistical techniques in the analysis of such data. Finally, there is a more basic problem, namely: just how reliable is a tooth as a genetic marker between two populations? These questions must all be

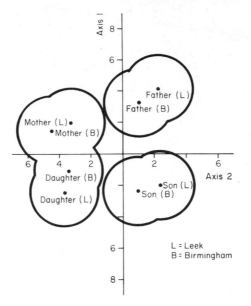

FIG. 11. First two canonical axes based on analysis of the mesoi-distal and bucco-lingual crown dimensions of all the upper and lower teeth combined together of parents and offspring derived from two different regions of England (Leek and Birmingham) separated by some 50–60 miles. The figure shows centroids and their 90% confidence limits.

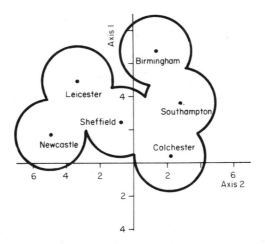

FIG. 12. First two canonical axes based on analysis of the mesoi-distal and bucco-lingual crown dimensions combined together of male adults from six different regions of England. The figure shows centroids and their 90% confidence limits.

FIG. 13 (facing page). Variation in odontometric dimensions
  A. identical dental casts measured with calipers and dividers,
  B. identical samples measured from casts derived from different impression materials.

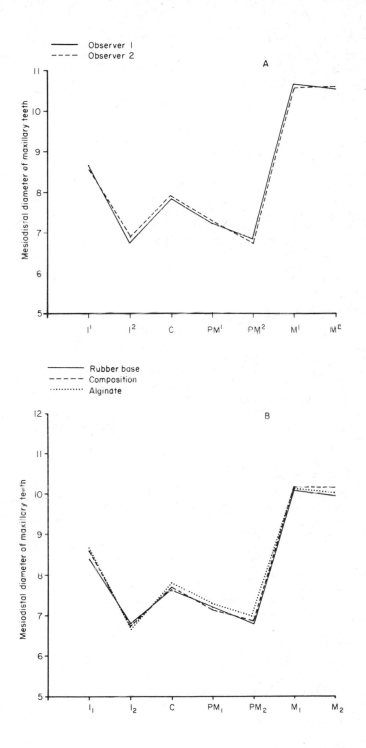

answered before undue reliance is placed on odontometric studies of primate evolution. Ultimately, however, objective examination and investigation of teeth will only be achieved by a metrical approach.

REFERENCES

ANDERSON, T. W. (1958). "An Introduction To Multivariate Statistical Analysis." John Wiley and Sons, New York.

ASHTON, E. H. and OXNARD, C. E. (1964). Functional adaptations in the primate shoulder girdle. *Proc. zool. Soc. Lond.* **142**, 49–66.

ASHTON, E. H., HEALY, M. J. R. and LIPTON, S. (1957). The descriptive use of discriminant functions in physical anthropology. *Proc. R. Soc.* **146**, 552–572.

BAILIT, H. L., DE WITT, S. J. and LEIGH, R. A. (1968). The size and morphology of the Nasioi dentition. *Am. J. phys. Anthrop.* **28**, 271–288.

BLACKITH, R. E. (1965). Morphometrics. In "Theoretical and Mathematical Biology" (Waterman, T. H. and Morowitz, H. J., eds.). Blaisdell, New York.

BRACE, C. L. (1962). Cultural factors in the evolution of the human dentition. *In* "Culture and the Evolution of Man" (Montagu, C. G. A., ed.). Oxford University Press, New York.

CAMPBELL, T. D. (1925). "Dentition and Palate of the Australian Aboriginal." Hassell Press, Adelaide.

CHMIELOWSKI, N. and VARNER, J. R. (1969). An application of holographic contouring in dentistry. *Biomed. Sci. Instr.* **6**, 72–79.

CORRUCCINI, R. S. (1973). Size and shape in similarity coefficients based on metric characters. *Am. J. phys. Anthrop.* **38**, 743–754.

DEMPSTER, A. P. (1969). "Elements of Continuous Multivariate Analysis." Addison-Wesley, Reading, England.

FISHER, R. A. (1938). The statistical utilization of multiple measurements. *Ann. Eugen.* **8**, 376–386.

GARN, S. M. (1964). Culture and the direction of human evolution. *In* "Culture and the Direction of Human Evolution" (Garn, S. M., ed.). Wayne State University Press, Detroit.

GARN, S. M. LEWIS, A. B. and KEREWSKY, R. (1965). Genetic, nutritional and maturational correlation of dental development. *J. dent. Res.* **44**, 228–242.

GARN, S. M., LEWIS, A. B., SWINDLER, D. R. and KEREWSKY, R. (1967). Genetic control of sexual dimorphism in tooth size. *J. dent. Res.* **46**, 963–972.

GARN, S. M., LEWIS, A. B. and WALENGA, A. (1969). Crown size profile patterns and presumed evolutionary trends. *Am. Anthrop.* **71**, 79–84.

GILBERT, E. S. (1969). The effect of unequal covariance metrices of Fisher's linear discriminant function. *Biometrics* **25**, 505–515.

GILES, E. (1956). Cranial allometry in the great apes. *Hum. Biol.* **28**, 43–58.

GOOSE, D. H. (1967). Preliminary study of tooth size in formation. *J. dent. Res.* **46**, 959.

HINE, K. R., FLINN, R. M. and LAVELLE, C. L. B. (1971). The analysis of tooth shape. *J. Anat.* **108**, 585.

HOLLOWAY, L. N. and DUNN, O. J. (1967). The robustness of Hotelling's T^2. *J. Am. statist. Ass.* **62**, 124–136.

HUNT, E. E. (1960). Malocclusion and civilization. *Am. J. Orthod.* **47**, 406–421.

HUNTER, W. S. and PRIEST, W. R. (1960). Errors and discrepancies in measurement of tooth size. *J. dent. Res.* **39**, 405.

KENDALL, M. G. (1957). "A Course in Multivariate Analysis." Hafner, New York.

KOWALSKI, C. J. (1972). A commentary on the use of multivariate statistical methods in anthropometric research. *Am. J. phys. Anthrop.* **36**, 119–132.

LAVELLE, C. L. B. (1972). The incisors of man and apes. *Bull. Group Int. Rech. Sc. Stomat.* **15**, 285–301.

LEAKEY, L. S. B. (1961). The juvenile mandible from Olduvai. *Nature, Lond.* **191**, 417–418.

LUNDSTROM, A. (1943). Intermaxillara Tandbreddsforhallanden och Tandstallningen *Svensk. Tandläkare-Tidskrift* **36**, 575–624.

MOSIMANN, J. E. (1970). Size allometry size and shape variables. *J. Am. statist. Ass.* **65**, 930–945.

RAO, C. R. (1952). Advanced Statistical Methods in Biological Research. John Wiley and Sons, New York.

ROBINSON, J. T. (1956). The dentition of the Australopithecinae. *Transv. Mus. Mem.* No. 9.

ROHLF, F. J. (1968). Stereograms in numerical taxonomy. *Syst. Zool.* **17**, 246–255.

SIMPSON, G. G. (1953). "The Major Features of Evolution." Columbia, New York.

SMITH, C. A. B. (1947). Some examples of discrimination. *Ann. Eugen.* **13**, 272–282.

SNEATH, P. H. A. (1967). Trend surface analysis of transformation grids. *J. Zool. Lond.* **151**, 65–122.

SOKAL, R. R. (1961). Distance as a measure of taxonomic similarity *Syst. Zool.* **10**, 70–79.

SWINDLER, D. R., GAVAN, J. A. and TURNER, W. M. (1963). Molar tooth size variability in African monkeys. *Hum. Biol.* **35**, 104–122.

TOBIAS, P. V. (1964). The early hominid remains from Tanganjika: *Australopithecus* and *Homo. Proc. VII Int. Cong. Anthrop Ethnol. Sci.* (Moscow, 1964).

VAN VALEN, L. (1963). Intensities of selection in natural populations. *Proc. 11th Int. Cong. Genet.* **1**, 153–166.

WOLPOFF, M. H. (1971). Metric trends in hominid dental evolution. *In* "Studies in Anthropology." Case Western Reserve University Press, Cleveland and London.

18. Molar Structure and Occlusion in Cretaceous Therian Mammals

A. W. CROMPTON

Museum of Comparative Zoology, Harvard University, Cambridge, Massachusetts, U.S.A.

and

ZOFIA KIELAN-JAWOROWSKA

Zaklad Paleobiologii, Polska Akademia Nauk, Warszawa, Poland

INTRODUCTION

The purpose of this chapter is to outline the main features of the molars and their occlusal pattern in Cretaceous therians. We will only be discussing forms which have tribosphenic molars, i.e. with a protocone on the uppers and a talonid basin on the lowers. Some of the Symmetrodonta and Pantotheria (Simpson, 1945) extend into the Cretaceous, and may be therians, but are not discussed in this chapter. We also wish to attempt to explain in functional terms the various patterns which are encountered. An understanding of the occlusal pattern of the molars can be an aid to systematic and phylogenetic studies on Cretaceous therians, because the classification of these forms has to a large extent in the past been based on molar structure. Although the structure of numerous molars, representing several genera of Late Cretaceous mammals have been known from North America and elsewhere for many years, it was difficult to describe occlusal relationships or to discuss the way the molars were used because matching occluding upper and lower molars from the same individual were virtually unknown. In 1926, Gregory and Simpson described the molars of the genera *Zalambdalestes*, *Deltatheridium* and *Hyotheridium* from the Late Cretaceous of Mongolia. Although the jaws of these forms were found in occlusion, the preservation of the molars is so poor that it was impossible to determine the occlusal pattern. The discovery of numerous articulated jaws of Mongolian Cretaceous mammals by the Polish–Mongolian Palaeontological Expeditions (Kielan-Jaworowska, 1969, 1975a, b) has made it possible for the first time to determine accurately the form–function relationships of upper and lower molars in several different types of Cretaceous mammals. This can be used as a basis for interpreting the structure and function of other Cretaceous therian molars of which matching occluding teeth are not known. A detailed description has been given of only one of the Mongolian Cretaceous therian mammals, i.e. *Deltatheridium* (Kielan-Jaworowska, 1975b) but preliminary descriptions have been given of the others (Kielan-Jaworowska, 1969, 1975a) and detailed descriptions of these are being prepared.

The basic structure of the Cretaceous therian molar pattern is retained in the American opossum (*Didelphis marsupialis*) and it is possible, by studying jaw movements, feeding behaviour and jaw muscles with the aid of techniques such as cinefluoroscopy and electromyography in the opossum (Hiiemae and Jenkins, 1969; Crompton and Hiiemae, 1970; Hiiemae and Crompton, 1971) to gain insight into the nature of therian mastication during Cretaceous times. A brief review of some of the published and recent results of this experimental work, which are applicable to molar structure is included in the discussion section.

Although the literature abounds with descriptions of the morphology of the molars of Mesozoic and Early Tertiary mammals, relatively few workers have attempted to analyse their structure in terms of occlusion or jaw movements. Notable exceptions are Butler (1952, 1961) and Mills (1964, 1966) who were, to a large extent, instrumental in initiating studies in this field. Subsequently, Clemens and Mills (1971), Crompton (1971, 1974), Crompton and Jenkins (1973), Krebs (1971) and Kermack et al. (1965) have studied Triassic and Jurassic therians, and Kay and Hiiemae (1974) have studied late Cretaceous therians in these terms. It is hoped that this chapter will serve as an introduction to the structure of therian molars known from the Cretaceous and help bridge the gap between the extensive studies either published or in the process of being published on Tertiary and Recent mammals on the one hand and those on Triassic and Jurassic mammals on the other. The terminology used in this chapter for numbering wear or shearing surfaces is the same as that introduced by one of us (Crompton, 1971) and adopted by Kay and Hiiemae in their papers (Hiiemae and Kay, 1973; Kay and Hiiemae, 1974) on occlusion and jaw movements in fossil and Recent primates.

In this chapter we will be referring to a large selection of Cretaceous therians. In the first section we have attempted to document the time and continental distribution of these mammals. These are summarized in Table I.

On the basis of our studies on Cretaceous therian molars we have attempted to determine the interrelationship of most Cretaceous therians, but as our conclusions are based on such limited information, because of the paucity of the record and total absence of therians from the Cenomanian, Turonian, Coniacian and part of the Santonian, our phylogenetic chart (Table II) is tentative. In order to facilitate the comparison of Cretaceous therian

TABLE I. List of Cretaceous therian genera (see footnote on p. 252).

STAGES[a]	EUROPE	ASIA	NORTH AMERICA	SOUTH AMERICA
MAESTRICHTIAN			Hell Creek Formation — *Alphadon Batodon Cimolestes / Didelphodon Gypsonictops Pediomys Glasbius Pediomys Protungulatum Purgatorius*	?Viquechico Formation — *Alphadon* and unnamed didelphid and pediomyid *Peratherium* marsupials
CAMPANIAN — Upper	?Champ-Garimond Beds[b] — unnamed eutherian lower molar		Upper Part of Edmonton F. — *Alphadon Batodon Cimolestes / Didelphodon Gypsonictops Pediomys* Lance Formation — *Alphadon Batodon Didelphodon Cimolestes Glasbius Gypsonictops Pediomys Pediomys* and unnamed therian teeth St. Mary River Formation — *Didelphodon? Pediomys Eodelphis?* unnamed therian	
CAMPANIAN — Middle		?Barun Goyo Formation[b] — *Deltatheridium Asioryctes Barunlestes*	El Gallo Formation — *Pediomys Gallolestes* Oldman Formation — *Boreodon* undescribed *Deltatheridium Didelphodon* eutherian *Eodelphis* teeth Mesaverde F. — ?	
CAMPANIAN — Lower			Judith River Formation — *Alphadon Boreodon Gypsonictops Pediomys* Upper Part of Milk River Formation — *Aquiladelphis Alphadon Eodelphis Pediomys / Potamotelses* and isolated upper molar, recognized by Fox as a eutherian	
SANTONIAN		?Djadokhta Formation[b] — *Deltatheroides Deltatheridium Hyotheridium Kennalestes Zalambdalestes*		
CONIACIAN				
TURONIAN				
CENOMANIAN				
ALBIAN			Trinity Sandstone — *Holoclemensia Pappotherium Kermackia* and several isola.e., unnamed therian teeth	
APTIAN		?Ausin Beds[b] ?Khovboor Beds — *Endotherium / Prokennalestes Prozalambdalestes Kielantherium*		
NEOCOMIAN	Lower Wealden of Cliff End — *Aegialodon*			

[a] The lengths of particular stages are not in proportion to their absolute age.

[b] Question mark in front of the name of the formation or beds indicate doubts as to their age.

[c] The generic names *Prokennalestes* and *Prozalambdalestes* are cited after Dr Trofimov's identifications in the PIN (Paleontological Institute in Moscow) collection.

TABLE II. Phylogenetic chart*.

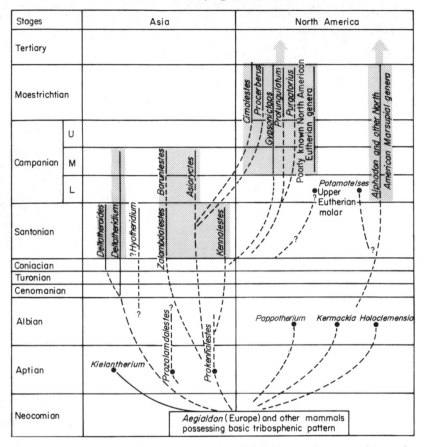

molars we have prepared illustrations in which the molars are shown from similar angles, i.e. occlusal, crown, anterior and posterior. In those cases where matching uppers and lowers are known we have also included a posterior view of the upper and lower second molars to show the relationship of the protocone to the talonid basin, and an internal view of upper molars and external surface of the lowers to illustrate the matching surfaces.

Records of Cretaceous Therian Mammals

The earliest known mammal with tribosphenic molars (see Table I) is *Aegialodon dawsoni* from the Wealden of Great Britain (Kermack *et al.*,

* Since this paper was submitted for publication, a paper by Gradziński *et al.* (1977) has been accepted for publication, in which the authors suggest that the Djadokhta Formation is of ?Late Santonian and/or ?Early Campanian age rather than ?Santonian as suggested earlier by Kielan-Jaworowska (1975b). It proved impossible to introduce the emendation of the age of the Djadokhta Formation to Tables I and II and throughout the text.

1965). From the late part of the Early Cretaceous the therian mammals are known from three places: from Manchuria (genus *Endotherium*—see Shikama, 1947; McKenna, 1969); from the Aptian (?) sandstone of Khovboor in the Gobi Desert, in the Mongolian People's Republic in Asia (Beliajeva *et al.*, 1974; Dashzeveg, 1975) and from the Trinity sandstone (Albian) of Texas in North America (Patterson, 1956; Slaughter, 1965, 1968a, b, c, 1971; Crompton, 1971; Turnbull, 1971).

Of the therian mammals from the Khovboor locality in the Gobi Desert only one genus, *Kielantherium*, has been described (Dashzeveg, 1975). It is a single lower molar, assigned to the Aegialodontidae. A description of the remaining part of the Khovboor fauna, currently investigated by Dr B. A. Trofimov in the Palaeontological Institute in Moscow, has not been published. It appears from the paper by Beliajeva *et al.* (1974) that in the Khovboor fauna there are two more therian genera designated by Trofimov as *Prokennalestes* and *Prozalambdalestes*, but they have not been described as yet.

After the Albian there is a long gap in record of therians from sites all around the world; this includes the Cenomanian, Turonian, Coniacian and possibly also a part of Santonian (see footnote on p. 252 regarding Tables I and II). Of the five monotypic therian genera found in the Djadokhta Formation (Gregory and Simpson, 1926, Kielan-Jaworowska, 1969, 1975a, b), with the exception of *Deltatheroides*, all were found with associated upper and lower jaws. The next Late Cretaceous formation yielding therian mammals is the Barun Goyot Formation (previously called also the Lower Nemegt beds), the age of which has been estimated as Middle (?) Campanian (Kielan-Jaworowska, 1974a). In the Barun Goyot Formation, three therian monotypic genera are represented by skulls with associated lower jaws (Kielan-Jaworowska, 1975a, b).

A fragmentary mandible with few teeth has been described (Bashanov, 1972) from the Coniacian of Kazakhstan (USSR) as *Beleutinus orlovi*. The specimen is so poorly preserved that in our opinion it must be regarded as *nomen dubium*. It is not shown in Table I.

In contradistinction to the conditions in the Late Cretaceous of Asia (Mongolia), the therian mammals of the Late Cretaceous of North America are represented by isolated teeth or fragments of upper and lower jaws with teeth. The only North American Cretaceous mammal represented by an associated upper and lower dentition is *Alphadon marshi*, described by Lillegraven (1969). The oldest Late Cretaceous formation yielding the therian mammals in North America is the upper part of the Milk River Formation of Alberta, which is of Early Campanian age (Fox, 1970, 1971, 1972). Above the Milk River Formation in North America there is a hiatus in the therian records, because the Milk River Formation is overlain by the marine Pakowki Formation. The next North American formations yielding the therian faunas are of the Middle Campanian age and these are: Judith River Formation (Sahni, 1972), Oldman Formation (Russell, 1952; Fox, personal communication) and Mesaverde Formation (McKenna, personal communication).

From the Belly River Formation of North America, which is also of the Middle Campanian age, the mammals are not known. Late Campanian is represented in North America by both marine (Bearpaw Formation) and continental formations (lower part of the Edmonton Formation, St. Mary River and El Gallo formations). The lower part of the Edmonton Formation has not yielded therian mammals. Therian mammals from the St. Mary River Formation were described by Russell (1962) and Sloan and Russell (1974). The trigonid assigned by these authors to the Miacidae, and referred by Clemens (1966, his p. 95) to *Alphadon* (?) is cited in Table I as an unnamed therian. Therian mammals from the El Gallo Formation of Baja California in northern Mexico, were described by Lillegraven (1972, 1976).

The three non-marine Maestrichtian formations of North America (upper part of the Edmonton Formation, Lance and Hell Creeks) have yielded a rich and differentiated fauna of therian mammals (Clemens, 1966, 1973; Clemens and Russell, 1965; Lillegraven, 1969; Simpson, 1951; Sloan and van Valen, 1965; van Valen and Sloan, 1965).

Outside of Asia and North America the Late Cretaceous therian mammals were found in the Viquechico Formation in Peru (Grambast *et al.*, 1967, Sigé, 1972) and in southern France (Ledoux *et al.*, 1966). The exact age of both the Late Cretaceous beds of Peru and France is dubious. McKenna (1969) referred to the Viquechico Formation of Peru as Paleocene (?), but in this chapter we regard it tentatively as Late Cretaceous possibly Maestrichtian. The Champ-Garimond beds of southern France have been referred to by McKenna as Campanian (?), and we have tentatively referred to them as Late Campanian (?).

DESCRIPTION OF A PRIMITIVE TRIBOSPHENIC MOLAR

In order to compare the morphology of the molars of the different Cretaceous therians a brief description of the structure and occlusion of an upper and lower molar with a primitive tribosphenic pattern is included (Fig. 1). These illustrations are, in part, based upon the structure of primitive Cretaceous therians such as *Aegialodon* from the Neocomian of England, *Kielantherium* from the Aptian of Asia, *Pappotherium*, *Holoclemensia* and *Kermackia* from the Albian of Texas and studies on the evolution of the tribosphenic molar. The description of the tribosphenic molar given below is essentially the same as that given by one of us (Crompton, 1971). However, it is repeated here for convenience because it provides a suitable model for comparison with the molars discussed in this chapter.

A primitive tribosphenic molar has six matching shearing surfaces, numbered from 1 to 6 (Crompton, 1971; Kay and Hiiemae, 1974) and a triangular-shaped area on the upper tooth (the trigon) which bites against a backward extension of the lower tooth (the talonid), Fig 1A. Molars of this type are well adapted for shearing on the one hand and puncturing on the other. The principal shearing surfaces (1 and 2) on the lower tooth are on the near vertical surfaces of a high triangular block, the trigonid, which fits into

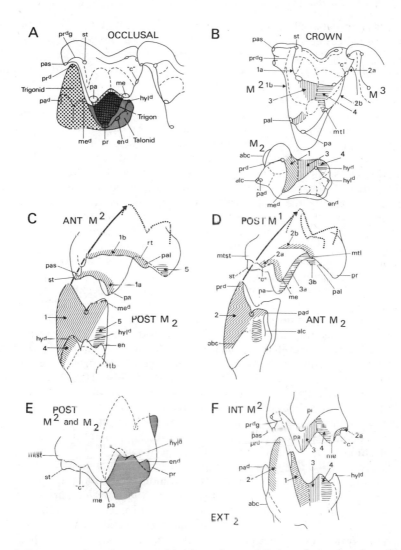

Fig. 1. Reconstruction of upper and lower molars and their occlusion in a hypothetical Early Cretaceous therian mammal. The reconstruction is based mostly on *Pappotherium*. The hypothetical molars here figured are more advanced than those in the Aegialodontidae, but less than in the Late Cretaceous eutherian and marsupial mammals. abc = antero-buccal cuspule (cingulum); alc = antero-labial cuspule; "c" = cusp "c" on metacrista (Crompton, 1971); en^d = entoconid; ft^b = floor of talonid basin; hy^d = hypoconid; hyl^d = hypoconulid; me = metacone; me^d = metaconid; mtl = metaconule; mtst = metastyle; pa = paracone; pa^d = paraconid; pal = paraconule; pas = parastyle; pr = protocone; pr^d = protoconid; pr^{d}g = groove for the protoconid; rt = roof of trigon area; st = stylocone; 1a,1b–6 = matching shearing surfaces.

an embrasure between succeeding upper teeth. The structure of these two shearing surfaces can be appreciated best if they are viewed either from the front or behind; for example, in Fig. 1C, shearing surface 1 on the back of the trigonid of M_2 and its matching shearing surface on the front of the upper trigonid of M^2. Shearing surface 1 on the lower trigonid lies below the ridge connecting a high protoconid to a slightly lower internal metaconid and the cutting edge of the matching surface (1a) on the upper trigonid lies between a high paracone and lower external stylocone. As the lower tooth moved upwards and inwards along the path indicated by the bold arrow, the leading edges of the shearing surfaces passed one another and food trapped between the cusps was sheared. As the lower tooth continued to move upwards the leading edge of shearing surface 1 on the lower trigonid passed a second shearing surface 1b, the leading edge of which extends outwards along the anterior surface of the tooth from a small cusp, the paraconule. In order to prevent food being forced into the gap between two succeeding molars, the protoconid moved in a deep groove ($pr^d g$), in an antero–external extension or parastylar region of the upper molar. This groove is bordered externally between the stylocone behind and a parastylar cusp in front. The parastylar region is hook-shaped in crown and occlusal views, and is extremely large in primitive therian molars. A small pointed protocone (Fig. 1E) fits into a shallow basin in the talonid when the teeth are in occlusion and when the talonid basin was in this position, further upward and inward movement of the lower jaw was prevented. As the lower tooth moved upwards and slightly inwards to reach this position the anterior edge of the protocone sheared down the posterior surface of the metaconid (5, Fig. 1C). The shearing surfaces on the front of the trigonid (2 of M_2, Fig. 1D) and the back of the upper trigonid of M^1 functioned the same way as shearing surface 1. The lower part lies below a ridge connecting a lower inner paraconid to a higher outer protoconid and the upper (2a) between the high internal metacone and a point slightly beyond a more laterally placed cusp "c". After the lower molar moved past this upper shearing surface it encountered a second shearing surface 2b lying above a ridge extending externally from a small metaconule. An oblique ridge or cingulum on the anterior surface of the trigonid (Fig. 1D, abc) protected food from being forced against the gum by the metacone. This ridge and a more internally placed cusp and/or ridge (alc) form the borders of a vertically orientated concave area in to which the hypoconulid of the preceding tooth fits. In occlusal view it can be seen that a V-shaped embrasure exists between a large anterior situated paracone and a more posteriorly situated and smaller metacone. A large hypoconid on the external surface of the talonid moved up the centre of this embrasure as the teeth came into occlusion. When the protocone fits tightly into the basin in the talonid, the hypoconid meets the domed roof of the trigon. The shearing surface or wear facet above the ridge connecting the centre of this embrasure with the paracone has been called shearing surface 3a. The matching surface on the lower tooth lies below the ridge (cristid obliqua) running antero–internally from the hypoconid to the deep groove for the paracone on the external surface of the lower tooth. Shearing surface 4a lies above the ridge connecting the centre of the embrasure to the metacone and the matching surface on the lower tooth lies below the ridge extending postero–internally from the hypoconid towards the hypoconulid. Shearing surfaces 3b and 4b lie above the ridges extending externo–posteriorly and externo–anteriorly from the paraconule and metaconule respectively. The paraconule and its wing are better developed than the metaconule and its wing. The ventral edge of the ridge connecting the protocone to the metaconule lies antero–externally to the hypoconulid and entoconid (Fig. 1A). As a result, small shearing surfaces (6) are present on the postero–lingual surface of the protocone and antero–external surface of the hypoconulid and entoconid.

MOLARS OF MAMMALS OF METATHERIAN–EUTHERIAN GRADE

Several Cretaceous mammals cannot be classified with certainty as either Eutheria or Metatheria. These have molars which have characteristics which can be regarded as slightly more advanced or less advanced than those of the primitive hypothetical tribosphenic molars described above.

Aegialodon and Kielantherium

The Wealden *Aegialodon* from Great Britain (Kermack *et al.*, 1965) and the

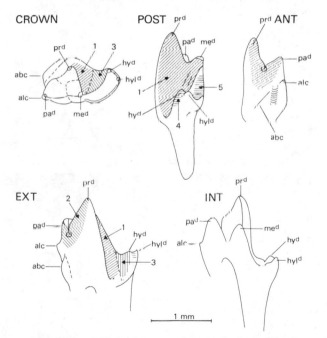

FIG. 2. Lower molar (?M$_2$ of *Kielantherium gobiensis*, Geological Institute, Academy of Sciences of Mongolia, Ulan Bator (IG) PST 10–4, from Dashzeveg (1975). In order to facilitate comparisons with the remaining drawings in this chapter, the posterior and external views have been reversed. See Fig. 1 for abbreviations.

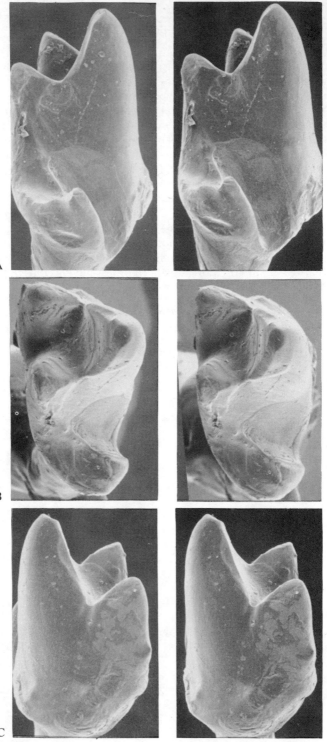

Aptian Mongolian *Kielantherium* (Figs 2 and 3) recently described by Dashzeveg (1975) are known only from isolated lower molars. In comparison with the hypothetical form the talonid is shorter, narrower bucco–lingually, shearing surface 4 is miniscule and the entoconid is apparently absent. The paraconid is slightly taller than the metaconid. This is associated with the fact that in primitive therians the paracone is higher and better developed than the metacone and a large paraconid was needed to form an inner border for the food "trap" (Crompton, 1974).

Kermackia

The Trinity *Kermackia* and the unnamed molar type 6 (Slaughter, 1965, 1971), are intermediate in structure between *Aegialodon* and *Kielantherium* on the one hand and *Pappotherium* on the other.

Pappotherium

The molars of the *Pappotherium* (Fig. 4) from the Albian Trinity sandstone have been discussed by several authors, including Patterson, 1956; Slaughter, 1965, 1971; Turnbull, 1971; Crompton, 1971. Slaughter considers them to be eutherian but we are not convinced and have, therefore, included them in this section (see Butler, 1977). Lower molars were collected from the same site as *Pappotherium* and have been described, figured and referred to as *Pappotherium* (Slaughter, 1971) but because they were not found in association, we have not included them in Fig. 4. *Pappotherium* upper molars differ from the hypothetical ancestral type in that the conules are not winged and, therefore, shearing surfaces 3b and 4b are absent but other than this they are almost identical to those of the hypothetical molars illustrated in Fig. 1.

Deltatheridium

In some aspects the molars of this genus (Fig. 5) from the ?Late Santonian and or ?Early Campanian and Middle Campanian of Mongolia (Gregory and Simpson, 1926; Butler and Kielan Jaworowska, 1973; Kielan-Jaworowska, 1975b; Gradziński *et al.*, 1977) are slightly less advanced than the hypothetical molar illustrated in Fig. 1, in that the conules are not winged, shearing surface 1b is poorly developed, shearing surface 2b is absent, the talonid is slightly smaller and lacks a medial wall external to the basin for the protocone and shearing surfaces 3 and 4 are slightly smaller. However, there is one important advance in *Deltatheridium* –shearing surface 2 is considerably larger and this has been achieved by extending the metastylar region much further postero–externally. Cusp "c" is absent and shearing surface 2 extends to the metastyle. A well developed shearing surface 1a is apparently a primitive feature and the enlargement of shearing surface 2 and slight enlargement of the metacone is, as already pointed out (Butler and Kielan-Jaworowska, 1973) reminiscent of the marsupials. *Deltatheridium*

FIG. 3. Scanning electron microscope stereo-photographs of ?M_2 of *Kielantherium gobiensis*, IG PST 10–4, × 45 (from Dashzeveg, 1975). A—posterior view, B—crown view and C—anterior view.

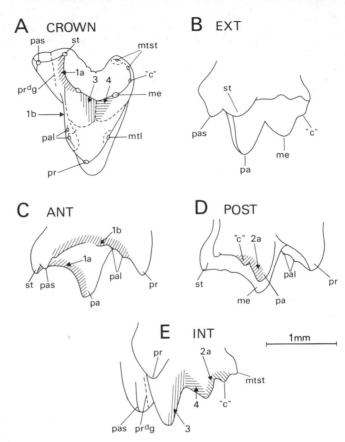

FIG. 4. Upper molar (?M²) of *Pappotherium pattersoni*, Shuler Museum of Paleontology, Southern Methodist University, Dallas (SMP-SMU) 71725. For abbreviations, see Fig. 1.

has an enlarged single-rooted canine and short skull, and this, and the powerful shearing surface 2 as well as the well developed shearing surface 1 indicate that *Deltatheridium* was specialized for a more carnivorous mode of life than the other Mongolian Cretaceous mammals. Although this genus possesses other features which are reminiscent of marsupials (Kielan-Jaworowska, 1975b) such as the dental formula and construction of the snout, it has been concluded that this genus should not be included in either the Eutheria or Metatheria. It is interesting to point out that the molars of some of the Tertiary paleoryctids such as *Didelphodus* (Crompton, 1971) and *Gelastops* are similar to those of *Deltatheridium* and to derive the molars of these paleoryctids from those of *Deltatheridium* it would only be necessary to increase the size of the talonid and protocone and develop wings to the conules. However, these paleoryctids have a eutherian dental formula and

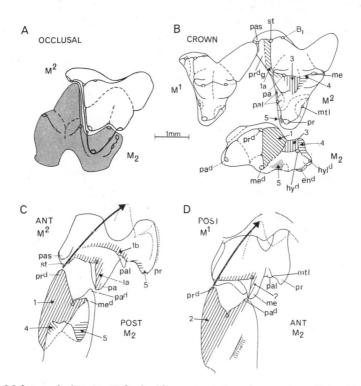

FIG. 5. Molar occlusion in *Deltatheridium pretrituberculare tardum*, Palaeobiological Institute of the Polish Academy of Sciences, Warsaw (ZPAL) MgM-I/91. (From Kielan-Jaworowska, 1975b). For abbreviations, see Fig. 1.

Deltatheridium cannot be regarded as ancestral to them. Fox (1974) designated *Deltatheroides* sp. an upper molar from the upper part of the Edmonton Formation of Alberta and a lower molar from the Lance Formation of Wyoming. As we do not know the dental formulae of forms to which these isolated teeth belong, and as very similar teeth may occur in some paleoryctids, the presence of the Deltatheridiidae in the Late Cretaceous of North America remains an open question.

EUTHERIAN MAMMALS

Asioryctes

In *Asioryctes* (Fig. 6) from the Campanian of Mongolia we pick up the initiation of a trend which is typical of most Late Cretaceous therians, namely a tendency to narrow the stylar shelf, so that in crown view the paracone and the metacone appear to have migrated towards the external border. Accompanying this is a tendency, especially in forms with a tall paracone, for shearing surface 1a to decrease in size and importance. This is the case in

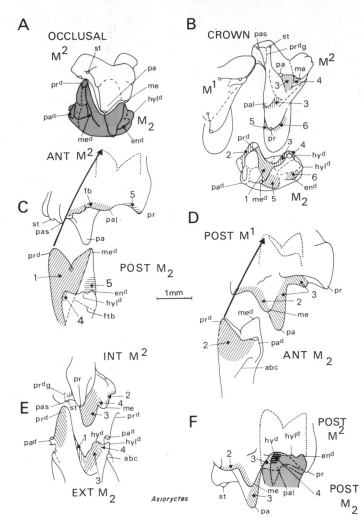

FIG. 6. Molar occlusion in *Asioryctes nemegetensis*, ZPAL MgM-I/73. For abbreviations see Fig. 1.

Asioryctes where the paracrista (Fig. 6C) shows no signs of wear and shearing on the front of the upper molar is limited to surface 1b. Because shearing surface 1a is absent, the metaconid is greatly increased in height so that food to be sheared could be effectively trapped between this cusp and the para-conule. The upper molar is relatively shorter antero–posteriorly and relatively transversely elongated in comparison with the hypothetical primitive molar (Fig. 1). This is presumably related to the well developed transverse shearing

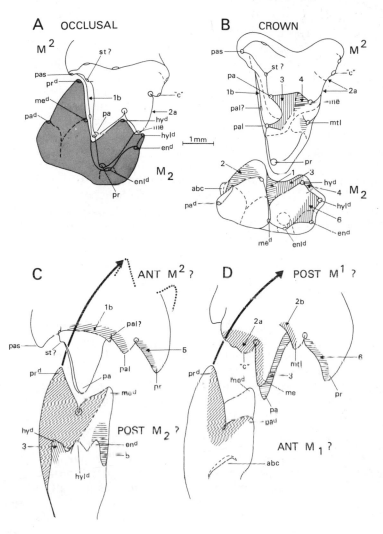

FIG. 7. Molar occlusion in *Cimolestes incisus*. Partially based upon M1, American Museum of Natural History, New York (AMNH) 58813; M2, AMNH 58802; M2, AMNH 59357. enl^d = entoconulid; for rest of abbreviations, see Fig. 1.

surfaces 1b and 5 and the small size of the metacone and associated shearing surfaces. Other than this, the only significant difference between *Asioryctes* and those of a hypothetical primitive molar is that the hypoconid bites against the edge of the trigon right at the point where a metaconule would be expected; consequently this conule is small and if it was present, was rapidly destroyed by wear. Accompanying the reduction or absence of the metaconule is the absence of shearing surface 2b. As a result of this contact, the hypoconid is visible in posterior view when the teeth are in occlusion (Fig. 6F). The metacone is exceptionally small and shearing surface 4 is very small. A medial wall to the talonid is absent and the protocone extends slightly beyond the internal edge of the talonid when the teeth are in occlusion. The entoconid and hypoconulid extend far above the medial floor of the talonid, and consequently shearing surface 6 on the antero–external surface of the hypoconulid and entoconid is well developed. The embrasure between two successive upper molars is narrow and the trigonid cusps, as seen in crown view, form a more acute angle than is the case in the hypothetical primitive molars. In the latter, the metaconule is fairly well developed and the hypoconid bites anterior to this cusp. *Asioryctes* may have been derived from forms which have molars similar to those shown in Fig. 1 of the hypothetical form simply by shifting the point of contact of the hypoconid. It is, however, possible that *Asioryctes* was derived from a form with molars slightly more primitive than those illustrated in Fig. 1 and in which a metaconule was not present and the metacone was still a minor cusp. *Asioryctes* appears to be closely related to the rather common North American Cretaceous genus *Cimolestes* (Fig. 7) and it is likely that these genera were derived from a common ancestor.

Cimolestes

Occluding upper and lower teeth of this genus (Figs 7 and 8) have not been described, but lower teeth have been assigned to this genus (Clemens, 1973; Lillegraven, 1969). In this genus all the shearing surfaces on the molars are well developed and the molars can be derived without difficulty from the hypothetical primitive molars shown in Fig. 1. As in *Asioryctes*, the paracone and the metacone are both extremely tall and situated fairly close to the outer edge of the tooth. The paracrista does not serve as a cutting edge for shearing surface 1a in slightly worn teeth and, as in *Asioryctes*, the functional shearing surface on the front of the molar is limited to 1b. In worn teeth a facet continuous with 1b spreads on to the anterior surface of the paracone. As would be expected, the metaconid is relatively high. The protocone extends only a short distance beyond the paraconule and fits into a deep pit in the talonid basin when the teeth are in occlusion. Shearing surface 2a is well developed and extends from the tip of the metacone to the metastylar region. A cusp "c" is still present on the leading edge of the shearing surface. Because the metacone is so tall and because its antero–posterior edge forms a large part of shearing surface 2a, the paraconid need not be as high as the metaconid. Shearing surface 2b and the metaconule are small. The molars of this genus accentuate vertical shear (surfaces 1 and 2) and judging from the high pointed cusps, including the paracone, puncture crushing was also important. The teeth were not well adapted for crushing, shearing surfaces 3 and 4 are present, and

FIG. 8. Stereo-photographs of the upper and lower molars in *Cimolestes incisus*. A—crown view of M², AMNH 58814; B—anterior view of M², AMNH 58802; C—posterior view of M¹, AMNH 58813; D—oblique (postero–external) crown view of M₂, AMNH 59357. All × 10.

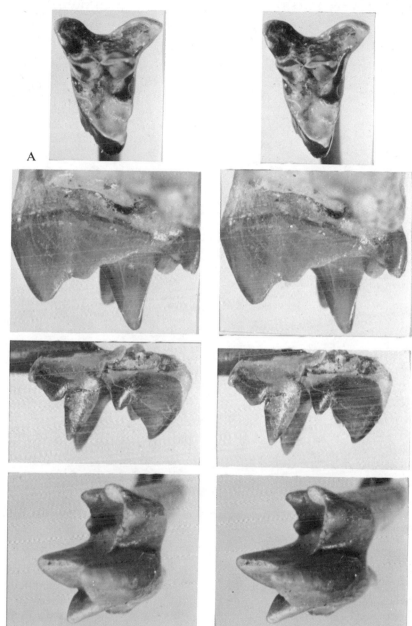

A

B

C

D

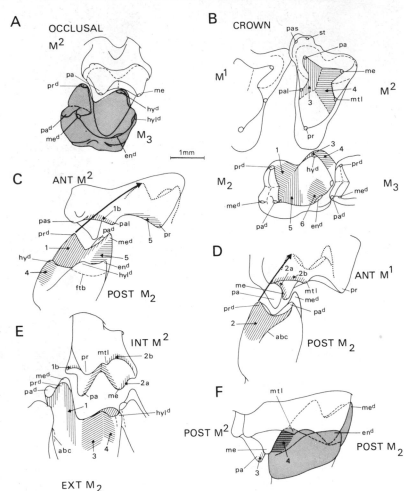

FIG. 9. Molar occlusion in *Zalambdalestes lechei*, ZPAL MgM-I/43. For abbreviations, see Fig. 1.

although the paraconule is winged, this does not always appear to be true for the metaconule. *Cimolestes* molars are well adapted for a carnivorous mode of life. The molars of this genus could well be derived from a mammal with molars of the type illustrated in Fig. 1 by slightly modifying the relative proportions and height of the cusps, and no major change in the pattern of jaw movements need be suggested. It does not seem possible to derive *Cimolestes* molars from those of *Asioryctes* because the molars of the latter

FIG. 10. Stereo-photographs of the upper and lower molars in *Zalambdalestes lechei*, ZPAL MgM-I/14 × 6.

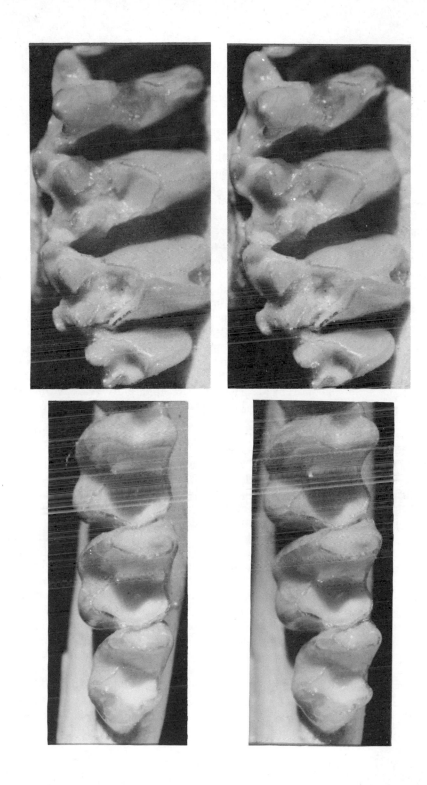

are a little too specialized in that the metaconid is considerably reduced and the metaconule is rapidly destroyed by wear. Unfortunately, we were not in a position to describe the occlusal pattern of *Procerberus* (Sloan¦and van Valen, 1965; van Valen, 1969, 1970) but it appears to be similar to that of *Cimolestes*.

Zalambdalestes

The molars of this genus (Figs 9 and 10) are the most aberrant of the Mongolian Late Cretaceous therian mammals (Gregory and Simpson, 1926; Simpson, 1928; Kielan-Jaworowska, 1969). The characteristic feature of these teeth is the enlargement of the talonid and matching area of the trigon. Coupled with this feature one finds a greatly enlarged hypoconid, which wears a wide groove (shearing surfaces 3 and 4) between the metacone and paracone, and a fairly high entoconid and medial wall to the talonid basin. The trigon and talonid basins are extensively worn and superficially it looks as if the lower talonid was drawn across the trigon during the power stroke. For this reason, the molars appear to be adapted for grinding. However, this is not the case. It is possible, based on the shape of the wear facets on the upper and lower molars to determine the path of movement of the lower molars during the power stroke. Although this path is considerably more oblique than in other ? Campanian Mongolian mammals, there is no evidence to support the view that the lower molars were dragged across the uppers after unilateral centric occlusion had been reached (Crompton and Hiiemae, 1970). Dorsomedial movement of the lowers apparently ceased when the molars came into this position. They are, therefore, adapted for crushing rather than for grinding. Nevertheless, shearing continues to play an important role. This is demonstrated by the fact that the trigonid is still fairly high relative to the talonid and fits into a deep embrasure between successive upper molars (see Fig. 10). The paracone and metacone are placed near the outer edge of the tooth and are lower than in other Campanian mammals. Shearing surface 1a is lost entirely, but 1b is retained. In order to form an efficient food trap for holding food to be sheared between 1b on the upper and 1 on the lower, the metaconid must be almost as high as the protoconid (see Fig. 9C). In order to provide the large crushing surface the protocone lies far medially of the paraconule and consequently the matching surfaces of the metaconid (5) are large. Shearing surface 2a is very small, because the metacone is situated so far laterally, but 2b is relatively well developed and the paraconid is nearly as high as the protoconid. In order for the matching surfaces to remain in contact during the power stroke, it was necessary for the upper surface of the lower jaws to rotate in a medial direction about their longitudinal axes (when viewed from behind) before the beginning of the power stroke. However, the path followed by the lower teeth during the power stroke was essentially the straight line. These early mammals presumably had mobile symphysis and symphysial movement was probably typical of all Cretaceous therians. The molars of the ?Middle Campanian Mongolian genus *Barunlestes* (Kielan-Jaworowska, 1974a) are almost identical to those in *Zalambdalestes* and the former was probably descended from the latter.

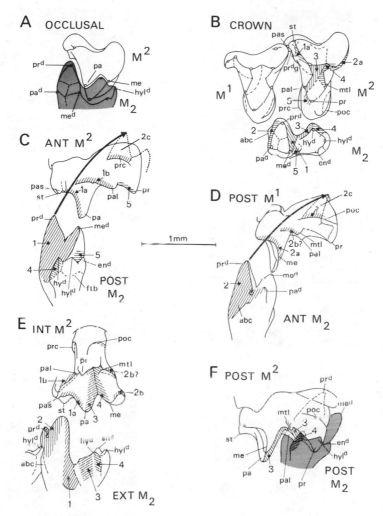

FIG. 11. Molar occlusion in *Kennalestes gobiensis*. The drawings are based on ZPAL MgM-I/1 and ZPAL MgM-I/5. poc = postcingulum; prc = precingulum; for rest of abbreviations, see Fig. 1.

Kennalestes

This genus (Figs 11 and 12) is perhaps the most interesting of the Mongolian Cretaceous mammals (Kielan-Jaworowska, 1969, 1975a). The basic structure of the molars, except for one notable advance, hardly differs at all from those of the hypothetical type illustrated in Fig. 1. The paracone and metacone are slightly nearer the external edge of the molar and considerably higher, and in this respect are not unlike those of *Cimolestes*. The advanced feature

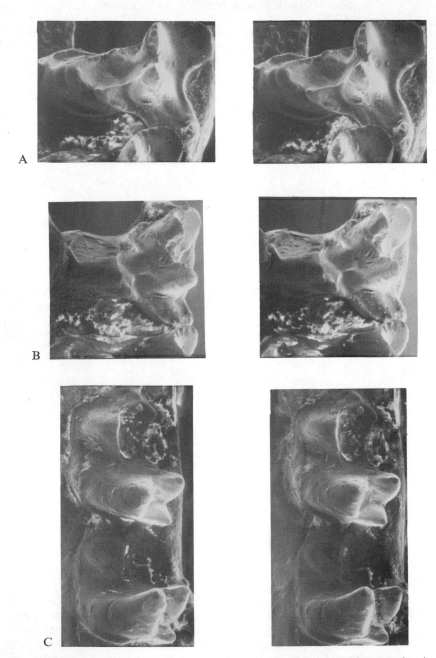

FIG. 12. Scanning electron microscope stereo-photographs of upper and lower molars in *Kennalestes gobiensis*. A—left M^2 in coronal view; B—the same in lingual view; C—right M$_1$ and M$_2$ coronal view; ZPAL MgM-I/1. All × 15.

of *Kennalestes* is the presence of pre- and postcingula, the postcingulum is considerably longer and wider than the precingulum. The postcingulum tends to widen in a medial direction, a shearing surface is present on the posterior surface of the external half of the postcingulum (Fig. 11D). The high protocone shears past this part of the cingulum, whereas the nearly flat occlusal surface of the paraconid appears to bite against the inner part of the postcingulum. The precingulum has a faint shearing surface on its anterior surface, this appears to have been formed by the posterior surface of the trigonid (shearing surface 1). In many of the Late Cretaceous therians of North America, such as *Gypsonictops*, *Protungulatum*, *Purgatorius* and the isolated molar from the upper part of the Milk River Formation figured by Fox (1970), molars with pre- and postcingula are considerably enlarged, and they could all be derived from ancestral forms which possessed molars of the *Kennalestes* type. There are, however, other Late Cretaceous forms such as *Procerberus* (Sloan and van Valen, 1965; van Valen, 1970) and some species of *Cimolestes* (Lillegraven, 1969) in which pre- and postcingula are present. The overall structure of the molars of these latter forms are not unlike those of *Kennalestes* and it suggests one of two possibilities: that the various *Cimolestes* species were derived from forms such as *Kennalestes* and some of the species retained the cingula, whereas the majority lost them, or that pre- and postcingula were independently developed in some species of *Cimolestes* and other genera such as *Procerberus*. Be this as it may, the molars of all species of *Cimolestes* and those of *Procerberus* and *Kennalestes* are so similar in basic structure that they could all be derived with little modification from the hypothetical molars illustrated in Fig. 1.

Gypsonictops

The upper molars of this genus (Figs 13 and 14) are characterized by a great increase, especially the medial part, in the size of the postcingulum. Based upon the orientation of the groove for the protoconid, the movement of the lower molar during the power stroke was far more horizontal than in *Kennalestes*. The reduction in the size of the parastylar region appears to be related to this change in direction. Consequently, *Gypsonictops*, like *Zalambdalestes*, lacks the large hook-shaped parastyle which was character-istic of the early hypothetical molars and most of the other Cretaceous molars with a vertically oriented power stroke. The paracone is reduced in height, is laterally placed, and shearing surface 1a is lost or rudimentary. However, 1b and the precingulum are extensively worn. The protocone in this genus is large and meets the floor of the talonid at the end of power stroke. The talonid floor and the matching surface on the upper crown are often exten-sively worn. The leading edge of shearing surface 2a is nearly vertical and situated near the outer edge of the tooth, and 2b is considerably reduced in extent. A groove for the protoconid is present in the lateral part of the postcingulum but the heavily worn occlusal surface of the more medial aspect of the postcingulum and the heavily worn tip of the paraconid, suggest that these two matching surfaces function as additional crushing areas.

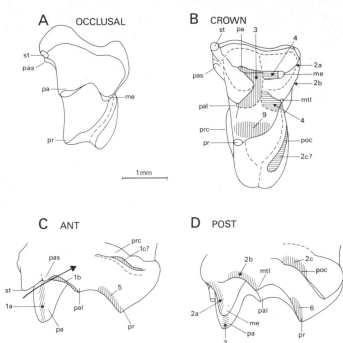

FIG. 13. Upper molar in *Gypsonictops hypoconus*, MCZ 188867. poc = postcingulum; prc = precingulum; for rest of abbreviations, see Fig. 1.

Shearing surfaces 3a and 4a are well developed and both the shearing surfaces on the inner surfaces of the conules are prominent features in moderately worn upper molars.

A detailed analysis of the morphology of the molars and occlusion in this form have been given by Kay and Hiiemae (1974). They have claimed that in this genus it is possible to divide the power stroke into two phases, Phases I and II. During Phase I, shearing surfaces 1–6 are used and this phase is terminated with the protocone being forced into the talonid basin (unilateral centric occlusion). During Phase II the teeth remain in contact but the direction of movement of the lower jaw changes to downwards and slightly antero–medially. During this phase new sets of wear facets are introduced and these involve the floor of the talonid being drawn across the trigonid (grinding) and the occlusal surface of the trigonid across the expanded part of the upper crown between shearing surface 6 and the medial part of the postcingulum. These new facets (surfaces 9 and 10) are only poorly developed in *Gypsonictops* because Phase II forms an insignificant part of the masticatory cycle. However, in *Purgatorius* (Sloan and van Valen, 1965; Clemens, 1974) and in later primates such as *Palenochtha*, *Pelycodus* and *Aegyptopithecus* (Hiiemae and Kay, 1973; Kay and Hiiemae, 1974) it is possible to observe an

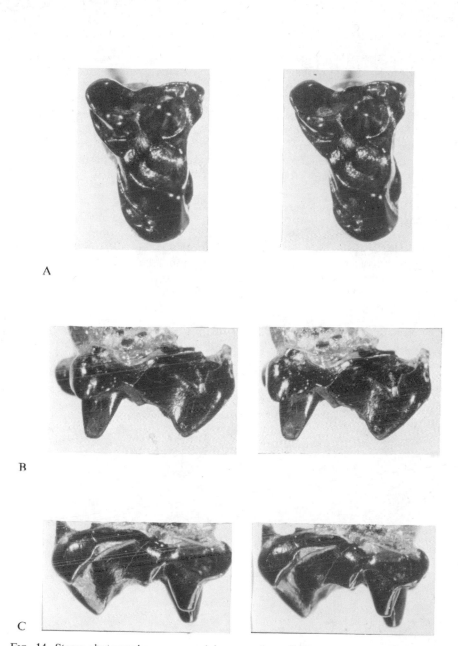

A

B

C

FIG. 14. Stereo-photographs, upper and lower molars of *Gypsonictops hypoconus*. A—crown; B—anterior; C—posterior view of M², Museum of Comparative Zoology, Harvard University (MCZ) 18867. All × 15.

increase in size of those features associated with both crushing and/or pulping (the talonid and trigonid) and grinding (Phase II, involving trigon and talonid, the postcingulum and expansion of the upper molar medial to the protocone and hypocone). Coupled with this is a decrease in the area of the molars involved with transverse shear (surfaces 1 and 2).

Gypsonictops molars can readily be derived from those of *Kennalestes* and we have in this form the initial development of features which were destined to be considerably enlarged in the molars of eutherian herbivorous and omnivorous mammals of the latest Cretaceous and later Tertiary.

Protungulatum

In this genus (Figs 15 and 16) we encounter a great increase in the complexity of the structure of the crown pattern of the upper molars comparable to that of *Purgatorius* (Sloan and van Vȧen, 1965; van Valen, 1969; Szalay, 1969). Shearing surfaces 1–6 are still the most important structures for the breaking down of food but their relative sizes and positions relative to one another have changed quite dramatically in this form. The pre- and postcingula are

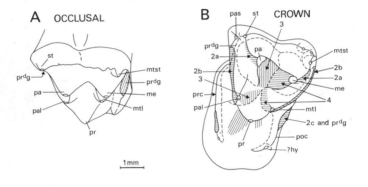

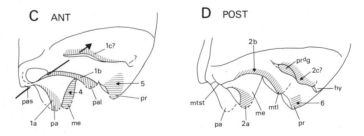

FIG. 15. Upper molar in *Protungulatum donnae*, Yale Peabody Museum (YPM) 21400. poc = postcingulum; = prc = precingulum; for rest of abbreviations, see Fig. 1.

FIG. 16. Stereo-photographs of M² and M₂ in *Protungulatum donnae*. A—crown; B—anterior; C—posterior view of YPM 21400; D—oblique (postero-external) crown view of YPM 24512. All × 10.

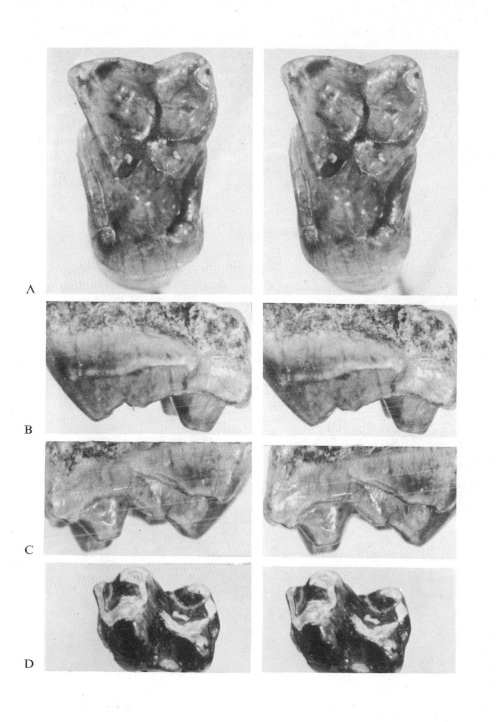

A

B

C

D

extremely large and a separate cusp, the hypocone, is present on the medial edge of the postcingulum. It is likely that, as in the case of *Gypsonictops*, this genus and a closely related form such as *Purgatorius* could both have been derived from a *Kennalestes* type. The major modifications of the crown structure in *Protungulatum* suggest jaw movements far more complex than the simple movements in the Cretaceous therians described above. *Gypsonictops*, *Purgatorius* and *Protungulatum* are the beginning of a complex radiation of molar types which are characteristic of the Paleocene and later Tertiary.

A detailed analysis of molar occlusion and jaw movement in *Purgatorius* and *Protungulatum* can only be undertaken when the abundant material of these genera has been described.

MARSUPIALS (METATHERIA)

Holoclemensia

Holoclemensia (Fig. 17) from the Albian Trinity Sandstone of Texas is regarded by Slaughter (1968b, c) as the oldest known marsupial (but see, Butler, 1977). Its identification as a marsupial is to a large extent based upon the presence of a large stylar cusp C (i.e. mesostyle, not to be confused with "c" on the metacrista), a slightly enlarged metasylar region (as compared with that of the contemporary *Pappotherium*) and a metacone also relatively larger than that of *Pappotherium*. In Fig. 17, an attempt has been made to reconstruct the penultimate molar of the genus *Holoclemensia*. Lower molars have been identified by Slaughter as belonging to this genus and these have been used

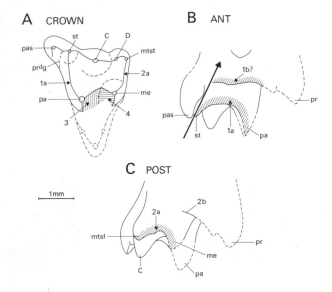

FIG. 17. Upper molar (?M³) of *Holoclemensia texana*, SMP-SMU 62009. C and D = marsupial stylar cusps (Bensley, 1906); for rest of abbreviations, see Fig. 1.

to reconstruct the penultimate upper molar. What is striking about the penultimate molar of *Holoclemensia* is that except for the special feature mentioned above, the general organization of the molars is not unlike that of *Pappotherium* or the hypothetical upper molar illustrated in Fig. 1. The parastyle is large and hooked, and the paracone is large and lingually situated, so that shearing surface 1a is extremely large. Shearing surface 1b was apparently also present, indicating the presence of a paraconule (present in the ultimate molar). Shearing surface 2a is moderately well developed and there is a suggestion of cusp "c" on shearing surface 2a. Shearing surface 2b appears to be rudimentary.

Alphadon

In Figs 18 and 19, the upper M^3 of the best known Cretaceous marsupial *Alphadon* is illustrated. This tooth is characterized by a relatively large

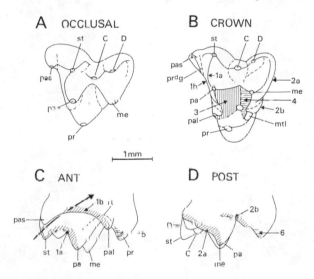

FIG. 18. Upper molar (?M³) of *Alphadon*, MCZ 8084. C and D = marsupial stylar cusps; for rest of abbreviations, see Fig. 1.

metacone, a well developed shearing surface 2 and a relatively wide trigon. This latter feature and the matching surface on the lower molar provide a crushing surface which is enlarged in later didelphids. This early marsupial, therefore, had teeth well adapted for both crushing and shearing, but with a tendency to develop shearing surface 2 to equal or surpass surface 1.

In Cretaceous marsupials this tendency is more marked in some species of *Alphadon* (i.e. *A. lulli* and *A. rhaister*) than in others (i.e. *A. marshi* and *A. wilsoni*) and is particularly marked in the genera of *Pediomys*, *Glasbius* and *Didelphodon*. In *Alphadon* the steep walls of shearing surfaces 3, 4, 5 and 6 form effective traps so that food was sheared and crushed between the trigon

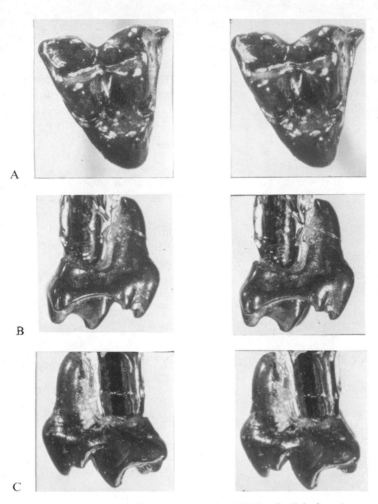

Fig. 19. Stereo-photographs of an upper molar (?M³) of *Alphadon*. A—crown; B—anterior; C—posterior view; MCZ 8085. All × 15.

roof and talonid floor and was prevented by these walls from being forced away from the impact areas. As would be expected, the ridges running medially from the hypoconid and laterally from the protocone are extensively worn before wear spreads onto the concave areas which those ridges border. The plunger type crushing and accentuating of shearing surface 2 sets the Cretaceous marsupials apart from the remaining therians. There is no evidence of Phase II facets (i.e. no grinding in the sense of a lower molar being dragged across an upper). It is of great interest to point out that the molars of *Alphadon* and their occlusal relationship are fairly close to

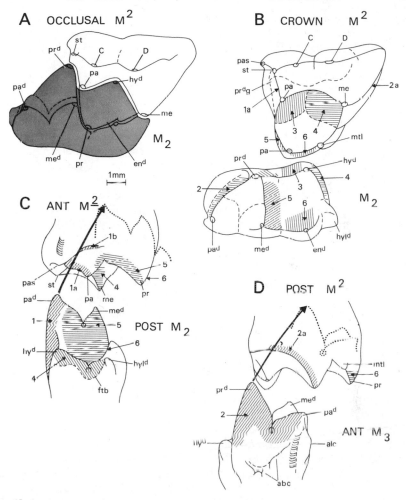

FIG. 20. Molar occlusion in *Didelphis marsupialis*, YPM 5500. C and D = marsupial stylar cusps; for rest of abbreviations, see Fig. 1.

those of the modern North American opossum *Didelphis marsupialis* (Fig. 20). Significant differences are, however, that in *Didelphis*, the paracone and shearing surface 1a are considerably reduced and the paraconule is lost, but a remnant of 1b remains. Because of the reduction of 1a and the paracone, the cristid obliqua on the lower molars has migrated outwards and most of the posterior wall of the trigonid meets the anterior surface of the enlarged protocone area (surface 5, Fig. 20C). The metacone is increased in size and shearing surface 2a is relatively larger than in *Alphadon*. Shearing surface 2b is lost and the metaconule is reduced or absent. The study of wear facets and extensive cinefluorographic studies have confirmed that in *Didelphis marsupialis* the lower jaw moves upwards and inwards at a steep angle during the power stroke of mastication and no further transverse movement takes place after the floor of the talonid basin has come to rest against the protocone (unilateral centric occlusion).

The molars of Late Cretaceous marsupials retain most of the features present in Early Cretaceous to Middle Cretaceous mammals.

CONCLUSIONS

In Table II an attempt has been made to present the tentative phylogeny of the known Cretaceous therian mammals. The oldest known therian mammal *Aegialodon* from the Lower Wealden of Great Britain (Kermack *et al.*, 1965) possesses a basic tribosphenic pattern, having a poorly basined talonid and presumably an incipient protocone. It is in some respects intermediate between the Jurassic pantotheres, such as *Peramus*, and the more advanced Cretaceous therians. The primitive structure characteristic of *Aegialodon* is retained in Aptian *Kielantherium* (Fig. 2) from Asia (Dashzeveg, 1975) and with some modifications in Albian therians from Texas, such as *Pappotherium* and *Kermackia* (Slaughter, 1971). In the Aptian beds of Asia (personal communication from Dr B. A. Trofimov), coeval with *Kielantherium*, there occur mammals, designated by Dr Trofimov as *Prokennalestes* and *Prozalambdalestes*, but they have not been described as yet. The molar teeth of these forms apparently lack marsupial features such as large stylar cusps and are tentatively considered as eutherians.

A primitive family of mammals, the Deltatheridiidae, occurs in the Late Cretaceous of Asia (?Santonian and ?Campanian) and although this family has a marsupial dental formula, it has been classified as belonging to Theria of a metatherian–eutherian grade (Butler and Kielan–Jaworowska, 1973; Kielan-Jaworowska, 1975b). The molars of the Deltatheridiidae can readily be derived from forms whose molars have the basic tribosphenic pattern such as that of *Aegialodon* or *Kielantherium*. Marsupials are not known from the Late Cretaceous of Asia. The Late Cretaceous Asian radiation of eutherian mammals could be derived from the Early Cretaceous Asian genera such as *Prozalambdalestes* and *Prokennalestes*. *Prokennalestes* (personal communication, Dr B. A. Trofimov), which lacks the pre- and postcingula may well be an ancestor of both *Kennalestes* and *Asioryctes*. Poorly known *Prozalambdalestes* is regarded by Dr Trofimov as an ancestor of the highly specialized Late Cretaceous genus *Zalambdalestes*; however, *Zalambdalestes* might also be derived from *Prokennalestes*. The descendants of the Zalambdalestidae are not known.

In the Albian of North America, in contradistinction to the conditions in Asia, there are no forms which can be unequivocally classified as belonging to the eutherian mammals. We do not accept Slaughter's (1968a, 1971) view to the contrary (see Butler, 1977). In addition to the primitive mammals with molars of a metatherian–eutherian grade, such as *Pappotherium*, *Kermackia* and unnamed lower molars, there also occurs in Texas the genus *Holoclemensia*, considered by Slaughter (1968b) to be the oldest known marsupial.

Marsupials appear to have evolved in North (Clemens, 1968) or South America (Tedford, 1974) or in Australia (Kirsch, 1977) during the early Cretaceous. *Holoclemensia* may be tentatively regarded as close to the ancestors of the Late Cretaceous North American marsupials. *Potamotelses* from the upper part of the Milk River Formation, described by Fox (1972) as a primitive therian might also be a marsupial. From the same formation Fox (1970) has also described a single upper molar which he classified as belonging to a eutherian mammal. This tooth has well developed pre- and postcingula and it cannot be ruled out that it is from a eutherian mammal; its origin is unknown. The better known Late Cretaceous North American eutherian genera make their appearance on that continent in the Middle Campanian; the oldest is *Gypsonictops* which is probably related to the Asiatic *Kennalestes*. The remainder of North American "eutherian" mammals are possibly also of Asiatic origin, although many of the known forms are slightly too specialized to be regarded as directly ancestral to North American forms, e.g. *Asioryctes* cannot be directly ancestral to *Cimolestes*, but it is very likely that this form and the closely related *Procerberus* could be derived from the Asian stock giving rise to *Asioryctes*. The latest Cretaceous North American eutherian radiation, represented by the genera *Gypsonictops*, *Protungulatum*, *Purgatorius* and others may be easily derived from forms closely related to the Asian *Kennalestes* or the ancestral stock.

It has been shown by one of us (Kielan-Jaworowska, 1970, 1974b) that during the Late Cretaceous, one-way migration of multituberculates took place from Asia to North America. It has been suggested in the same paper that in addition to the multituberculates some eutherian mammals also invaded North America from Asia during the Late Cretaceous. The Asiatic origin of North American eutherian mammals had been suggested earlier by Lille graven (1969). Our current studies on the molar occlusion of Cretaceous therian mammals support the previous hypothesis on the Asian origin of the North American Late Cretaceous eutherian mammals. Whether all the North American eutherians are of Asiatic origin remains, however, for the time being an open question. The distinction drawn between marsupials and placentals is based upon reproduction rather than minor differences in dental structure (Lillegraven, 1974) and we agree with his view that it is extremely difficult for this reason to unequivocally assign the earliest therians to either the Eutheria or Metatheria and that some of the Cretaceous mammals may have evolved features which are not characteristic of either of these groups.

If one views the evolution of therians (excluding pantotheres and symmetrodonts) during the Cretaceous, what is so remarkable is that the basic tribosphenic pattern of the molar teeth underwent so little change during a period of over 100 million years. It is only in some of the more advanced forms occurring during the Late Cretaceous, such as *Gypsonictops*, *Protungulatum* and *Purgatorius*, that the molar structure was modified and even in these forms the basic pattern is still clearly recognizable. This appears to indicate that jaw movements and the way in which molar teeth were used remained much the same during most of this period and it is only towards the Cretaceous and during the early part of the Tertiary that several advanced types of feeding patterns can clearly be recognized by the structure of the molar teeth such as specializations for grinding and shearing.

Tribosphenic molars are ideal for an omnivorous diet which involves a combination of puncturing, shearing and crushing; they are not highly specialized and do not appear to be capable of shearing/grinding. The basic tribosphenic pattern has been retained in the Northern American marsupial *Didelphis marsupialis*. Feeding of this form has been extensively studied with the aid of cinefluoroscopy and electromyography.

On the basis of these studies it is possible to divide the masticatory cycle when the molars are being actively used, into four somewhat arbitrary divisions. During the first division (preparatory stroke) the jaws close rapidly and are brought into contact with the food. During the second division (power stroke) the food is punctured, crushed or sheared. During the third division the jaw opens slightly and during the fourth (recovery) it opens further and at a faster rate. The movement of hyoid and tongue are closely correlated with these divisions which are based upon jaw positions during the masticatory cycle. Also, when the molar teeth are brought into unilateral centric occlusion (i.e. with the protocone engaging the talonid basin), no further lateral movement of the jaw takes place, i.e. there is no evidence for a grinding phase (i.e. Hiiemae and Kay's (1973) Phase II is absent). In the recent work of one of us (Crompton) on opossum mastication, we were able to correlate the electrical activity of individual muscles with specific portions of the masticatory cycle. During rhythmic chewing and at the end of the second division (i.e. the power stroke) in the case of both puncture crushing, when the molars do not come into occlusion, and shearing when they reach unilateral centric occlusion, there is an abrupt cessation of electrical activity in all the adductor musculature from which recordings have been made (i.e. several parts of the temporalis, the superficial masseter and internal ptery-goids). This abrupt cessation of electrical activity is thought to coincide with a sudden termination of an adductor force across the molars.

These EMG recordings confirm the observations based on cinefluoroscopy that after unilateral centric occlusion has been reached in the opossum the lower molars are not dragged across the uppers in a grinding stroke. Hiiemae and Kay (1973) and Kay and Hiiemae (1974) have recorded the presence of Phase II wear facets in the Late Cretaceous therian mammals, *Gypsonictops* and *Protungulatum*. Phase II facets can also be observed in other Early Tertiary herbivores and primates but they are not as marked and as deeply scarred as shearing surfaces 1–6. If Phase II facets are associated with grinding (i.e. further medial movements of the active mandible), it would imply a continuation of the contractile force of the adductor musculature beyond unilateral centric occlusion during rhythmic mastication. Modification of the basic tribosphenic pattern for grinding involves not only a reduction and modification of Phase I facets but changes those parts of the crown associated with Phase II facets, i.e. the protocone area, the talonid and the pre- and postcingula areas of the crown. It is possible that the conservative nature of the molars and jaw movement in Cretaceous therians may, in part, be related to the abrupt cessation of power stroke once unilateral centric occlusion was reached and that it was only possible to develop effective grinding when it was possible to maintain pressure between the molars while at the same time dragging the active lower jaw medially. This change in the programming of the muscles of mastication may have evolved only in the Late Cretaceous and may prove to be an important factor in the diversity of molar structure and feeding patterns which characterize mammalian evolution during the Tertiary. What is needed are accurate data correlating occlusal relations and jaw positions with simultaneous EMG recordings from the jaw musculature on several herbivorous and carnivorous mammals during normal mastication.

SUMMARY

The structure and occlusal details of most of the Cretaceous therian mammalian molars have been described and discussed. The distribution of therians in time and space during this period has been summarized. It is virtually only in the vast collections of therian skulls from the ?Santonian and Campanian that matching upper and lower molars are known. The description of the molars of these mammals formed the bulk of this chapter and provided a model for the description of isolated molars of other Cretaceous therians. On the basis of molar structure alone tentative suggestions about the relationships and phylogeny of Cretaceous therians were made. It was concluded that although early therian mammals probably had a near world-wide distribution during Late Jurassic and Early Cretaceous times, metatherians (i.e. marsupials) appeared to have evolved in North or South America or Australia during this period, whereas eutherians (i.e. placentals) appeared to have evolved in Asia and migrated to Europe and North America sometime during the later half of the Cretaceous. It cannot, however, be proven at the present time that all American eutherians are of Asiatic origin. It was shown that the basic tribosphenic pattern of the therian molar, except for that of a few genera occurring towards the end of the Cretaceous (i.e. *Gypsonictops*, *Protungulatum* and *Purgatorius*) underwent relatively little change during this period. The changes in these Late Cretaceous genera appeared to be related to a shift from molars capable only of puncturing, shearing and crushing to those capable also of grinding (i.e. moving the lowers in a medial direction across the uppers.). It was suggested that this advance might be related not only to a modification of the crown structure, but also to important modifications in the control and organization of the muscles of mastication.

ACKNOWLEDGEMENTS

The following persons and institutions provided one or both of us with facilities to study the specimens in their charge: Professor A. W. Clemens (University of California, Berkeley), Dr D. Dashzeveg (Laboratory of Stratigraphy and Paleontology, Geological Institute, Academy of Sciences of the Mongolian People's Republic, Ulan Bator), Professor R. C. Fox (University of Alberta, Edmonton), Professor M. C. McKenna (American Museum of Natural History, New York), Professor B. H. Slaughter (Southern Methodist University, Dallas), Dr B. A. Trofimov (Paleontological Institute USSR Academy of Sciences, Moscow) and Dr W. D. Turnbull (Field Museum of Natural History, Chicago).

Professors A. W. Clemens, R. C. Fox, J. A. Lillegraven and M. C. McKenna kindly read the section "Records of Cretaceous Therian Mammals" and offered useful criticism. When this contribution was read at the IV International Symposium on Dental Morphology, Cambridge, in September, 1974, we learned that Professor P. M. Butler (Royal Holloway College, London) had been working on the problem of interrelations of Cretaceous eutherian mammals on the basis of their dentition, and had reached conclusions which in most points agreed with ours. Professor P. M. Butler kindly sent us his notes, but it was too late to introduce discussions of his views into our chapter.

The line drawings were inked by Mrs P. Chaudhuri (Museum of Comparative Zoology, Harvard University, Cambridge), the scanning electron microscope photographs published as Figs 3 and 12 were taken by Mr G. R. Pierce and Mr. E. Seling (Harvard University), and the remaining photographs by Mr A. Coleman (Harvard University).

To all these persons and institutions we wish to express our deep gratitude.

REFERENCES

BASHANOV, V. S. (1972). First Mesozoic Mammalia (*Beleutinus orlovi* Bashanov) from the USSR. *Teriologiya*, Akademiya Nauk SSR, Sibirskoe Otdelenie. **1**, 74–80 (in Russian with English summary).

BELIAJEVA, E. I., TROFIMOV, B. A. and RESHETOV, V. J. (1974). General stages in evolution of late Mesozoic and early Tertiary mammalian fauna in central Asia. *In* "Mesozoic and Cenozoic faunas and biostratigraphy of Mongolia" (Kramerenko, N. N. *et al.*, eds), Vol. 1, pp. 19–45. The Joint Soviet-Mongolian Paleontological Expedition, Moscow (in Russian with English summary).

BENSLEY, A. B. (1906). The homologies of the stylar cusps in the upper molars of the Didelphidae. *Univ. Toronto Stud. Biol. Ser.* **5**, 148–159.

BUTLER, P. M. (1952). The milk-molars of Perissodactyla, with remarks on molar occlusion. *Proc. Zool. Soc. Lond.* **121**, 777–817.

BUTLER, P. M. (1961). Relationships between upper and lower molar patterns. International Colloquium on the evolution of lower and non specialized mammals. *Kon. Vlaamse Acad. Wetensch. Lett. Sch. Kunsten Belgie.* Part I, 115–126.

BUTLER, P. M. (1977). The Trinity therians reconsidered. *Breviora* (in press).

BUTLER, P. M. and KIELAN-JAWOROWSKA, Z. (1973). Is *Deltatheridium* a marsupial? *Nature, Lond.* **245**, 105–106.

CLEMENS, W. A., Jr. (1966). Fossil mammals of the type Lance Formation, Wyoming. Part II. Marsupialia. *Univ. Calif. Publ. Geol. Sci.* **62**, 1–222.

CLEMENS, W. A., Jr. (1968). Origin and early evolution of marsupials. *Evolution* **22**, 1–18.

CLEMENS, W. A., Jr. (1973). Fossil mammals of the type Lance Formation, Wyoming. Part III. Eutheria and Summary. *Univ. Calif. Publ. Geol. Sci.* **94**, 1–102.

CLEMENS, W. A. Jr. and MILLS, J. R. E. (1971). Review of *Peramus tenuirostris* Owen (Eupantotheria, Mammalia). *Bull. Br. Mus. nat. Hist. (Geol.)* **20**, 89–113.

CLEMENS, W. A., Jr. (1974). *Purgatorius*, an early paromomyid primate (Mammalia). *Science, N. Y.* **184**, 903–905.

CLEMENS, W. A., Jr. and RUSSELL, L. S. (1965). Mammalian fossils from the Upper Edmonton Formation. *In* "Vertebrate Paleontology in Alberta". *Univ. Alberta Bull. Geol.* **2**, 32–40.

CROMPTON, A. W. (1971). The origin of the tribosphenic molar. *In* "Early mammals" (Kermack, D. M. and Kermack, K. A. eds). *Suppl. No. 1. Zool. J. Linn. Soc.* **50**, 65–87.

CROMPTON, A. W. (1974). The dentitions and relationships of the Southern African Triassic mammals, *Erythrotherium parringtoni* and *Megazostrodon rudnerae*. *Bull. Brit. Mus. nat. Hist. (Geol.)* **24**, 7, 397–473.

CROMPTON, A. W. and HIIEMAE, K. M. (1970). Molar occlusion and mandibular movements during occlusion in the American opossum, *Didelphis marsupialis* L. *J. Linn. Soc. (Zool.)* **49**, 21–47.

CROMPTON, A. W. and JENKINS, F. A. (1973). Mammals from reptiles: a review of mammalian origins. *In* "Annual Review of Earth and Planetary Sciences", Vol. 1, pp. 131–155. Annual Reviews Palo Alto, U.S.A.

DASHZEVEG, D. (1975). *Kielantherium gobiensis*, a primitive therian from the Early Cretaceous of Mongolia. *Nature, Lond.* **256**, 402–403.

FOX, R. C. (1970). Eutherian mammal from the Early Campanian (Late Cretaceous) of Alberta, Canada. *Nature, Lond.* **227**, 630–631.

FOX, R. C. (1971). Marsupial mammals from the Early Campanian Milk River Formation, Alberta, Canada. *In* "Early Mammals" (Kermack, D. M. and Kermack, K. A. eds). *Suppl. No. 1 Zool. J. Linn. Soc.* **50**, 145–164.

FOX, R. C. (1972). A primitive therian mammal from the Upper Cretaceous of Alberta. *Can. J. Earth Sci.* **9**, 11, 1479–1494.

FOX, R. C. (1974). *Deltatheroides*—like mammals from the Upper Cretaceous of North America. *Nature, Lond.* **249**, 5455, 392?

GRADZINSKI, R. KIELAN-JAWOROWSKA, Z. and MARYANSKA, T. (1977). Upper Cretaceous Djadokhta, Barun Goyot and Nemegt formations of Mongolia, including remarks on previous subdivisions. *Acta Geol. Poloncia* **27**, no. 3 (in press):

GRAMBAST, L., MARTINEZ, M., MATTAUER, M. and THALER, L. (1967). *Perutherium altiplanense*, nov gen., nov. sp., premier Mammifere Mesozoique d'Amerique du Sud. *C. r. Acad. Sci. Ser.* D. **264**, 5, 707–710.

GREGORY, W K. and SIMPSON, G. G. (1926). Cretaceous mammal skulls from Mongolia. *Am. Mus. Novit.* **225**, 1–20.

HIIEMAE, K. M. and CROMPTON, A. W. (1971). A cinefluorographic study of feeding in the American opossum *Didelphis marsupialis*. *In* "Dental Morphology and Evolution" (Dahlberg, A. A. ed.). University of Chicago Press, Chicago, U.S.A.

HIIEMAE, K. M. and JENKINS, F. A., Jr. (1969). The anatomy and internal architecture of the muscles of mastication in *Didelphis marsupialis*. *Postilla* **140**, 1–49.

HIIEMAE, K. M. and KAY, R. F. (1973). Evolutionary trends in the dynamics of primate mastication. *Symp. Int. Cong. Primatol.* **3**, 28–64.

KAY, R. F. and HIIEMAE, K. M. (1974). Jaw movement and tooth use in recent and fossil primates. *Am. J. phys. Anthrop.* **40**, 227–256.

KERMACK, K. A., LEES, P. M. and MUSSETT, F. (1965). *Aegialodon dawsoni*, a new trituberculosectorial tooth from the lower Wealden. *Proc. R. Soc. Lond.* B. **162**, 535–554.

KIELAN-JAWOROWSKA, Z. (1969). Preliminary data on the Upper Cretaceous eutherian mammals from Bayn Dzak, Gobi Desert. Results Pol. Mong. Palaeontol. Exped. I. *Palaeontol. Pol.* **19**, 171–191.

KIELAN-JAWOROWSKA, Z. (1970). New Upper Cretaceous multituberculate genera from Bayn Dzak, Gobi Desert. Results Pol. Mong. Palaeontol. Exped. II. *Palaeontol. Pol.* **21**, 35–49.

KIELAN-JAWOROWSKA, Z. (1974a). Multituberculate succession in the Late Cretaceous of the Gobi Desert (Mongolia). Results Pol. Mong. Palaeontol. Exped. V. *Palaeontol. Pol.* **30**, 23–44.

KIELAN-JAWOROWSKA, Z. (1974b). Migrations of the Multituberculata and the Late Cretaceous connections between Asia and North America. *Ann. S. Afr. Mus.* **64**, 231–243.

KIELAN-JAWOROWSKA, Z. (1975a). Preliminary description of two new eutherian genera from the Late Cretaceous of Mongolia. Results Pol. Mong. Palaeontol. Exped. VI. *Palaeontol. Pol.* **33**, 5–16.

KIELAN-JAWOROWSKA, Z. (1975b). Evolution of the therian mammals in the Late Cretaceous of Asia Part I. Deltatheridiidae. Results Pol. Mong. Palaeontol. Exped. VI. *Palaeontol. Pol.* **33**, 103–132.

KIRSCH, J. A. W. (1977). The six-percent solution: second thoughts on the adaptedness of the Marsupialia. *Am. Scient.* **65**, 276–288.

KREBS, B. (1971). Evolution of the mandible and lower dentition in dryolestids (Panthotheria, Mammalia). *In* "Early Mammals" (Kermack, D. M. and Kermack, K. A. eds). *Suppl. No. 1. Zool. J. Linn. Soc.* **50**, 89–102.

LEDOUX, J. C., HARTENBERGER, J. L., MICHAUX, J., SUDRE, J. and THALER, L. (1966). Découverte d'un Mammifère dans le Crétacé supérieur a Dinosaures de Champ-Garimond près de Fons (Gard). *C. r. Acad. Sci.* Sér. D. **262**, 18, 1925–1928.

LILLEGRAVEN, J. A. (1969). Latest Cretaceous mammals of the upper part of the Edmonton Formation of Alberta, Canada and review of marsupial-placental dichotomy in mammalian evolution. *Paleont. Contr. Univ. Kansas* **50**, 1–122.

LILLEGRAVEN, J. A. (1972). Preliminary report on late Cretaceous mammals from the El Gallo Formation, Baja California del Norte, Mexico. *Contr. Sci. nat. Hist. Mus. Los Angeles*, **232**, 1–11.

LILLEGRAVEN, J. A. (1974). Biogeographical considerations of the marsupial-placental dichotomy. *A. Rev. Ecol. Syst.* **5**, 74–95.

LILLEGRAVEN, J. A. (1976). A new genus of therian mammal from the Late Cretaceous "El Gallo Formation", Baja California, Mexico. *J. Paleont.* **50**, 437–443.

MCKENNA, M. C. (1969). The origin and early differentiation of therian mammals. *Ann. N. Y. Acad. Sci.* **167**, 1, 217–240.

MILLS, J. R. E. 1964. The dentitions of *Peramus* and *Amphitherium*. *Proc. Linn. Soc. Lond.* **175**, 2, 117–133.

MILLS, J. R. E. 1966. The functional occlusion of the teeth of Insectivora. *J. Linn. Soc. (Zool.)* **47**, 1–25.

PATTERSON, B. (1956). Early Cretaceous mammals and the evolution of mammalian molar teeth. *Fieldiana (Geology)* **13**, 1, 1–105.

RUSSELL, L. S. (1952). Cretaceous mammals of Alberta. *Ann. Rep. Nat. Mus. Canada Bull.* **126**, 110–119.

RUSSELL, L. R. (1962). Mammal teeth from the St. Mary River Formation (Upper Cretaceous) at Scabby Butte, Alberta. *Nat. History Papers Nat. Mus. Canada.* **14**, 1–4.

SAHNI, A. (1972). The vertebrate fauna of the Judith River Formation, Montana. *Bull. Am. Mus. nat. Hist.* **147**, 6, 325–412.

SHIKAMA, T. (1947). *Teilhardosaurus* and *Endotherium*, new Jurassic Reptilia and Mammalia from the Husin coal-field, South Manchuria *Proc. Jap. Acad.* **23**, 76–84.

SIGÉ, B. (1972). La faunule de mammifères du Crétacé supérieur de Laguna Umayo (Andes péruviennes). *Bull. Mus. nat. Hist. Nat.* Sér. 3 **99**, 375–405.

SIMPSON, G. G. (1928). Further notes on Mongolian Cretaceous mammals. *Am. Mus. Novit.* **329**, 1–9.

SIMPSON, G. G. (1945). The principles of classification and a classification of mammals. *Bull. Am. Mus. nat. Hist.* **85**, 1–350.

SIMPSON, G. G. (1951). American Cretaceous Insectivores. *Am. Mus. Novit.* **1541**, 1–9.

SLAUGHTER, B. H. (1965). A therian from the Lower Cretaceous (Albian) of Texas. *Postilla* **93**, 1–18.

SLAUGHTER, B. H. (1968a). Earliest known eutherian mammals and the evolution of premolar occlusion. *Texas J. Sci.* **20** (1), 3–12.

SLAUGHTER, B. H. (1968b). Earliest known marsupials. *Science, N.Y.* **62**, 254–255.

SLAUGHTER, B. H. (1968c). *Holoclemensia* instead of *Clemensia*. *Science, N.Y.* **162**, 1306.

SLAUGHTER, B. H. (1971). Mid-Cretaceous (Albian) therians of the Butler Farm local fauna, Texas. *In* "Early Mammals" (Kermack, D. M. and Kermack, K. A., eds). *Suppl, No 1 Zool. J. Linn. Soc.* **50**, 131–143.

SLOAN, R. E. and RUSSELL, L. S. (1974). Mammals from the St. Mary River Formation (Cretaceous) of Southwestern Alberta. *Life Sci. Contr. R. Ont. Mus.* **95**, 1–20.

SLOAN, R. E. and VAN VALEN, L. (1965). Cretaceous mammals from Montana. *Science, N.Y.* **148**, 220–227.

SZALAY, F. S. (1969). Origin and evolution of function of the mesonychid condylarth feeding mechanism. *Evolution* **23**, 703–720.

TEDFORD, R. H. (1974). Marsupials and the new paleogeography. Paleogeographic provinces and provinciality. *Soc. Econ. Paleont. Mineral.* Spec. Publ. **21**, 109–126.

TURNBULL, W. D. (1971). The trinity therians: their bearing on the evolution of marsupials and other therians. *In* "Dental Morphology and Evolution" (Dahlberg, A. A. ed.) pp. 151–179. University of Chicago Press, Chicago, U.S.A.

VAN VALEN, L. (1969). The multiple origins of the placental carnivores. *Evolution* **23**, 118–130.

VAN VALEN, L. (1970). An analysis of developmental fields. *Devl. Biol.* **23**, 3, 456–477.

VAN VALEN, L. and SLOAN, R. E. (1965). The earliest primates. *Science, N.Y.* **150**, 3697, 743–745.

19. Relationship between Natural Selection and Dental Morphology: Tooth Function and Diet in *Lepilemur* and *Hapalemur*

DANIEL SELIGSOHN

and

FREDERICK S. SZALAY

Hunter College, City University of New York, U.S.A.

INTRODUCTION

If biologists (in the broadest sense) were to give one overriding reason for the study of an organism, then surely an "ultimate" explanation of a species would not lie in its genetics, morphology, function or physiology only. It would probably involve an explanation which would (a) first place into causal relationships the specific biological features of this species and the selective forces responsible for their evolution, and (b) the sum total of these interactions, i.e. the role of this organism in its environment would become defined. Generally speaking, this is the "ultimate" goal of many evolutionary biologists, and the proper order of the questions asked is what, how, why and when. When one is asking a series of questions, however, it is a rare instance indeed that the biological role of various aspects of an organism can be understood before the varied attributes are recognized and described, and explained on a functional (i.e. either chemical or physical–mechanical) level. Only after the mechanical functions of character complexes are understood can the study of the biological roles of these features proceed based on adequate foundations (Bock and von Wahlert, 1965).

The separation of the study of mechanical functions and biological roles of any character on an operational level is clearly artificial. An organism is a unit, and any one part of it is unable to function independently. Rather, it should be viewed in relation to the whole, function always occurring in a given experimental context. Yet the practice of asking questions on different levels of organization and studying different aspects of characters is a necessary prerequisite to understanding the whole.

This study of two lemurids ideally illustrates the relationships between morphology, mechanical function and biological roles. *Lepilemur* and *Hapalemur* represent closely related, small herbivores in which the noted morphological differences cannot be explained in terms of either "zoophagy" or "phytophagy," but rather by differences in consistency between their respective preferred food substances and their manner of food handling and mastication. The morphological differences of the cheek teeth and the corresponding inferred mechanical divergence in the masticatory cycle is distinctive. Another important reason for the study of these closely related taxa is that their feeding habits are reasonably well established. Additional reasons, rather than being general in nature, are more specific to the study of phylogenetic reconstruction within the Strepsirhini and will be viewed in another context elsewhere. Taking living species, with due consideration given to recent studies of mammalian jaw movements and tooth morphology (worn and unworn), we can perform a mechanical analysis of dried specimens and, in turn, these studies can be effectively correlated with diet in the species. Eventually, through similar studies, prediction about fossil taxa can be made more reliable than it is possible at present.

We believe there is one simple, but major lesson to be learned from an increasingly greater awareness of the adaptive aspects of dentition. Rather than being concerned with a crown pattern or dentition being "herbivorous," "insectivorous," or whatever the student might more profitably concentrate on the paths of adaptive shifts and, consequently, on the causality for these changes. This forces an awareness of the genealogy of the taxon studied and therefore necessitates the inquiry to be within the confines of the most plausible phylogenetic hypothesis. The fullest explanations we suggest, therefore, lie within the grasp of those efforts which attempt to deal with phylogenetic reconstruction, mechanical function, and associated biological roles.

Of the living Strepsirhini, the family Lemuridae (*sensu stricto*) is perhaps the most primitive in overall morphology when compared to other living strepsirhines or to the Holarctic fossil Adapidae. All the four known groups of lemurids (*Lepilemur*, *Hapalemur*, *Lemur* and *Varecia*) are primarily phytophagous (Jolly, 1972; Martin, 1972), taking relatively little animal food in their habitats. In a previous study of *Lemur* spp. and *Varecia* sp. (Seligsohn and Szalay, 1974) we attempted to show how differing emphasis in aspects of the chewing stroke in the two groups can be correlated with hardness of the bulk of the diet, known in most species of *Lemur* and predicted, at that time, in the only living species of *Varecia*. In that study we attempted to test the reliability of utilizing morphology, wear patterns and inferred masticatory function of the dentition to predict, at least broadly, the texture of preferred foods.

As in the previous study, our aim in examining *Lepilemur* and *Hapalemur* is to sharpen a method of predicting diet in fossils by the study of tooth morphology and facets via the inferred mechanical function emphasized in a given species.

The size of the animal is only a very general guide to broad dietary prediction of living or fossil forms. The immense number of small, phytophagous rodent specialists; the equally small, varied, yet similar-sized metatherian carnivorous and insectivorous species which are primarily zoophagous; the extreme specializations among similar-sized chiropterans; the folivory of *Lepilemur* and *Gorilla*, differing greatly in size; and the habitual bamboo diet of *Ailuropoda* as well as *Hapalemur*, equally divergent in size, are all remarkable examples casting doubt on overall size as a predictive tool for fossils. Although tooth size relative to body size may be utilized for predictive purposes, the notorious lack of record for the latter parameter among fossils, particularly for small forms, limits the significance of this approach.

MATERIALS AND METHODS

Dietary data on *Lepilemur* and *Hapalemur* were obtained from the published field studies of Petter and Peyrieras (1970) and Hladik and Charles-Dominique (1972) and will be summarized below.

Molar and premolar morphology and wear were studied by stereomicroscopy on the following dry specimens from the collection at the American Museum of Natural History: *Lepilemur mustelinus leucopus:* AMNH 170553, 170554, 170567, 170572, 170563, 170575, 170576 and 170573; *Hapalemur griseus olivaceous:* AMNH 170689, 170682, 100629, 100628 and 170672. Drawings in occlusal and distal view were made using a camera lucida attached to a Wild M5 stereoscope.

Hiiemae and Kay (1973) and Kay and Hiiemae (1974) have recently reliably correlated wear features with mandibular movements during the puncture-crushing and chewing phases of mastication. This facilitated occlusal analyses which involved superimposing scale drawings of the upper and lower dentitions over a light box and moving the lowers in directions suggested by the faceted wear. This method was checked against hand-simulated "mastication" with dried skulls.

DIETARY SPECIALIZATIONS IN *Lepilemur* AND *Hapalemur*

The diet of *Lepilemur mustelinus leucopus* is nutritionally quite marginal, consisting mainly of the highly fibrous leaves of *Alloudia* and *Tamarindus indicus* (Charles-Dominique and Hladik, 1971). The flowers of *Alloudia* are also eaten during the dry season. Since the initial nutritive content of its ingested food is very low, *Lepilemur* must resort to caecotrophy to assimilate additional nutrients made available during the first digestive phase.

Hapalemur griseus griseus was reported (Petter and Peyrieras, 1970) to subsist mainly on young shoots and leaves of bamboo. These authors suggest that this animal displays a distinctive manner of feeding which includes running a bamboo stem across the tooth rows and, with rapid jaw movements, initially puncture-crushing the stem with the last premolar teeth.

Milton (personal communication) has observed that when captive *Hapalemur* at the Duke University Primate Research Facility feed on bamboo shoots provided them, they initially run the stems across the back of their upper canines, stripping off the tough outer layers of tissue. The remaining stem is then conveyed to the premolars and molars, where, with a rapid "champing" action of the jaw, the stem is finally "crushed".

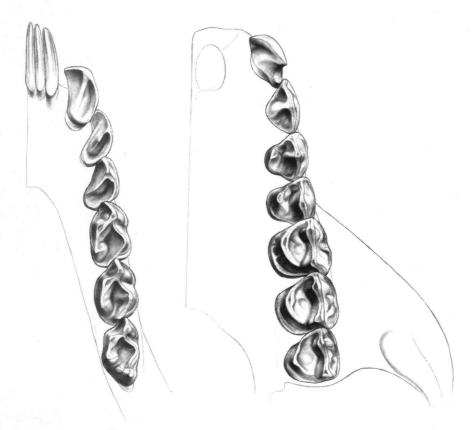

FIG. 1. Occlusal view of the relatively unworn upper and lower dentitions of *Lepilemur*. Both figures are from AMNH 170575. Right: entire upper left dentition. Left: entire lower right dentition. See text for discussion of morphology.

POSTCANINE MORPHOLOGY

The antemolar and molar dentitions of both *Lepilemur* and *Hapalemur* are fully illustrated in Figs 1 and 2. We will only discuss below those dental features which apparently reflect significant functional differences between the dentitions of the two taxa.

Lepilemur mustelinus

The upper and lower tooth rows as well as the ectoloph and ectolophid

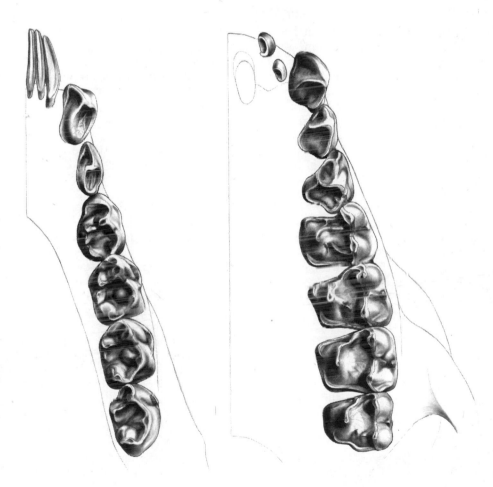

FIG. 2. Occlusal view of the relatively unworn upper and lower dentitions of *Hapalemur*. Both figures are from AMNH 170672. Right: entire upper left dentition. Left: entire lower right dentition. See text for discussion of morphology.

crests of this species are virtually linearly arranged, while PM^4 and PM$_4$ are premolariform. The molar teeth are characterized by: cusps which are of moderate relief and acuity, squat and mesio-distally elongated; crests which are extensive, emphasize a mesio-distal orientation, and which, during occlusion, emphasize a pattern of reciprocal curvature and/or differential orientation characteristic of *horizontal point cutting* (see p. 307); and basins which are mesio-distally broad and unconfined with planar surfaces. During centric occlusion, there is relatively little overlap of the ectolophids by the ectolophs.

Hapalemur griseus

In this species, the upper and lower tooth rows, along with their ectoloph and ectolophid crests, assume a more curvilinear arrangement. The PM^4 and PM$_4$ are highly derived and are the most molariform of the postcanine teeth. The teeth within the PM$_4^4$–M$_3^3$ region emphasize: cusps which are conical and of greater relief and acuity; crests which are less extensive, emphasize a more bucco-lingual orientation, and which, during occlusion, emphasize a pattern of reciprocal curvature and/or differential orientation more characteristic of *vertical point cutting* (see p. 307); and basins that are basically deep, round, well confined and concave. With centric occlusion, there is relatively extensive ectoloph overlap of the ectolophids.

Dental Wear

Figures 3 and 4 illustrate the relief and effect of wear on the molar dentitions of *Hapalemur* and *Lepilemur*, while Fig. 5 shows the patterns of faceted wear. Both dental abrasion and faceted wear differ in these two genera. In *Lepilemur*, buccal phase faceted wear is strikingly evident. Throughout ontogeny this faceted wear maintains and generates very extensive and finely honed enamel cutting edges as it transects the very well developed system of molar crests. Buccal phase faceting does not maintain crown relief ontogenetically, however.

Dental abrasion in *Lepilemur*, by contrast, is not very evident. Very light scratches and fine pitting may be found for example in the molar basins, but this wear has no appreciable adverse impact on the enamel cutting edges, nor does it mask the faceted wear. Consistent with these observations, dentine exposures are only shallowly recessed from the enamel surrounding them.

In *Hapalemur*, buccal phase faceting is somewhat less extensive. Because of the molar morphology, this faceted wear often fails to either maintain or generate well honed leading edges of enamel, especially on the lower molars and on the upper molar protocones. Buccal phase faceting, however, does appear to contribute towards the maintenance of crown relief throughout ontogeny.

Dental abrasion in *Hapalemur* is most dramatically evident. Leading edges of enamel are rounded off, and heavily and coarsely pitted while the slopes beneath them are vertically scratched. Basins are also heavily pitted and

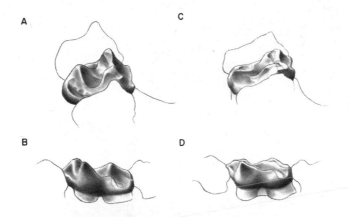

FIG. 3. This figure illustrates the relief and effect of wear in the molar dentition of *Lepilemur*. A. Distal view of lightly worn upper left M^2 of AMNH 170576. B. Lingual view of lightly worn lower right M_2 of AMNH 170576. C. Distal view of more heavily worn upper left M^2 of AMNH 170553. D. Lingual view of more heavily worn lower right M_2 of AMNH 170553.

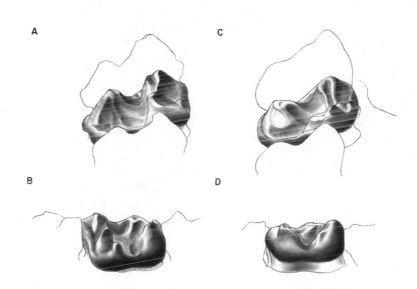

FIG. 4. This figure illustrates the relief and effect of wear in the molar dentition of *Hapalemur*. A. Distal view of lightly worn upper left M^2 of AMNH 170672. B. Lingual view of lightly worn lower right M_2 of AMNH 170672. C. Distal view of more heavily worn upper left M^2 of AMNH 100629. D. Lingual view of more heavily worn lower right M_2 of AMNH 100629.

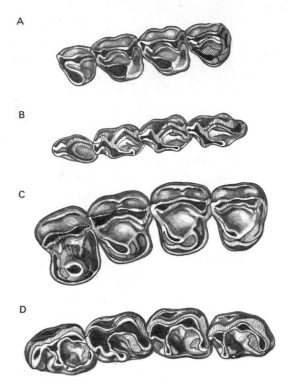

Fig. 5. Patterns of faceted dental wear in *Hapalemur* and *Lepilemur*. Faceted enamel wear is indicated by hatching, the direction of the hatching reflecting the direction of the striations found on these facets. Exposed dentine is shown as solid black. All figures are from moderately worn specimens and are in occlusal view. From top to bottom: *Lepilemur*: A. a composite of faceted wear seen in left PM^4–M^3 of AMNH 170553 and AMNH 170567; B. a composite of faceted wear seen in right PM$_4$–M$_3$ of AMNH 170553 and 170554. Note the extensive development of enamel cutting edges around exposures of dentine, created by buccal phase faceting. *Hapalemur*: C. pattern of faceted wear seen in left PM^4–M^3 of AMNH 100629; D. pattern of faceted wear seen in right PM$_4$–M$_3$ of AMNH 100629. Note the failure of many buccal phase facets to either transect exposures of dentine, or intersect leading edges of enamel.

scratched. The magnitude of dental abrasion is also evident in the nature of exposed dentine, which is greatly recessed beneath the surrounding enamel, and in the relatively greater extent to which buccal phase faceting is obliterated.

FUNCTION

With their recent cinefluorographic studies Crompton and Hiiemae (1970), Hiiemae and Crompton (1971), Kallen and Gans (1972), Hiiemae and Kay (1973), and Kay and Hiiemae (1974) have demonstrated that mammals possessing relatively primitive molar morphology consistently exhibit two definable phases of mastication, which may be called puncture-crushing and chewing. The basic kinematic characteristics of these two phases are fairly stereotyped among those primates thus far investigated. Puncture-crushing involves a relatively more orthal movement of the mandible, and results in the more vertical apposition of cusps and basins. This phase is associated with the preliminary reduction of an ingested mass of food, and basically involves the point penetration and incusion of ingested material. Tooth–food–tooth contact is the rule during this phase. Dental abrasion, consisting of rounded, pitted and scratched enamel and "basined-out" exposed dentine, has now been reliably correlated (Kay and Hiiemae, 1974) with tooth function during the puncture-crushing phase of mastication. Chewing involves a more transverse movement of the mandible and includes two phases: the buccal phase, during which the lower molars initially contact the uppers and then move dorso-lingually, ultimately achieving centric occlusion; and the lingual phase, in which the lower molars move ventro-linguo-mesially out of centric occlusion until occlusal contact with the upper molars is terminated. Chewing ultimately involves tooth–tooth contact and results in the occlusion of molar cutting edges (and possibly grinding surfaces). During this phase, food is thus more finely reduced by cutting and possibly grinding. Striated and faceted dental wear (variously called attritional or thegotic), especially along the leading molar crests, has now been strongly correlated with the cine-fluorographically observed movements of the mandible during chewing (Kay and Hiiemae, 1974).

With this background of information, it is possible to reliably establish the relative movements of the upper and lower premolars and molars in *Lepilemur* and *Hapalemur*, thereby opening the way for a sound functional interpretation of the dental morphology in these two genera. Puncture-crushing may be performed by both genera, but the dental abrasion bearing evidence of this is markedly different in each taxon. In *Hapalemur*, as previously mentioned, abrasion is most dramatic, appearing as coarse pitting along the leading edges of enamel and at the bottoms of the basins of the premolars and molars. The slopes of cusps are vertically scored, while dentine exposures are greatly ablated, so that they recede dramatically from surrounding walls of enamel. Leading edges of enamel are invariably blunt and rounded. This evidence certainly strongly indicates a heavy reliance on relatively orthal mandibular movements during puncture-crushing.

Signs of abrasion in *Lepilemur* are, by contrast, minimal. The dentine exposed at the apices of the protocones are only shallowly basined out, and pitting of enamel, if it does occur, is extremely fine. Leading enamel cutting edges are not discernibly affected by abrasion. We can conclude that puncture-crushing in *Lepilemur* plays only an incidental role in mastication.

Striated, faceted dental wear in these two genera also differs, and in some respects quite dramatically. Nonetheless, this wear indicates that buccal and lingual phase chewing movements in both *Lepilemur* and *Hapalemur* are essentially similar. Buccal phase faceting, as described and illustrated above, bears striations which indicate a basically dorso-lingual movement of the mandible in both genera, while discernibly striated lingual phase faceting indicates a ventro-mesio-lingual shift in mandibular movement in each genus. When viewed in the occlusal plane, mandibular movement during the lingual phase is deflected from that of buccal phase by about 45° in both *Hapalemur* and *Lepilemur*.

FUNCTIONAL MORPHOLOGY
Mechanical Function

The data on dental morphology and movement were combined so that a full functional appreciation of the dentitions of *Lepilemur* and *Hapalemur* could be obtained. To facilitate this, the scale drawings of the dental batteries, including those indicating faceted wear, were consulted. Using a light box, scale drawings of the upper and lower dentitions were superimposed over and moved relative to each other, on the basis of the kinematic data given above. The dried skulls of each genus were also used in simulated mastication as a check against the functional patterns that emerged from the "occlusion diagram" technique.

The following functional patterns emerged for the postcanine dentitions of *Hapalemur* and *Lepilemur*.

Hapalemur: Puncture-Crushing. During this phase, the apposing, and relatively steep-sided, cusps, crests and basins are optimally aligned. As the mandible closes in nearly orthal fashion the tall conical protocones are driven into the spacious and well defined talonid basins, while the cristid obliquas drive upwards past the steep, notched, lingual walls of the ectolophs, ultimately penetrating the trigon basins. At the same time the extraordinarily prominent and robust entoconids are thrust past and fit snugly against the distal slopes of the rotated protocones, ultimately lodging in disto-lingual extensions of the trigon basins situated at the bases of the distal slopes of the protocones. The very tall, steep-sided protocristids meanwhile course vertically past the relatively sharp-edged preprotocristas and ultimately lie against the steep mesial walls of the latter feature.

The mechanical actions produced during the "puncture-crushing" phase in *Hapalemur* may be interpreted as exaggerated point penetration, crushing and, especially, crest penetration (or punching).

Chewing. During chewing, the occlusal relationships indicated above are modified by the greater transverse component in the movement of the mandible. The buccal phase possesses enough of a transverse component to upset the fine engagement of cusps and basins seen during the more orthal "puncture-crushing" phase. Ironically, however, the buccal phase in large part only repeats the mechanical actions seen in the "puncture-crushing" phase. While the ectolophs and ectolophids, and protocones and metaconids occlude along areas bearing buccal phase faceting, relatively little of this occlusion involves well honed cutting edges. Hence, the buccal phase results, not in efficient cutting, but in point and crest penetration or punching. Because of the greater bucco-lingual orientation of occluding crests and their

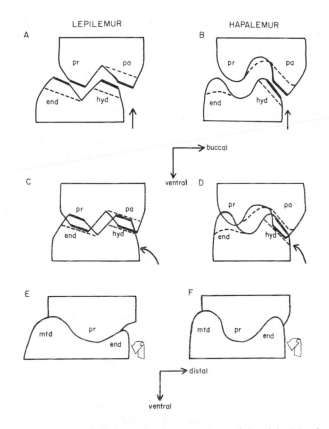

FIG. 6. A, C and B, D represent schematic cross-sections of the right M^1_1 of, respectively, *Lepilemur* and *Hapalemur* as viewed distally.

A and B indicate the apposition of M^1_1 in these two taxa during the puncture-crushing phase of mastication. C and D indicate the pattern of occlusion of M^1_1 in these two taxa during the buccal phase of chewing. E and F represent schematic lingual views of the same teeth during the buccal phase of chewing, E referring to *Lepilemur*, F to *Hapalemur*. A, C and E demonstrate that in *Lepilemur*, the cheek teeth emphasize the development of extensive enamel cutting edges, which are continually generated and honed by buccal phase faceting. Cusp relief and basin confinement are reduced. B, D and F demonstrate that in *Hapalemur*, the cheek teeth emphasize cusp relief and extensive basin development. Crests are tall and steep-sided, but do not always bear cutting edges honed by buccal phase faceting. Apposing cusps and basins are greatly defined, and demonstrate a high level of congruity.

Arrows roughly indicate path taken by lower M_1. Dotted lines indicate crown features outside the plane of the cross-section. Thickened, straight lines on tooth diagrams indicate buccal phase faceting. Abbreviations in alphabetic order: end—entoconid; hyd—hypoconid; mtd—metaconid; pa—paracone; pr—protocone.

pattern of reciprocal curvature and/or differential orientation, that cutting which is performed more closely resembles *vertical point cutting* (see p. 307). Centric occlusion may result in inefficient crushing in a manner similar to that seen in the "puncture-crushing" phase, while some grinding is inefficiently performed during the lingual phase.

Chewing, in *Hapalemur*, thus apparently results in very little efficient cutting, but does appear to emphasize point and crest penetration (or punching) and some crushing and grinding. Perhaps consistent with this pattern is the observation that both buccal and lingual phase faceting appear to result, not in extensive and well honed cutting edges, but in cusps and crests which demonstrate relatively great relief.

As dental wear ultimately reduces the crown relief of the postcanine dentition (especially in the upper teeth), the puncture-crushing phase may involve more crushing and the chewing phase more grinding, while both phases perhaps lose their point penetration and/or punching capabilities. *Hapalemur*, thus, appears to be one genus whose premolars and molars are primarily adapted to efficiently perform functions during the puncture-crushing phase of mastication.

Lepilemur: Puncture-Crushing.   This phase in *Lepilemur* is apparently not heavily relied upon or as functionally derived as in *Hapalemur*.

Chewing.   It is during chewing, and specifically during the buccal phase, that the molar teeth of *Lepilemur* appear to functionally come into their own.

During the buccal phase, the very extensive and finely honed leading enamel cutting edges along the ectolophs and ectolophids and along the protocones, and the unusually extensive and well-honed entocristids respectively occlude, and perform very efficient and very extensive cutting. Because of the largely mesio-distal orientation of occluding crests, and their pattern of reciprocal curvature and/or differential orientation, the cutting performed is basically *horizontal point cutting* (see p. 307). It should be emphasized here that progressive dental wear (except in extremely gerontic conditions) appears, not to reduce, but maintain cutting efficiency during the buccal phase in *Lepilemur* (Seligsohn, 1977). This is made possible because the upper molars buccally erupt while the lower molars lingually erupt at a rate commensurate with that of molar wear. This permits an ontogenetic increase in the horizontal component of buccal phase faceting. Fresh bevels and rejuvenated leading edges are thus continually being put on molar crests as molar wear progresses. What is emphasized then during the buccal phase in *Lepilemur* is the generation and functional utilization of finely honed enamel cutting edges.

Centric occlusion no doubt produces some crushing while the lingual phase, as indicated by the configuration of the lingual phase faceting, may result in grinding to an extent perhaps greater than that seen in *Hapalemur*. The relatively derived nature of the molars in *Lepilemur* thus appears to relate to their function during the chewing phase of mastication.

Biological Role

We may establish that *Hapalemur* divides its diet of young bamboo shoots and leaves essentially by means of puncturing, punching and crushing. As such the functional efficiency of the "puncture-crushing" phase of mastication appears to be most emphasized in this genus. Such a means of food division may or may not seem intuitively "suitable" for the diet in question. One of the aims of this chapter, however, is to merely establish the high probability that *Hapalemur* processes its distinctive diet in the manner described, and not to "second guess" natural selection by questioning the functional suitability of this evolutionary choice.

Hapalemur is known to initially divide (puncture-crush) the thick and fibrous stems of bamboo with the aid of the PM_4^4 region of its upper and lower tooth rows. It is perhaps not surprising that PM_4^4 in *Hapalemur* is highly molariform, and functionally the most derived of the postcanine teeth. The very specialized mode of initial food division habitually carried out in this limited region of the tooth row is apparently consistent with the highly derived nature of PM_4^4.

We may similarly conclude that *Lepilemur* divides its diet of tough, fibrous leaves and flowers primarily be means of buccal phase cutting. Apparently the functional efficiency of the "chewing phase" of mastication is crucial to food processing in this genus. Although the admonition given above relating to intuitive notions of functional suitability pertains equally well to the situation in *Lepilemur*, the following observations may be tentatively offered.

Lepilemur feeds almost solely on tough, leafy material which is very low in nutritive value. It would appear that the pattern of molar occlusion outlined above for *Lepilemur* would maximize the efficiency with which this animal divides sheets of fibrous, compliant material by not only recruiting the longest cutting edges possible at any given period of time, but also by distributing effective food division over as much of the length of the tooth row as possible at any given instant. This intuitively would appear to be a sound adaptive answer to the relatively severe problem of energy budgeting faced by this animal.

This functional analysis has shown, it is hoped, that two totally herbivorous and relatively closely related strepsirhine primates can demonstrate dramatically different means of oral food division, as a consequence of masticatory adaptations related to their specific diets.

DISCUSSION

Two major areas of inquiry form the foundations to the construction of selectional hypotheses and testing of dental function. Major studies in species specific diets, on the one hand, and studies of jaw movements, on the other, in both dried and live specimens, have yielded some solid predictive bases for studies of biological roles of specific dentitions.

We believe that the study of differences between species is the most powerful generating force of new ideas and insights. The last decade has been a time of uniquely sophisticated eco-ethological field studies of primates. In particular, many of these have concentrated on the diet and manner of feeding of subject species in their natural environments. These studies (for literature summary see Jolly, 1966) have increasingly put an end to such zoo-fed ideas as, for example, that many primates are merely opportunistic feeders. What comes to light is a general picture that each species of mammals has a habitual although often season-specific dietary regime which, when averaged out yearly, is a highly specific and characteristic aspect of a population. Such findings are a necessary prerequisite for the rigorous study of causal relationships between dietetic requirements and adaptational change of the feeding mechanism. With the feeding habits of a species established, adaptational models can be constructed and morphology explained in terms of specific phylogenetic changes.

The widespread occurrence of a very similar masticatory cycle for therians in general has emerged (Crompton and Hiiemae, 1970; Kallen and Gans, 1972; Kay and Hiiemae, 1974). What is probably of relatively limited significance are the differences, if any, between the preparatory and recovery strokes from species to species. Adaptive modifications have occurred primarily in the power phases of the puncture-crushing stroke (Crompton and Hiiemae, 1970) and the chewing stroke; the latter has long been recognized as having buccal and lingual components.

Bock and von Wahlert (1965, pp. 276–277 in this reference), in their powerful reassessment of the meaning of evolutionary adaptation, stated the following:

> Each utilized faculty [form–function complex] of a feature is controlled by a different set of selection forces and hence, each would have a separate evolution so far as possible. Hence, it is obvious that the feature cannot be perfectly adapted to all the selection forces acting upon it, but must be a compromise between all of these selection forces. In the case of the feature having only one form, then that particular form would be a compromise so that each of its faculties satisfies as best as possible the demands of the selection force (or forces) acting upon it. A feature with one or a few utilized functions would be better adapted to each selection force as fewer faculties enter the compromise. Features that are important "functionally" would be generally less well adapted to each selection force as more faculties are involved in the compromise, and more likely at least some of these faculties and the corresponding selection forces would conflict with one another.

The dentitions of *Lepilemur* and *Hapalemur* appear to conform rather nicely to the above mentioned generalizations. *Hapalemur* has evolved a dentition which apparently emphasizes (among other things) the efficient puncture-punching of bamboo stems especially during the puncture-crushing phase of mastication. Natural selection in this direction has, however, severely compromised the cutting and grinding efficiency of these teeth during chewing. *Lepilemur*, by contrast, has evolved a dentition which apparently emphasizes the very efficient cutting of tough, leafy material during the buccal phase of chewing. While such a dentition does not preclude efficient puncture-crushing, it does place a definite limit on the spectrum of possible functions which can be efficiently performed during the puncture-crushing phase of mastication.

It is most likely that species have specific dietetic strategies and use a basically similar masticatory cycle, employed by most therians. It now becomes possible, in particular lineages, to view aspects of whole dentitions, but more particularly crown patterns of teeth, as specifically maximizing the efficiency of certain mechanical functions which in some cases may affect the relative efficiency of puncture-crushing and chewing (either buccal or lingual phases).

Evolutionary changes are the result of selective forces derived from a specific dietary regime. Thus, the recognition of the derived morphological-functional aspect of a dentition can be attributed to specific functional changes, and consequently the deciphering of "fossil diets" is placed on a more precise basis, basically rooted in the recognition of analogous mechanical solutions. The greatest difficulties will still rest in the explanation of the biological roles to which otherwise functionally well-understood dentitions were adapted. Understanding the causal factors for evolutionary change, the performance of biological roles, however, whether in the dentition or other osseous remains, will supply us with the most powerful models to test new and imaginative hypotheses.

Attempts to overemphasize the differences between "shear" and "grind" as always distinct functions of the occluding cutting edges obscure the mechanical principles involved in food cutting, as pointed out and discussed by Every (1972). It would appear that past explanations of the acquisition of new elements of molar crowns (such as hypocones, cingula etc.) being the result of changes from "shearing" to "grinding," as stated by Szalay (1968) or recently by Kay and Hiiemae (1974), obscure the fundamental relationship between

(a) the kind of edge on the tooth,
(b) the consistency of the food material, and
(c) the optimal relationships between edges and edges, or edges and platforms, reflecting actions of forces along different planes, to cut food substances of given mean consistency in the most efficient manner possible.

We believe that the selection forces, responsible for different morphologies from species to species, may act primarily to emphasize one or several of a spectrum of possible mechanical functions, as well as the directions in which these functions can most efficiently be performed. Thus, hypocones, for example usually of recognizably different construction, can evolve to perform one of a variety of functions (i.e. puncturing, crushing, cutting) with their greatest effectiveness in more derived cases limited to specific portions of the mastica-tory cycle. Furthermore, the mere presence of similar dental morphology in different species does not necessarily imply similarity in either mechanical emphasis or biological role. The pointed hypocone of the metatherian *Cercartetus*, for example, modified and used differently from that of a more primitive phalangerid ancestor and that of the small indriid *Avahi* hold neither mechanical function nor biological role for specific diet in common.

A vast spectrum of specializations exists among mammals as far as diet is concerned. Although the temptation is always present to draw much needed generalizations for urgently sought after deductive theories, the science of dental morphology has not as yet reached the stage where we can adequately explain the adaptive significance of most dentitions. This is partly due to the fact that

(a) the exact genetic mechanisms underlying changes in tooth morphology are not fully explained yet,

(b) most often we are ignorant of the morphology preceding an adaptive shift,

(c) we do not know the precise mode in which the morphology of the skull, influenced by non-masticatory requirements, affects the chewing mechanism, and

(d) we are not certain as to the exact nature and combination of selective forces from the food substances responsible for one as opposed to another course taken by selection.

Kay and Hiiemae (1974, p. 255 in this reference) noted in their outstanding cinefluorographic study that:

the manner in which the food is treated is a direct function of consistency . . .

and that the different forms they worked with, irrespective of their characteristic dental morphology, treated the same food substances in a nearly identical manner. They also imply that a given food consistency will require a particular approach to the opposition of the teeth to cut up the food in the most efficient manner. We agree with them and it follows therefore that an "innate-learned" recognition of the physical properties of food through proprioceptors in the teeth and mouth is probably a basic mechanism in mammals. Given that each species has a typically mammalian chewing cycle as well as genetically stringently controlled dental occlusion and a behavioural propensity for a particular diet, selection would rapidly maximize a tooth design most suited for the optimum division of a diet of a given mean consistency. With these phylogenetic possibilities, natural selection will favour those mechanical functions of the teeth which most efficiently divide preferred diets.

As we hinted in this study, highly divergent specializations in both the morphology and mastication do not necessarily depict shifts from zoophagy to phytophagy or vice versa but signify specializations in one as opposed to another type of food substance. It may be added that often minor morphological specializations are all that are necessary to change the mechanical function of cheek teeth to cope with dietary shifts from largely animal to primarily plant foods or vice versa.

SUMMARY

The dental morphology and wear of two lemurids, *Hapalemur griseus olivaceous* and *Lepilemur mustelinus leucopus*, were examined and a functional model for each species was established in the light of data from recent studies on mandibular kinematics.

With the aid of dental wear features (now reliably correlated with the various phases of mastication) and occlusal analyses, inferences of post-canine function for *Lepilemur* and *Hapalemur* were made possible.

Lepilemur appears to emphasize very efficient point cutting during buccal phase chewing, while possibly performing efficient crushing and grinding during centric occlusion and the lingual phase. respectively. Dental function during the puncture-crushing phase appears less extensive and far less derived.

Hapalemur appears to emphasize extensive point and crest penetration (or "punching") during both the puncture-crushing and chewing phases of mastication. Efficient point cutting is clearly not emphasized in mastication, however.

The functional differences apparent in the postcanine dentitions of *Lepilemur* and *Hapalemur* appear to derive from their different biological roles in each genus. *Lepilemur* habitually feeds on and prepares sheets of tough and compliant food material having low nutritional value (e.g. leaves). The several efficient but low penetrative functions performed by the postcanine teeth appear to be adaptations to this biological role. The extensive and efficient system of cutting edges appears to allow *Lepilemur* to prepare its marginal diet with the least possible expenditure of energy.

Hapalemur habitually feeds on and prepares more rigid and relatively thicker food material (e.g. stems). The relatively highly penetrative functions performed by the postcanine teeth appear to be adapted to the ingestion and processing of material from such a food source. Perhaps significantly, PM^4 and PM_4 are the most derived and molariform postcanine teeth. According to accounts of feeding in the wild, it is precisely this region of the tooth row which carries out the initial (and presumably most demanding) preparation of bamboo stems.

This study strongly suggested that a given dentition is definitely limited with respect to the number of mechanical functions it can optimally perform. A number of conclusions that are applicable to the function of all mammalian dentitions have emerged as a result:

(a) Using the concepts of evolutionary adaptation developed by Bock and von Wahlert, it is possible to postulate that (within the constraints of the mammalian feeding mechanism) natural selection will favour those mechanical functions of teeth which most efficiently divide preferred food having a given set of physical properties. Thus dental specializations can change the spectrum of mechanical functions which can be efficiently performed during the puncture-crushing and chewing phases of mastication.

(b) The two genera studied illustrate how natural selection will favour a tooth design which wears in such a manner as to best rejuvenate functions emphasized in the unworn condition.

(c) Two closely related and totally phytophagous taxa can demonstrate dramatically different patterns of food division, with the physical properties of preferred food appearing to be a crucial selective factor. It is emphasized that as great a range of dental function may be found between two phytophagous species which subsist on foods of very different consistency, as between phytophagous and zoophagous species.

ACKNOWLEDGEMENTS

Figures were prepared by Anita J. Cleary, and technical assistance was rendered by Miriam Siroky. Research was supported by NSF Grant GS-32315 and a CUNY Doctoral Research Grant.

REFERENCES

BOCK, W. J. and VON WAHLERT, T. (1965). Adaptation and the form–function complex. *Evolution* **19**, 269–299.

CHARLES-DOMINIQUE, P. and HLADIK, C. M. (1971). Le *Lepilemur* du sud de Madagascar: ecologie, alimentation et vie sociale. *Terre et Vie*, **1**, 3–66.

CROMPTON, A. W. and HIIEMAE, K. M. (1970). Functional occlusion and mandibular movements during occlusion in the American opossum, *Didelphis marsupialis* *J. Linn. Soc. (Zool.)* **49**, 21–47.

EVERY, R. G. (1972). "A New Terminology for Mammalian Teeth." Pegasus Press, Christchurch, New Zealand.

HIIEMAE, K. and CROMPTON, A. W. (1971). A cinefluorographic study of feeding in the American opossum, *Didelphis marsupialis. In* "Dental Morphology and Evolution" (Dahlberg, A. A., ed.), pp. 299–334. University of Chicago Press, Chicago and London.

HIIEMAE, K. M. and KAY, R. F. (1973). Evolutionary trends in the dynamics of primate mastication. *In Symp. 4th Int. Cong. Primatol.* **3**, 28–64. Karger, Basel.

JOLLY, A. (1966). "Lemur Behavior." University of Chicago Press, Chicago and London.

JOLLY, A. (1972). "The Evolution of Primate Behavior." Macmillan, New York.

JONES, F. W. (1929). "Man's Place among the Mammals." Edward Arnold, London.

KALLEN, F. C. and GANS, C. (1972). Mastication in the little brown bat, *Myotis lucifugus. J. Morph.* **136**, 385–420.

KAY, R. F. and HIIEMAE, K. M. (1974). Jaw movement and tooth use in Recent and fossil primates. *Am. J. phys. Anthrop.* **40**, 227–256.

MARTIN, R. D. (1972). Adaptive radiation and behaviour of the Malagasy lemurs. *Phil. Trans. R. Soc. Ser.* B **264**, 295–352.

PETTER, J. J. and PEYRIERAS, A. (1970). Observations eco-ethologiques sur les lemuriens Malgaches du genre *Hapalemur. Terre et Vie* **24**, 356–382.

SELIGSOHN, D. (1977). Analysis of species-specific molar adaptations in Strepsirhine primates. *Contr. Primatol.* **11**, 1–116.

SELIGSOHN, D. and SZALAY, F. S. (1974). Dental occlusion and the masticatory apparatus in *Lemur* and *Varecia:* their bearing on the systematics of living and fossil primates. *In* "Prosimian Biology" (Martin, R. D., Doyle, G. A. and Walker, A. C., eds). Duckworth, London.

SZALAY, F. S. (1968). The beginnings of primates. *Evolution*, **22**, 19–36.

NOTES ADDED IN PROOF

Horizontal point cutting—is a means of dividing food at very high pressures by interposing food between two occluding sharp-edged crests whose orientations strongly emphasize both horizontal and mesio-distal components, and which are reciprocally curved and/or differentially oriented primarily in a plane parallel with that of the crown cervix. Division of food involves the movement of these crests past each other. The space between the two sets of crests diminishes as these crests cross at only one or two points at any given instant. Point cutting is thus capable of progressing relatively extensively along a horizontal (mesio-distal) axis, while still utilizing the mandibular movements characteristic of primitive therian chewing.

Vertical point cutting—is a means of dividing food at very high pressures by interposing food between two occluding sharp-edged crests whose orientations strongly emphasize a component perpendicular to the cervical plane of the molar, and which are reciprocally curved and/or differentially oriented primarily in a plane which is both normal to that of the crown cervix and parallel with the bucco-lingual axis of the molar. Division of food involves the movement of these crests past each other. The space between the two sets of crests diminishes as these crests cross at any given instant at only one or two points. Point cutting is thus capable of progressing relatively extensively along a vertical axis, while still utilizing the mandibular movements characteristic of primitive therian chewing.

20. Molar Structure and Diet in Extant Cercopithecidae

RICHARD F. KAY

Department of Anatomy, Duke University Medical Center, Durham, North Carolina, U.S.A.

INTRODUCTION

The Old World monkeys, the Cercopithecidae, offer an unusual opportunity for the study of dental mechanics, allometry and dietary adaptation. There are essentially three reasons for this opportunity. First, the molar structure of the group is very uniform; although species differ in the size and proportions of molar crushing, grinding and shearing mechanisms, the pattern and sequence of contacts between cusps, crests and basins are identical. Thus we have in this group a conservative structural organization reflecting an ancestral heritage. Superimposed differences in molar structure between members of the group can be unambiguously attributed to phenotypic responses to environmental pressure.

Second, it is a rather diverse family that is represented by about 17 genera and some 73 species. Furthermore, although all species are predominantly herbivorous, considerable differences are present in the proportions of fruits and leaves eaten. This has the advantage that hypotheses relating dental structure to behaviour can be tested in a number of independent cases.

Third, the size range of the extant species (from 1000 g to about 37 000 g) is adequate for the study of changes in shape in response to body size, and the testing of hypotheses relating tooth size changes to metabolic rates and diet. The present study has three purposes. The first is to further test the hypothesis that tooth size increases proportionally to metabolic rate in mammals. The second is a quantitative and qualitative assessment of molar occlusion and function among Cercopithecidae. Special attention is paid to the functional significance of the cercopithecid bilophodont molar pattern and how it differs from other anthropoids. This has been derived from a study of the pattern and size of molar structures which puncture, shear, crush and grind food during mastication. The third purpose is the examination of these functional characters as they relate to feeding behaviour in extant Cercopithecidae.

MATERIALS AND METHODS

Altogether, 285 osteological specimens were examined from the American Museum of Natural History, the United States National Museum and the British Museum of Natural History. The material was sampled from 49 species and 57 subspecies representing all the subgenera of Cercopithecidae recognized by Napier and Napier (1967), Hill (1966, 1970 and 1974), and Thorington and Groves (1970). Since body mass data are often unavailable for osteological specimens, some of the body mass estimates required for allometric studies were taken from the literature. A summary of most of this information has been published (Kay, 1973). For all species where body mass was estimable, the samples were segregated by sex and separate body mass figures were used. Eight measurements were made on second upper and lower molars. These dimensions and the anatomical landmarks on which they are defined are illustrated in Fig. 1 and the mean dimensions for each species are presented in Table I. Four tooth dimensions are the same as those used in previous studies (Kay, 1973, 1975b). These are the mesio-distal lower second molar length (LM_2), the length of the cristid obliqua on the second lower molar (c.o.), the cusp height of the second molar hypoconid (h.h.), and the total surface of crushing (s.a.), which is the sum of all the areas on the lower molars coming into contact at or near centric conclusion. Four new measurements were used: the length of the entocristid (e), a crest running anteriorly and ventrally from the entoconid tip to a groove on the medial surface on the crown; the length of the postmetacristid (p.m.), the crest running posteriorly and ventrally from the metaconid tip to a groove on the medial side of the crown; the metaconid cusp height (m.h.), measured from the tip of the metaconid to the ventral-most extent of the cemento–enamel junction at its base; and the crown width (c.w.), the distance on M^2 from the junction of the premetacrista with the postmetacrista to the medial lingual notch.

Linear measurements were made in millimetres with a helios dial caliper, or, when specimens were too small to be measured accurately in this manner, with a calibrated reticle mounted on a binocular microscope. Surface areas were estimated by orienting each surface parallel to the focal plane of the microscope, and drawing its outline using a camera lucida. The area within each outline was measured with a polar planimeter; the areas of all tooth surfaces were summed, and corrected for magnification.

Specimens were used in which the upper and lower second molars were intact so a complete set of dimensions could be obtained. The antero-posterior dimensions of the exposed dentine on the tips of the hypoconid and entoconid were measured. When the sum of these measurements exceeded 25% of the antero-posterior second molar diameter, the specimen was rejected.

In addition to simple univariate and bivariate statistics, two variations of

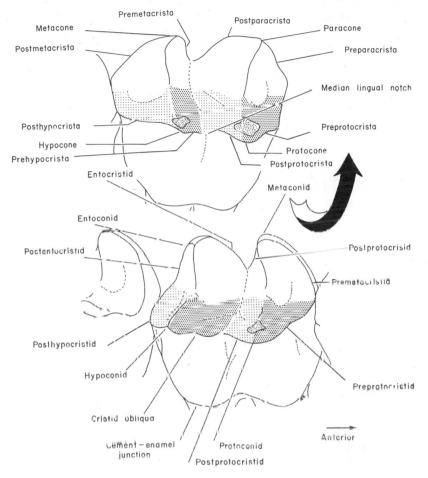

FIG. 1. The upper (top) and lower (bottom) right molars of *Presbytis johni* based on several specimens to illustrate the terminology used in the text. The upper molar is viewed from a ventral and medial aspect, the lower molar from the dorsal and lateral aspect. The solid lines are crests, and the dashed lines are valleys. The areas with large stippling are dentine windows in the enamel. Fine stippling indicates crushing–grinding surfaces: the areas of light stipple occlude with areas of dark stipple at the termination of Phase I of mastication such that the protocone fits in the embrasure between the hypoconid and protoconid.

principal components analysis were used: principal components analysis and principal coordinates analysis. For details concerning these methods see Wahlstedt and Davis (1968) and Blackith and Reyment (1971).

    The measurements used in multivariate analyses were regression adjusted to minimize the effects of changes in tooth shape due to body size using a procedure outlined by Kay (1973, 1975b) in his studies of other primates. The use of tooth length as the basis for allometric adjustment (and the

TABLE I. Means of tooth measurements taken from dental specimens (mm and mm²). The number in parenthesis to the right of the species is the sample size. Species are arranged alphabetically within each subfamily. Symbols: LM₂, length of the second lower molar; h.h., hypoconid height; m.h., metaconid height; s.a., surface area of crushing; c.w., crown width (upper second molar); c.o., cristid oblique length; e, entocristid length; p.m., postmetacristid length. Measurements were all made on second lower molars except where indicated.

Taxon and Sample Size	Tooth Dimensions							
	LM_2	h.h.	m.h.	s.a.	c.w.	c.o.	e	p.m.
Allenopithecus nigroviridis (4)	6·30	5·25	4·49	10·86	2·37	1·73	1·67	2·34
Cercocebus albigena (8)	6·79	4·62	4·25	11·78	3·04	1·86	1·67	2·14
Cercocebus atys (1)	8·30	6·90	6·00	17·21	3·60	2·20	2·20	2·40
Cercocebus torquatus (8)	7·97	6·62	5·31	15·76	3·29	2·26	2·14	2·78
Cercopithecus aethiops (5)	6·34	4·48	4·37	12·73	3·70	1·90	1·76	2·08
Cercopithecus ascanius (6)	5·33	3·61	3·43	9·37	2·70	1·60	1·48	1·78
Cercopithecus cephus (9)	5·59	3·90	3·52	9·87	2·49	1·53	1·39	1·77
Cercopithecus diana (4)	6·10	3·80	3·35	10·16	2·59	1·50	1·48	2·02
Cercopithecus lhoesti (4)	6·42	4·46	4·34	13·85	3·10	2·08	2·11	2·73
Cercopithecus mitis (19)	6·52	4·15	3·92	12·71	3·29	1·99	1·77	2·21
Cercopithecus pogonias (4)	5·55	4·00	3·27	9·30	2·65	1·65	1·50	1·42
Cercopithecus neglectus (11)	6·19	4·21	3·82	12·62	3·00	1·80	1·75	2·05
Cercopithecus nictitans (7)	6·39	3·86	3·73	11·13	2·89	1·90	1·60	1·84
Erythrocebus patas (6)	7·55	5·35	4·47	16·76	3·36	2·27	2·34	2·72
Macaca cyclopis (7)	7·73	5·34	4·44	14·73	3·17	2·20	2·17	2·26
Macaca fuscata (3)	8·73	6·58	5·67	22·12	3·66	2·60	2·37	3·10
Macaca maura (2)	8·00	6·34	5·17	17·11	2·91	2·29	2·26	2·68
Macaca sylvanus (5)	9·56	6·94	5·77	23·99	4·84	3·20	2·62	3·20
Macaca fascicularis (15)	6·95	4·69	4·07	12·45	3·25	2·07	1·92	2·38

Macaca mulatta	(4)	8·27	5·64	4·72	17·33	3·31	2·43	2·47	2·80
Macaca nemestrina	(9)	8·57	5·74	5·58	16·80	3·32	2·35	2·42	2·89
Macaca nigra	(10)	8·04	5·31	4·92	16·55	3·45	2·27	2·00	2·67
Macaca philippensis	(8)	7·37	5·15	4·56	14·17	3·06	2·12	1·96	2·25
Macaca speciosa	(4)	9·17	7·04	6·31	21·19	3·60	3·17	2·86	2·94
Mandrillus sphinx	(6)	12·28	8·87	7·39	36·60	4·63	3·46	3·41	3·86
Miopithecus talapoin	(4)	4·04	2·70	2·41	5·07	2·10	1·32	1·11	1·26
Papio anubis	(4)	12·00	7·81	6·94	35·13	5·25	3·70	3·11	3·87
Papio cynocephalus	(6)	12·03	8·45	6·45	35·51	4·77	3·33	3·60	3·81
Papio hamadryas	(5)	12·60	8·76	7·40	37·07	4·76	3·66	3·58	4·16
Papio ursinus	(5)	15·18	8·58	7·65	41·60	5·13	3·77	4·02	4·57
Theropithecus gelada	(4)	13·23	9·68	7·60	41·05	4·60	3·88	4·00	4·38
Colobus badius	(8)	7·31	5·23	4·75	16·37	3·55	2·76	3·18	3·61
Colobus guereza	(12)	7·24	5·34	5·08	17·31	3·72	2·52	2·78	3·35
Nasalis concolor	(7)	7·00	5·40	4·89	16·67	3·73	2·72	2·71	3·06
Nasalis larvatus	(8)	8·17	5·91	5·80	21·07	4·05	3·08	3·65	3·99
Presbytis aygula	(4)	5·52	3·50	3·75	9·95	2·95	1·77	2·27	2·52
Presbytis cristatus	(9)	6·17	4·48	3·98	11·48	3·28	2·10	2·32	2·72
Presbytis entellus	(10)	8·23	6·08	5·47	20·32	3·99	2·82	3·43	3·41
Presbytis frontata	(5)	5·70	3·64	3·72	11·14	3·10	1·64	1·92	2·30
Presbytis johni	(4)	5·95	5·46	4·62	16·09	3·52	2·50	2·95	3·19
Presbytis melalophos	(2)	6·00	4·59	4·23	12·33	3·09	2·16	2·42	2·49
Presbytis obscurus	(6)	6·62	4·77	4·74	14·09	3·12	2·34	2·59	3·22
Presbytis rubicundus	(1)	5·60	3·69	3·56	12·58	3·10	2·26	2·00	2·33
Presbytis potenziani	(7)	6·61	4·36	4·17	14·21	3·52	2·40	2·23	2·88
Procolobus verus	(5)	5·56	3·79	3·92	10·35	2·85	2·04	2·24	2·46
Pygathrix nemaeus	(1)	7·40	5·82	4·85	17·36	3·88	2·39	2·91	3·69
Pygathrix nigripes	(2)	7·35	5·43	4·69	16·62	3·78	2·75	3·17	3·52
Rhinopithecus avunculus	(2)	7·50	5·00	5·23	16·64	4·05	3·00	3·40	3·52
Rhinopithecus roxellanae	(4)	9·04	6·50	5·97	25·61	4·59	2·91	3·61	4·16

corresponding abandonment of body mass used by Kay, 1973, 1975b) is discussed below.

RESULTS

Metabolism and Tooth Size

The size of the postcanine teeth have long been thought to be tied to an animal's energy needs (Cuvier, 1863; Romer, 1945; Gould, 1966; Szalay, 1972). One simple hypothesis is that since the metabolic rate of mammals increases by the 0.75 power of body mass (Kleiber, 1961) for metabolic scaling, tooth surfaces (or even linear dimensions) might be expected to increase by the 0.75 exponent. Several authors have sought recently to test the hypothesis that tooth surfaces are so scaled. Pilbeam and Gould (1974) give the exponents of power functions relating postcanine tooth surface and body size, but were unable to demonstrate that these surfaces increase disproportionately with increasing body mass despite Gould's (1974) statement to the contrary. Kay (1973, 1975b) looked at tooth dimensions in non-cercopithecid primates and concluded that in a vast majority of cases tooth dimensions are scaled by simple isometry: areas increase by the two-thirds power of body mass and linear dimensions by the one-third power. For example, he found an exponent of 0.65 ± 0.06 (95% confidence interval) for the equation relating body mass and second molar crushing surfaces. For Cercopithecidae, the exponent of the equation relating body mass to second molar surface areas is 0.62 ± 0.08, not significantly different from isometry but significantly different at the 95% confidence level from 0.75, the exponent of metabolic change with body mass (Fig. 2). Primate molar surfaces do not increase proportionally to changes in energy needs. A similar finding holds for Artiodactyla. The exponent of the equation relating the total surface of the grinding battery to body mass for ten genera of Bovidae ranging in size from 2 kg to 900 kg is 0.53 for the uppers and 0.51 for the lowers. Both of these exponents are significantly different from 0.75 at their 95% confidence interval (Kay, 1975a). The exponents of the power functions relating body mass to the linear dimensions examined for this study range from 0.26 to 0.40 (Table II). Again, these are usually isometric with simple body size scaling except that crown width is negatively allometric and several shearing blades are positively allometric. It is premature to place much significance on these exceptions. They could be the result of uneven sampling of dietary groups at different sizes.

Since in mastication food is broken down into small pieces, increasing its surface area to volume ratio (to facilitate chemical breakdown), why shouldn't the mechanisms which perform this function increase proportionally to the amount of food which must be handled? The explanation may lie in a number of other factors which presumably would affect food preparation scaling. These would include changes in the food volume to energy ratio, the consistency of the food eaten, the size and shape of food items, the life span of the individual, the speed of chewing and the number of chews possible in

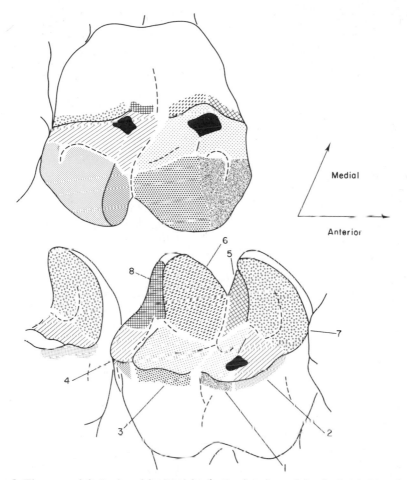

FIG. 2. The upper left (top) and lower right (bottom) molars of *Presbytis johni* based on several specimens to illustrate the wear facets produced in the two phases of mastication. The system of numbering used to identify wear facets is the same as that of Kay and Hiiemae (1974). The cross-hatching indicates the surfaces which are ground across one another in Phase II of mastication. Surface 9 is situated on the antero-medial facing surface of the hypoconid and the postero-medial facing surface of the protoconid. Surface 10 is situated on the antero-medial facing surface of the protoconid and on the postero-medial facing surface of the hypoconid. Matching surfaces are found on the hypocone and protocone.

preparing a food item. Possibly the influence of one or more of these factors explains why there is no simple relationship between tooth size and metabolic rate.

Female Cercopithecidae have larger molars for a given body size than do males. Data in Tables III and IV show that in six of eight cases at a given body size female Cercopithecidae have larger tooth dimensions than males.

TABLE II. Male and female Cercopithecidae. Slopes (x) and intercepts (b) of equations relating body mass to eight tooth dimensions. The form of the equation is $Y = x(M) + b$, where Y is the $\log_e$ of the tooth dimensions, and M is the $\log_e$ of the body mass. Symbols are as in Table I. Figures in parenthesis represent the 95% confidence interval for the slope or intercept.

Dimension	Slope	Intercept	Coefficient of Correlation
LM$_2$	0·34(0·05)	−1·05(0·03)	0·838
h.h.	0·37(0·06)	−1·70(0·04)	0·844
m.h.	0·35(0·05)	−1·56(0·03)	0·852
s.a.	0·62(0·08)	−2·81(0·05)	0·889
c.w.	0·26(0·04)	−1·07(0·02)	0·834
c.o.	0·37(0·05)	−2·41(0·03)	0·848
e	0·42(0·05)	−2·89(0·03)	0·855
p.m.	0·40(0·05)	−2·54(0·03)	0·847

TABLE III. Male Cercopithecidae. Slopes (c) and intercepts (b) of equations relating body mass to tooth dimensions. The form of the equation is $Y = x(M) + b$, where Y is the $\log_e$ of the tooth dimension, and M is the $\log_e$ of body mass. Symbols are as in Table I. Figures in parenthesis represent the 95% confidence interval for the slope or intercept.

Dimension	Slope	Intercept	Coefficient of Correlation
LM$_2$	0·38(0·07)	−1·44(0·04)	0·870
h.h.	0·41(0·08)	−2·04(0·05)	0·845
m.h.	0·35(0·06)	−1·66(0·04)	0·865
s.a.	0·70(0·09)	−3·54(0·05)	0·926
c.w.	0·28(0·04)	−1·29(0·03)	0·888
c.o.	0·40(0·07)	−2·79(0·04)	0·872
e	0·46(0·07)	−3·31(0·04)	0·898
p.m.	0·38(0·07)	−2·47(0·04)	0·865

Possibly females need large teeth because at certain times they have a higher metabolic rate; pregnant female mammals have higher metabolic rates than adult non-pregnant females (Hylander, personal communication). For example, Marine *et al.* (1924) showed that pregnant rabbits have a 30% higher metabolic rate than non-pregnant controls.

A coherent theory which accounts for molar size must explain why tooth dimensions are negatively allometric with respect to "metabolic body size" (mass $^{\frac{3}{4}}$), why all dimensions do not follow the same regressions (see Table II) and why females have consistently larger molars for their body size than do

Table IV. Female Cercopithecidae. Slopes (x) and intercepts (b) of equations relating body mass to tooth dimensions. The form of the equation is $Y = x(M) + b$, where Y is the $\log_e$ of the tooth dimension, and M is the $\log_e$ of body mass. Symbols are as in Table I. Figures in parenthesis represent the 95% confidence interval for the slope of intercept.

Dimension	Slope	Intercept	Coefficient of Correlation
LM$_2$	0·35(0·08)	−1·05(0·05)	0·831
h.h.	0·39(0·07)	−1·78(0·04)	0·882
m.h.	0·39(0·08)	−1·92(0·04)	0·870
s.a.	0·65(0·11)	−2·92(0·06)	0·900
c.w.	0·26(0·07)	−1·06(0·04)	0·775
c.o.	0·38(0·07)	−2·53(0·04)	0·872
e	0·43(0·10)	−2·99(0·06)	0·840
p.m.	0·50(0·08)	−3·34(0·06)	0·891

males. The hypothesis of Gould (1974) and Pilbeam and Gould (1974) that tooth size in mammals is scaled according to metabolic body size does not accord with the data from this study and that of Kay (1973, 1975a, b). However, larger teeth for females may result from elevated energy requirements during pregnancy.

Occlusion in Cercopithecidae

The upper and lower molars of *Presbytis johni* are illustrated in Figs 1 and 3. The terminology used is based on that of van Valen (1966) and Szalay (1969). Several additional crests have been given names in accordance with their system. Matching upper and lower wear facets are numbered after Crompton (1971) and Kay and Hiiemae (1974a). The upper second molars of *Presbytis johni* are four-cusped. Two medial cusps, the protocone and the hypocone, are situated directly transverse to two cusps on the lateral edge of the tooth (paracone and metacone, respectively). Long, trenchant crests extend anteriorly and posteriorly from paracone and metacone to form a sharp lateral edge on the crown. An additional crest extends medially from each cusp to the centre of the tooth. Shorter and lower crests extend antero-laterally and postero-laterally from protocone and hypocone to delineate the inner margin of the crown. Two low ridges extend laterally from protocone and hypocone to join the transverse crests from paracone and metacone. Two basins are present on upper molars, one in the centre of the tooth and one between adjacent teeth. The former is bordered medially by crests running antero-laterally from the hypocone and postero-laterally from the protocone; laterally by the bases of paracone and metacone; anteriorly by the ridge running laterally from the protocone; and posteriorly by one running laterally from the hypocone. The second basin is a composite of the posterior basin of a molar and the contiguous anterior basin of its immediately posterior successor. It is bordered medially by the protocone and the hypocone; laterally by the bases of paracone and metacone and anteriorly and posteriorly by crests running laterally from the protocone and hypocone. The lower second molars of *P. johni* are practically mirror images of the uppers with four cusps at the edges of the tooth arranged in transverse pairs. The two medial cusps (metaconid and entoconid) are higher and have better developed crests than the lateral cusps. Three crests run antero-laterally, postero-laterally, and directly laterally from each medial cusp. Lower and less trenchant crests run antero-medially and postero-medially from the lateral

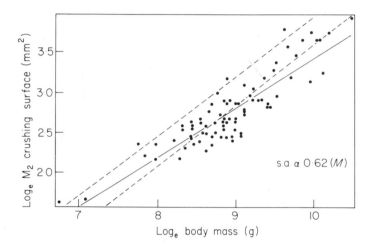

Fig. 3. The $\log_e$ of the second molar crushing surfaces (mm²) is proportional to the 0·62 power of the $\log_e$ body mass (g). The best-fit axis is the solid line fit to 89 subspecies and sexes of cercopithecids. The two dashed lines are slopes of 0·75 fit to the grand mean and to the smallest species studied, *Cercopithecus talapoin*. These lines miss the trend for the small species and large species respectively.

cusps (protoconid and hypoconid). In addition, ridges run medially from each lateral cusp to join the crests originating from the medial cusps. Again, two basins are present, one in the centre of each molar and the other formed from contiguous portions of adjacent molars. Each is bordered medially by the bases of metaconid and entoconid, laterally by the crests running antero-medially and postero-medially from the lateral cusps, and antero-posteriorly by transverse ridges from lateral to medial cusps.

Preliminary results of a cineradiographic study of *Macaca* show that chewing usually occurs on only one side of the jaw at any given time. When the molars first come into contact in the power stroke, the lower teeth are displaced to the chewing side so that their lateral crests are vertically aligned. From this position the lower molars are moved upwards, slightly anteriorly, and medially until the protoconid and hypoconid rest in upper molar basins. There follows a medial, slightly anterior, and slightly downward jaw movement before tooth contact terminates. In other primates the two jaw movements have been termed respectively Phase I and II (Hiiemae and Kay, 1972). At the beginning of Phase I nearly simultaneous contacts occur between eight pairs of upper and lower molar crests, producing eight wear facets on their slopes. These are labelled in Fig. 3. Each of the eight numbered lower molar wear surfaces has a leading edge or crest which is moved across a matching upper molar crest in the course of the upward medial movement in Phase I. Food trapped between the blades is sheared. Sharp transverse crests running laterally from the metaconid and entoconid on the lower molars engage notches between the cusps on the upper medial edge of the upper molars and act as guides for the shearing action of the lateral upper and lower molar blades. A similar action occurs on the medial edge of the tooth, with crests running medially from the paracone and metacone engaging lateral notches on the lower molars. Thus Phase I is primarily a shearing phase involving engagement of upper and lower crests and their movement across each other. The upper and antero-medial Phase I movement terminates when protocone and hypocone are brought into contact with food in the lower molar basins; a corresponding crushing action occurs between hypoconid and protoconid and the upper molar basins. Crushing at the termination of Phase I would be accompanied by the production of bending forces in structurally rigid foods since contact surfaces are continuous and uneven. Immediately following Phase I, opposing washboard-like surfaces are ground across each other in an antero-medial and horizontal or slightly downward direction producing wear facets 9 and 10 on these surfaces.

Cercopithecid molar function resembles other higher primates in having nearly simultaneous shearing occurring in Phase I along the medial and lateral edges of two crushing surfaces. But several striking differences make Old World monkey molars unique (see Fig. 4). In ceboids, crushing surface 9 on the surface of the M_2 hypoconid is separated anteriorly from the protoconid crushing surface 10 by the shearing edges of wear surfaces 1 and 5 and posteriorly from surface 10 on the M_3 in one of several ways. In *Saimiri*, the posterior margin of the M_2 is raised so that the leading edges of wear surfaces 4 (on the hypocristid) and 8 (on the postentocristid) are nearly continuous, separating the M_2 hypoconid crushing surface (9) from the M_3 protoconid crushing surface (10). In some ceboids, such as *Callicebus*, the protoconid crushing surface (9) is prolonged anteriorly on to the posterior margin of the anteriorly adjacent molar. The postentocristid is incorporated into the wall of the crushing basin and the M_3 protoconid crushing surface (10) is separated from the M_2 crushing basin (9) by the leading edge of wear surface 6, running from the M_2 hypoconid through the M_3 hypoconulid, and the leading edge of surface 2, running anteriorly and medially from the M_3 protoconid. Other ceboids such as *Ateles* and *Alouatta* have no effective separation between medial facing crushing surface (9) on the M_2 hypoconid and (10) on the M_3 protoconid. In extant Hominoidea wear surface 9 on the hypoconid has been extended anteriorly and is continuous with surface 10 on the posterior aspect of the trigonid; a crest is still present between surfaces 9 and 10, but it

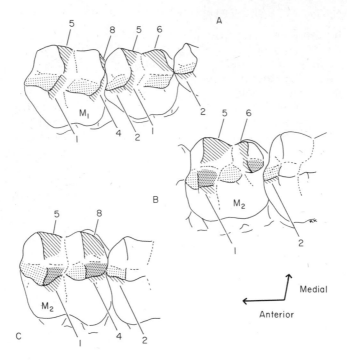

Medial

Anterior

FIG. 4. Lateral views of part of the lower molar dentitions of (A) *Saimiri sciureus* (Ceboidae); (B) *Dryopithecus indicus* (Pongidae) AMNH 19413; and (C) *Cercocebus albigena* (Cercopithecidae). Cross-hatching indicates several of the shearing blades; stippling indicates crushing surfaces. There are two crushing basins on the lower molars of ceboids and Old World anthropoids; one on the antero-medial face of the hypoconid (9) (talonid basin) and one on the same face of the protoconid (10) (trigonid basin). The latter occasionally extends on to the heel of its anteriorly adjacent tooth. Among primitive anthropoids, trigonid and talonid crushing basins are set apart from one another by the steep posterior edge of the trigonid supporting the leading shearing edges of wear surfaces 1 and 5. This condition is preserved in most Ceboidea (A). The posterior margin of the talonid crushing basin is also set apart by shearing blades from the trigonid crushing basin of its posteriorly adjacent molar. This separation is accomplished in a variety of ways, two of which are shown in A and B. In A, the leading shearing edges of wear surfaces 8 and 4 across the back of the talonid of M_1 provide the separation of the M_1 talonid from the M_2 trigonid. In B, the leading shearing edges of wear surfaces 6 on the M_2 talonid and 2 on the M_3 trigonid combine to separate the M_2 talonid crushing surface from the M_3 trigonid crushing surface. Old World Anthropoidea progressively abandon the system of separating crushing basins with shearing blades.

Among pongids (B) wear surface 5 and its corresponding leading edge are restricted to the medial part of the tooth. Wear surface 1 is rotated antero-laterally. The lateral part of the posterior face of the trigonid is flattened out and the talonid crushing surface is extended on to it. This is represented in (B) by dark stippling. Thus, although a low ridge separates the trigonid and talonid basins, that ridge does not perform a shearing function. Pongids maintain the shearing blade separation of molar talonid basins from the trigonid crushing basins of their posteriorly adjacent teeth.

Cercopithecids (C) are similar to pongids but have gone one step further: wear surface 6 and its leading edge are confined to the medial part of the tooth; wear surface 2 and its does not support a Phase I shearing blade. The crest supporting lower molar wear surface 1 is antero-posteriorly orientated and wear surface 5 does not reach across the tooth to join surface 1. Crushing surface 9 of M_2 and surface 10 on M_3 are separated by the leading edges of wear surfaces 6 and 2 between the protoconid of M_3 and the entoconid of M_2. Cercopithecids are unique among extant primates in having continuity between crushing surfaces 9 and 10 both anteriorly and posteriorly. As among hominoids, wear surface 9 on the M_2 is prolonged forward to contact M_2 surface 10 across a low ridge running medially from the protoconid. Lower molar surface 6 is short and a hypoconulid is absent. Wear surface 10 on the lower molars is extended anteriorly to contact surface 9 across a ridge running medially from the hypoconid. Lower molar surface 8 is well developed and forms part of the medial shearing margin of the crushing basin. These morphological differences affect the way food is prepared. Antero-posteriorly in cercopithecid molars, valley and crest are followed successively by a valley and crest producing a continuous wash-board surface which can be used to produce bending moments in food at the termination of Phase I. This system is quite different from that of other higher primates in which shearing crests which occlude in Phase I separate the basins. Discrete particles of food are trapped in compression chambers by shearing in Phase I and are crushed at the termination of Phase I, but little bending is possible. The molar design adapted by cercopithecids is one mechanically efficient way of preparing a variety of plant foods but it clearly is not the only efficient system since other plant-eating extant primates have not chosen it.

Phase II jaw movement produces in cercopithecids a cusp in groove grinding action between molar cusps and grooves. It is similar to that found in other primates.

The term "bilophodonty" used to describe cercopithecid molars might lead one to suppose that two cross lophs or crests move across each other producing shearing in the power stroke. Such is not the case. The medial lower molar and lateral upper molar lophs produce bending forces when brought into contact late in Phase I; the lateral lower and medial upper cross lophs function as guides for the shearing movement between medial and lateral shearing crests in Phase I and presumably strengthen these cusps against breakage.

Molar Function and Allometry

To facilitate more rigorous functional comparisons between cercopithecid molars, molar size, shearing, crushing, grinding and wear resistance, dimensions were measured on the second molars of 49 species. From the description of molar occlusion it is clear that the leading edges of many crests shear past

---

leading edge are shortened and rotated antero-laterally. The crushing surface of the trigonid is prolonged forwards on to the heel of its anteriorly adjacent tooth. The crushing surface on the molar talonid is continuous across a low ridge with the crushing surface of its posteriorly adjacent molar. Thus, all crushing surfaces are continuous rather than being compartmentalized by shearing blades.

one another in Phase I. The dimensions of three of these important crests (cristid obliqua, entocristid and postmetacristid) were taken as measures of the importance of this function. The sum of the surfaces of contact of hypoconid and protoconid with hypocone and protocone estimates the total crushing and grinding surface. The cusp height of hypoconid and metaconid measure the total tooth material available for resistance to wear during the individual's life. Higher cusps may also be linked with elongation of shearing crests on their sides and thus may be an indirect measure of shearing. The distance across the upper molar crown from buccal to lingual median notches estimates the movement of the M_2 hypoconid across the M^2 in the power

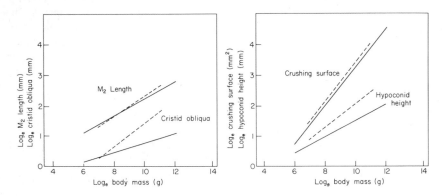

FIG. 5. Plots of tooth measurements and body mass for Cercopithecidae (dashed line) and non-cercopithecid primates (solid line). The ends of the lines indicate the size range for these groups.

stroke. Finally the length of the second molars were used to measure molar size. Four of the dimensions were used by Kay (1973, 1975b) in a study of non-cercopithecid primates and *Tupaia*. These are compared graphically in Fig. 5a and b. Second molar size (as expressed by M_2 length) is virtually the same in cercopithecid species as among other primate species of the same body mass. There is a slight tendency for cercopithecids to have larger M_2 crushing surfaces than other primates although the slopes are not significantly different. This does not confirm the suggestion by Mills (1955) that the lingual phase (Phase II) is greatly abbreviated in cercopithecids. Within the size range of extant species (about 800 g to about 60 000 g) cercopithecids have comparatively longer cristid obliqua shearing blades at any given body size. This trend becomes most evident at larger body sizes because of the comparatively large exponent in the equation (0.37 for cercopithecids compared with 0.18 for other primates). Within their size range, cercopithecids have relatively higher hypoconids than other primates of the same size (except the smallest, *Miopithecus talapoin*). The height of the M_2 metaconid in cercopithecids follows a similar slope to that of the hypoconid, but comparable data are not available for other primates. Several species of non-cercopithecids have cristid obliqua lengths comparable to Old World monkeys. Each of these species takes significant proportions of leaves in its diet. They are the ceboid *Alouatta*, the indriids *Indri*, *Avahi* and *Propithecus*, and the lemurine, *Hapalemur*. Folivorous non-cercopithecid primates have higher hypoconids than frugivorous species of the same body size (Kay 1973, 1975b). All of these features emphasize the general similarities between cercopithecids and folivorous non-cercopithecid primates.

The lengths of the entocristid and postmetacristid—the leading shearing edges of wear surfaces 5 and 6—are roughly the same length as the cristid obliqua within the size range of Cercopithecidae. The rate of size increase of these crests is significantly positively allometric with respect to body mass (see Table II). Although these crests were not measured in other primates, visual observations suggest that these are relatively longer in Old World monkeys. Among non-cercopithecid primates these crests appear to be best developed among folivorous primates such as *Alouatta* and the indriids.

The distance traversed by the M_2 hypoconid across M^2 is negatively allometric with body mass; large cercopithecids have relatively shorter hypoconid traverses than do small species. In visual terms, large cercopithecid species have more restricted upper molar crowns than do their smaller relatives. In summary, the allometric changes in second molars of cercopithecids would fit a model for primates which consume high proportions of folivorous materials. Cercopithecids share with non-cercopithecid primate folivores the emphasis on shearing crests, having high cusps which reflect increased wear potential and perhaps reflect a shearing emphasis. All of these features are packed into a second molar which is roughly the same size as in other primates.

Molar Shape and Diet

Molar dimensions described above were adjusted for tooth length based on regression equations presented in Table V. A principal components analysis was run on regression adjusted molar dimensions for 49 species. The factor loadings show that species values for the first component, which accounts for 36% of the total variance of the system, are strongly and about equally influenced by the length of shearing crests (-0.41 to -0.45), the size of crushing surfaces (-0.42), the breadth of the upper molars (-0.36) and the height of the metaconid (-0.34). The height of the hypoconid is a much less significant factor (-0.13). Since all the factor loadings are negative, species with proportionately large crushing surfaces, long shearing blades and high cusps have comparatively low values in this component.

The results of a principal coordinates analysis of the regression standardized tooth dimensions are illustrated in Figs 6 and 7. Although only one analysis was undertaken the results are represented in two figures; the first and second principal coordinates are plotted for African cercopithecids in Fig. 6, while Fig. 7 shows the results for the Asian species. The first principal coordinate derived from this analysis accords well with the first component of the

TABLE V. Forty-nine species of Cercopithecidae. Slopes (x) and intercepts (b) of regression equations relating the length of the lower second molar to the tooth dimensions described above. The equations take the form $Y = x(LM_2) + b$ where LM_2 = tooth length, and Y is a tooth dimension. Figures in parenthesis are the 95% confidence intervals for slope and intercept. Symbols are as in Table I.

Dimension	Slope	Intercept	Coefficient of Correlation
h.h.	1·05(0·08)	−0·96(0·03)	0·964
m.h.	0·91(0·08)	−0·27(0·02)	0·955
s.a.	1·64(0·11)	−0·51(0·03)	0·974
c.w.	0·68(0·11)	−0·14(0·03)	0·876
c.o.	0·90(0·13)	−0·96(0·03)	0·900
e	0·92(0·21)	−1·00(0·05)	0·786
p.m.	0·88(0·19)	−0·77(0·05)	0·801

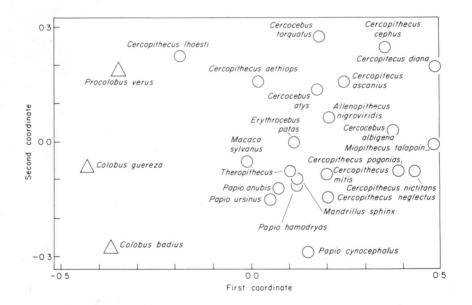

FIG. 6. The first two coordinates of a principal coordinates analysis of the molar dimensions of African cercopithecid primates (all measurements standardized for tooth length). The first coordinate accounts for 37% of the variability of the system. Second and subsequent coordinates account for 11, 7 and 4% respectively. Diamonds represent colobines; circles represent cercopithecines.

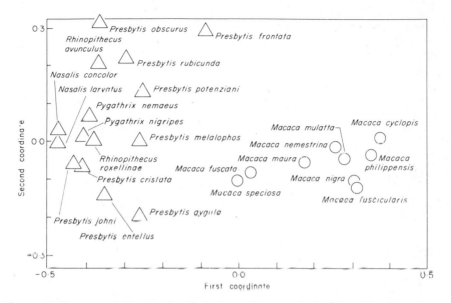

FIG, 7 The first two coordinates of a principal coordinates analysis of the molar dimensions of Asian cercopithecid primates. Symbols are as in Fig. 6.

principal components analysis described above. A Spearman's rank correlation of 0·97 was obtained between the species values of the first principal component and the first principal coordinate. This implies a nearly equal influence of all tooth dimensions in the result; if a species consistently has significantly larger tooth dimensions than empirically expected from its tooth length then it will have a negative value on the first coordinate. Body size or tooth size by itself does not influence the result; large and small species are dispersed throughout.

The first coordinate value for each species for this analysis is a clear and consistent indicator of its diet in the wild; the higher the value on the first coordinate, the more fruit and less leaves a species has in its diet. Leaf-eating species have small values and are clustered to the left in Figs 6 and 7. For example, of the African species studied, the colobines have the most purely folivorous diets while some of the cercopithecines have diets composed almost entirely of fruits. As expected, species of *Colobus* have low values, while frugivorous cercopithecines like *Cercopithecus talapoin* and *Cercocebus albigena* have very high values. Closer examination of the values of the first coordinate shows that this finding can be refined by comparison of species within family, subfamily or generic groupings. Among the folivorous African cercopithecids, the colobines *Colobus guereza* and *C. badius* are the best known and have similar diets. Clutton-Brock (1974) observed that *C. guereza* preferred mature leaves even when shoots, flowers and fruits were available. Other authors list leaves and some fruit in this species' diet (Malbrant and

Maclatchy, 1949; Booth, 1956b quoted in Tappen, 1960). *C. badius* has a
more varied diet with somewhat greater amounts of fruit although in some
seasons the animals spent up to 60% of their time feeding on mature leaves
(Clutton-Brock, 1974). There are several reports of *C. badius* feeding on a
variety of tree species, preferring young leaves, flowers and floral buds
(Kano, 1971; Struhsaker, 1974). The morphology of the second molars of
the species is similar: *C badius* has just about the same value on the first
principal coordinate as *C. guereza. Procolobus versus* is comparable to *C.
badius.* A high fibre diet with some fruit would be inferred. Booth (1957)
found leaves but no fruit in the stomach contents of 30 specimens of
P. verus.

Cercopithecines which are primarily found in riverine forests, semi-arid.
savannas and woodland savannas eat high proportions of grass stems,
rhizomes, leaves, buds, hard beans and the like. Since much of this food is
taken from the ground, a high grit component would be expected. Soft fruits
and other low grit, low fibre content foods are less common in their diets.
Species in this group whose diets are fairly well known are *Cercopithecus
aethiops, Papio spp., Erythrocebus patas, Mandrillus sphinx* and *Theropithecus
gelada.*

In Uganda gallery forests, Rowell (1964, 1966) found the diet of *Papio
anubis* to consist largely of green and often extremely bitter fruits, but also
included considerable leaves, shoots, flowers and roots. *P. anubis* also ate
some animal food. According to Washburn and DeVore (1961) and DeVore
and Washburn (1963), in Kenya woodland savannas, seeds and stems of
grasses amount to 90% of the diet for many weeks during the dry season.
In the middle of the dry season the species dug up and ate rhizomes. Buds,
blossoms and beans of the acacia tree were second in importance. A variety
of other plant and animal foods accounted for a small quantitative proportion
of the diet.

In Uganda forest patches and riverine forests, Hall (1965) noted that the
diet of *P. anubis* included grasses, leaves, pods and berries. In Ethiopian
gallery forests and woodland savannas the species spent roughly 43% of its
feeding time eating folivorous materials, mainly grass leaves but also flowers,
roots and bark. The remaining feeding time was divided between fruits
(55%) and insects (3%) (Dunbar and Dunbar, 1974). Aldrich-Blake *et al.*
(1971) reported that *P. anubis* will eat termites, birds, goats and rabbits.

In a study by Altmann and Altmann (1970) the diet of Kenyan *Papio
cynocephalus* living in semi-arid savannas consisted mainly of grass parts,
fever tree blossoms and green fruits. A variety of other foods were eaten
including a limited amount of animal food.

According to DeVore and Hall (1965) *Papio ursinus*, the chacma baboon,
fed on roots, tubers, bulbs, flowers, seeds, leaves, leaf bases and stems. A
staple food item in some places were the beans of the exotic wattle trees. In
some areas bark was the major item. Vegetables formed 90% of the Cape
baboon's diet. The remaining diet consisted of insects, lizards, caterpillars
and scorpions. Black mussels and limpets were eaten where encountered.

Ethiopian *Papio hamadryas* ate grasses and the flowers, leaves and fruits of shrubs and trees. Cactus fruits of a recently introduced species were eaten in quantity. Acacia trees provided the main subsistence in both wet and dry seasons. At the end of the dry season, hamadryas baboons ate large amounts of beans and dry leaves from this tree together with leaves and roots. In the rainy season, grass seeds provided 44% of the food; acacia flowers, 43%; other foods picked up off the ground plus acacia shoots and fruits accounted for the remainder. This species occasionally ate locusts and an isolated case of small mammal predation was reported (Kummer, 1968; Kummer and Kurt, 1973; Nagel, 1973).

In Uganda, Hall (1966) saw *Erythrocebus patas* eat mainly grasses together with berries, fruits, beans and seeds. These were supplemented by occasional finds of mushrooms, ants, grasshoppers, lizards, eggs and chunks of red mud.

According to Dunbar and Dunbar (1974) based on activity counts, almost 97% of the diet of *Theropithecus gelada* consisted of grass parts. The rest of the feeding time was spent on leaves, flowers and fruits of herbs, shrubs, bushes and trees. The preferred part of grasses were the leaves (91%) while seeds and roots of grasses represented about 6%. Crook (1966) and Crook and Aldrich-Blake (1968) noted that geladas occasionally ate flying ants.

In Ethiopia Dunbar and Dunbar (1974) saw *Cercopithecus aethiops* eat fruits (especially soft fruits) and seeds just over 50% of the time. The remainder of the diet consisted of leaves (19%), flowers (18%), bark (6%) and insects (7%). Reports of the feeding of this species by Struhsaker (1967), Gartlan and Brain (1968), Booth (1956b), Kano (1971), Hall and Gartlan (1965), Jackson and Gartlan (1965) and Malbrant and Maclatchy (1949) are similar to the Dunbar's findings.

Mandrillus sphinx searches on the ground for fallen fruits, berries, shoots and insects (Forbes, 1894; Jeannin, 1935 quoted in Tappen, 1960; Malbrant and Maclatchy, 1949; Gartlan and Struhsaker, 1972). It is a devastating raider of native crops in the dry season and eats cassava (manioc root).

Species of *Papio, Erythrocebus patas, Mandrillus sphinx* and *Theropithecus gelada* cluster together with much lower values than African cercopithecines which have diets with much more fruit (*Cercopithecus talapoin* and *Cercocebus albigena*). Of the group, *Theropithecus* eats the most grass. But although geladas have long shearing blades and extremely high crowns which would tend to make them have low values on the first coordinate, they also have unusually long molars. Thus, regression adjustment for tooth length gives a higher value on the first principal coordinate than would be expected on the basis of behavioural information. *P. cynocephalus* is the furthest right on the graph of *Papio spp.* suggesting that it has the most frugivorous diet.

Macaca sylvanus, the sole representative of this genus in Africa and Gibraltar, inhabits mixed conifer and oak forests often dissected with grasslands (Deag and Crook, 1971). Winters are wet and cold and there is snow; summers are dry with little rainfall. In Gibraltar, barbary apes eat acorns, juniper berries and conifer shoots as well as other shoots and roots and insects (Rumsey and Whiten, 1927). Additional food items listed by Sanderson

(1957), Deag and Crook (1971) and Forbes (1894) include the kernels of pine cones, grasses, cultivated plants, walnuts and figs. *M. sylvanus* not surprisingly falls to the left of all but one cercopithecine in Fig. 6, indicating a coarse diet.

Cercocebus albigena and *Cercopithecus talopin* appear to be the most frugivorous of the well known African species and the two species also have extremely high first coordinate values. In one study *Miopithecus talapoin* ate an overwhelming preponderance of fruit and berries; leaves and shoots accounted for only about 8 % of the plant foods. Cultivated foods were important at some times of the year in some regions. Large amounts of insect remains were also found in their stomachs (Gautier, 1966; Gautier-Hion, 1971). In an earlier study, Gautier and Gautier-Hion (1969) found 33 % insects by weight in the stomachs of four specimens. Jones (1970) found insects in five of the nine stomachs he analysed.

Cercocebus albigena in Uganda eats oil-palm nuts, although other fruits and green shoots were sometimes found in the stomach contents (Haddow *et al.*, 1947). Malbrant and Maclatchy (1949), Jones and Sabater-Pi (1968), Jones (1970), Chalmers (1968) and Gartlan and Struksaker (1972) indicated a diet of secondary forest berries and fruit and some leaves.

Cercopithecus ascanius eats high proportions of leaves and not surprisingly falls intermediate between *Cercopithecus aethiops* and *Cercopithecus talapoin*. By far the most common foods found by Haddow (1952) in the 100 stomachs of *C. ascanius* analysed were leaves, flowers and green shoots. Frequency of occurrence was often associated with abundance in quantity. Fruits were the next most important food item after leaves. Red-tailed monkeys did not eat the hard kernels contained within soft fruits, in contrast to *Cercocebus*, which broke up and swallowed kernels. Crops were often raided.

The diets of the remainder of African species are much less well known. On the first axis, *Cercopithecus cephus*, *C. pogonias*, *C. nictitans* and *C. diana* cluster with the fruit eaters *Cercopithecus talapoin* and *Cercocebus albigena* and are probably primarily frugivorous. This seems to be supported by the available dietary evidence. *Cercopithecus cephus* is said to be absent from forests which lack oil-palms because of its adaptation to subsist on the pulp of the oil-palm nut. The diet also includes flowers, buds, seeds, fruits and a few insects (Malbrant and Maclatchy, 1949; Hill, 1966; Gautier and Gautier-Hion, 1969; Jones, 1970).

According to Malbrant and Maclatchy (1949) *Cercopithecus pogonias* is largely frugivorous. Jones (1970) found leaves and fruit in the stomachs of six individuals. Gartlan and Struhsaker (1972) have observed that the fruiting of two plant species and the flowering of a third are coincident with seasonal troop movements of *C. pogonias*. It ate fruits, arils of fruit and flowers.

Cercopithecus nictitans probably eats largely fruit but also some leaves, flowers, bark and insects as well judging by stomach contents and behavioural observations (Malbrant and Maclatchy, 1949; Gautier and Gautier-Hion, 1969; Jones, 1970; Gartlan and Struhsaker, 1972).

Cercopithecus diana is an arboreal species with an almost entirely frugivorous diet based on the stomach content of 14 specimens (Booth, 1956a).

Cercopithecus mitis and *C. neglectus* cluster with *C. ascanis* and therefore may be more folivorous than other forest dwelling cercopithecines. *C. mitis* was reported by Haddow (1956) to eat fruits, leaves and shoots; it did not ordinarily raid crops. Gartlan and Brain (1968) recorded both fruit and leaves in the food and suggested that the staple diet of *C. mitis* included a large proportion of leaves and also flowers. Instances of feeding on fruit, leaves and bamboo have been reported (Aldrich-Blake, 1966 quoted in Nisihda, 1968; Kano, 1971; Stott, 1960; Ansell, 1964 quoted in Hill, 1966).

Malbrant and Maclatchy (1949) observed *Cercopithecus neglectus* eating fallen fruit. Gautier and Gautier-Hion (1969) analysed the stomach contents of two individuals and found 83% fruits and the remainder consisted of flowers, buds and insects. Jones (1970) analysed two stomachs containing leaves and fruit.

Allenopithecus nigroviridis, *Cercocebus torqatus* and *C. atys* all have distinctively lower values on the first axis than *Cercocebus albigena* and may therefore be found to have more folivorous materials in their diets. Dietary data on these species is sketchy. *A. nigroviridis* inhabits swampy country in the Congo. Pournelle (1959) suggested that they ate fish, shrimp and snails in addition to fruit, nuts and insect larvae. Beyond this nothing is known of their behaviour in the wild.

Cercocebus torquatus is largely vegetarian, eating mostly fruit, but may ingest limited amounts of leaves and animal matter (Jones and Sabater-Pi, 1968; Jones, 1970). The species raids crops (Malbrant and Maclatchy, 1949). The remaining *Cercocebus* species are very poorly known. See MacKenzie and Jones (1952) for *C. atys* and Gautier and Gautier-Hion (1969) for *C. galeritus*.

Perhaps the most interesting African cercopithecine studied is *Cercopithecus lhoesti*. Practically nothing is known of the diet of this species. It is confined to montane forests, where it is commonly seen on the ground. It was observed to eat the fruits of *Musanga cecropioides* (in the fig family) and reportedly plundered banana plantations (Haddow *et al.*, 1947, 1951; Haddow, 1952; Gartlan and Struhsaker, 1972). Its molar morphology suggests that it is by far the most folivorous of all extant cercopithecines; with its long shearing blades it falls within the range of Asian colobines.

Asian species conform generally to the pattern which has emerged from African species (Fig. 7); the colobines have lower values on the first principal coordinate than cercopithecines in conjunction with more folivorous diets. Most of the Asian colobines belong to the widespread and diverse genus *Presbytis*. The most thoroughly studied are the Indian and Ceylonese *P. johni* and *P. entellus*. *P. johni* is highly folivorous; in Ceylon its diet is 60% mature leaves and shoots by weight, and these were eaten along with 12% flowers and 28% fruits (Hladik and Hladik, 1972). Other reports on Indian and Ceylonese populations show that mature leaves, flowers, buds, seeds, bark, stems and some fruit are eaten (Jerdan, 1867; Poirier, 1970; Ripley,

1970; Horwich, 1972). *P. entellus* takes more fruit in its diet; quantitative analysis by Amerasinghe *et al.* (1971) and Hladik and Hladik (1972) show that leaves, shoots and flowers are most important (55 % by weight) but that a high proportion of fruits are eaten (45%). Other reports indicate a variety of foods are eaten including native crops (often in high percentages), grain, fruit, tree pods, flower nectar and inflorescences, but leaves and young shoots are the most common food item (Jerdan, 1867; Forbes, 1894; Hingston, 1920; McCann, 1928, 1934; Phillips quoted by Pocock, 1939; Yoshiba, 1967, 1968; Mohnot, 1972). Blandford (1888) says that they appear to be immune from strychnine since they eat quantities of fruit from *Nox vomica* from which this poison is extracted. More detailed recent observations on Ceylonese *P. entellus* indicates that mature leaves were eaten throughout the year but that seasonal abundances of buds, shoots, fruits and seeds were important (Ripley, 1970). Multivariate analysis of the second molars of *P. johni* suggest a high foliage component comparable to that of *Colobus guereza* whereas the molars of *P. entellus* have higher values suggestive of slightly more fruit in the diet.

Of the remaining Asian colobines studied here, *Nasalis larvatus* is extremely folivorous. Banks (1949) and Davis (1962) listed the young leaves, buds and shoots of mangrove and pedata trees as primary dietary items. Kern (1964) noted that at least 95 % of the diet consisted of leaves in all stages of growth as well as tender vines and shoots. Fruits and flowers were also probably eaten, but this was never observed in the wild. Not surprisingly, *N. larvatus* has the smallest score of any species on the first coordinate.

In addition to *N. larvatus*, specimens of three other Bornean species were studied. Not very much is known about their diets. *Presbytis frontatus* is said to take leaves, buds and fruits (Banks, 1949). *P. rubicundus* is known to eat leaves (Harrison, 1954). *P. aygula* takes leaves, buds, fruits and berries (Banks, 1949; Davis, 1962). Molar structure suggests that *P. frontatus* is the most frugivorous of all the colobines. Two other species, *P. rubicundis* and *P. aygula* are similar in having higher values than *P. entellus* and presumably a considerable amount of fruit in the diet. It is interesting that while *P. rubicundus* is most frequently found in hilly, upland primary forests, *P. aygula* is more commonly seen in lowland primary forest (Banks, 1949; Stott and Selsor, 1961). Potential dietary competition between these species suggested by dental evidence, would therefore be avoided. Bornean *P. cristata* was not measured but looks similar to Sumatran *P. cristata* (see below).

As among most other Bornean species, comparison of *P. melalophos* and *P. cristatus* from Sumatra must rest solely on molar morphology since both are said to eat leaves and fruit (Banks, 1949; Fooden, 1971; Medway, 1970). Molar morphology suggests that the latter eats more leaves than the former. *P. cristatus* is comparable in molar structure to extreme leaf-eaters such as *P. johni* and *Colobus guereza*. The molar morphology of *Presbytis obscurus* is indicative of a more folivorous diet than that of sympatric *P. melalophos*.

Two endemic colobines on the Mentawai Islands are quite distinct from one another in their molar morphology and presumably also in their diet.

Nasalis (*Simias*) *concolor* is very like Bornean *N. larvatus* and may be almost wholly a leaf eater; *Presbytis potenziani* has a larger first coordinate value than *P. entellus* and is comparable to that of Bornean *P. aygula*. It presumably supplements its leaf-eating diet with fruit.

Specimens of the remaining Asiatic colobines studied are largely or wholly geographically isolated from each other and are almost unknown ecologically. *Rhinopithecus avunculus*, *R. roxellinae*, *Pygathrix nemaeus*, and *P. nigripes* all have about the same values for the first coordinate. All fall intermediate between *Presbytis johni* and *P. entellus*. Moderate to high percentages of leaves in the diets are indicated for all species.

Nine species of the genus *Macaca* were studied. *Macaca sylvanus* was discussed with the African species. Of the remaining eight, (*M. speciosa*, *M. fuscata*, *M. cyclopis*, *M. mulatta*, *M. nemestrina*, *M. fascicularis*, *M. nigra* and *M. maura*), only the diet of *M. fuscata* has been adequately reported. The Japanese macaque reportedly has a diet consisting of more than 75 % grass, leaves, bark, twigs and flowers during some parts of the winter season; folivorous materials account for about half of its yearly diet (Izawa, 1971, 1972; Suzuki, 1965). The molar structure is consistent with these findings; *M. fuscata* has a first coordinate value which falls with the African cercopithecines *Papio*, *Erythrocebus*, *Theropithecus* and *Cercopithecus aethiops*, and with its little known relative *M. sylvanus*. Information on the other macaques studied is inadequate to allow certain dietary assignment. Inferred from molar structure, the diet of *M. speciosa* must be similar to *M. fuscata*, in containing significant portions of leaves, bark and buds. This is supported by McCann (1933) who stated that they fed largely on leaves, roots and fruit, and that some of the specimens he secured had their cheek pouches crammed with leaves. Bertrand (1969) commonly saw this species eating leaves and fruits as well as cultivated plants. But in Thailand, Fooden (1971) observed that the stomachs of four specimens contained exclusively fruit.

M. speciosa is widely sympatric with *M. mulatta*. Lindburg (1971) reported that the diet of *M. mulatta* included fruits, berries, leaves, bark, flowers, seeds, birds and insects. Southwick *et al.* (1965), Neville (1968), Fooden (1971), Mukherjee and Gupta (1965) and Mandal (1964) listed similar foods but suitable quantitative assessments are unavailable. The species is almost universally known as a crop raider (Blanford, 1888; Hingston, 1920; McCann, 1933; Pocock, 1939; Neville, 1968; Mukherjee, 1969). As is the case for bonnet macaques, rhesus are common inhabitants of temples, roadsides and towns where they feed on whatever they can forage (Mukherjee, 1969; Neville, 1968). The molar structure of the rhesus indicates a diet containing more fruit than that of *M. speciosa*.

Molar differences suggest that *M. speciosa* eats more leaves than *M. fascicularis* and *M. nemistrina* where the three are sympatric. None of the species are well enough known to firmly establish a quantitative dietary pattern. In Thailand, Fooden (1971) found the major dietary component of *M. fascicularis* to be fruit with a minor component of invertebrates on the basis of a large number of stomach contents. Pocock (1939) quoted several authors who found that molluscs, crustaceans and other marine animals were eaten by coastal populations as a supplement to vegetable material. In Malaysia, Kawabe and Mano (1972) noted that nuts and fruits were eaten. On Timor, Kurland (1973) observed the species eating fruits, young leaves and flowers as well as insects and other larvae. Fooden (1971) reported that the stomachs of seven specimens of *M. nemestrina* collected in Thailand contained predominantly fruit pulp although caterpillars and adult insects were a minor component in six cases. In Malaya, Bernstein (1967) reported a diet of fruits, seeds, young leaves and leaf stems, fungus, insects and spiders. In Borneo, Davis (1962) found cheek pouches of pigtails filled with palm fruits. The molar morphology of *M. nemestrina* and *M. fascicularis* suggests that these widely sympatric species have similar diets: predominantly fruit with some leaves. Habitat separation would be indicated for the two species on the basis of differences in body size and tail length.

Molar structure suggests that the diet of the Formosan *M. cyclopis* is extremely frugivorous. Swinhoe's (1862) account of their feeding neither confirms nor denies this. Of the Celebes species, *M. maura* may have more leaves in its diet than *M. nigra*. Again, reports by Wallace (1869), Hickson (1889) and Forbes (1894) make substantive conclusions impossible.

Second and subsequent principal coordinates of the multivariate analysis account for a high percentage of the total variability of the system but have no apparent value as indicators of feeding habits. The current analysis has used data which were regression adjusted for tooth length. In a study of non-cercopithecid primates (Kay 1973, 1975b), a similar regression adjustment was attempted using body mass rather an M_2 length. The results of an analysis of cercopithecid molars using body-mass-adjusted data will not be reported here, since no consistent behavioural information resulted. One thing that is apparent is that cercopithecines tend to have larger molars than do colobines of the same body size. Since the former tend to have more frugivorous diets, this result is the reverse of the findings of Kay (1973, 1975b) that frugivorous non-cercopithecid primates tend to have smaller molars than folivores of the same size. No explanation can presently be advanced to account for this surprising discrepancy. Nevertheless, the successful use of molar length regression adjustment of tooth length for the purposes of dietary prediction now opens the way for a similar analysis of fossil Cercopithecoidea.

In a recently completed study of incisor size in Cercopithecidae, Hylander (personal communication) has shown that species with broad incisors are more frugivorous than their relatives with narrow incisors. Interestingly enough, his independently derived diet–species grouping are virtually identical to those reported here.

CONCLUSIONS

Among cercopithecids there is no simple relationship between tooth size and changes in metabolic rate; molar surfaces are not scaled by the 0·75 power of body mass. That female cercopithecids have proportionately larger teeth than males suggests that metabolic scaling may be operating at the species level since females undergo periodic metabolic elevations during pregnancy.

Occlusion in Old World monkeys begins with an upward, medial Phase I movement of the molars such that eight matching shearing blades on upper and lower teeth contact. Crushing surfaces which are brought together at the termination of Phase I are antero-posteriorly continuous throughout the molar series, producing an undulating surface where bending moments can be applied to the food. During Phase II, a slightly downward and antero-medial movement, cusps are ground across basins.

The paired lophs of the "bilophodont" cercopithecid molars do not serve a shearing function: the medial part of the lower molar lophs engage medial embrasures on the upper molars acting as guides for shearing in Phase I; a similar action occurs between the lateral part of the upper molar lophs and the lateral lower molar embrasures. The lateral part of the lower molar lophs do not support shearing crests—they occlude into upper molar basins at the termination of Phase I, producing bending moments and crushing forces. A similar action characterizes occlusion between the medial part of the upper molar lophs and their corresponding lower molar basins.

Old World monkeys have higher cusps and crowns, longer shearing blades and slightly larger crushing surfaces on second molars than do comparably

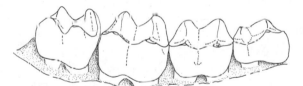

Cercocebus albigenu

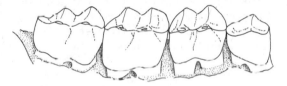

Cercopithecus lhoesti

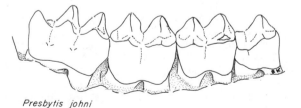

Presbytis johni

FIG. 8. Lower PM4–M3 of representative cercopithecids viewed from the lateral aspect.

sized non-cercopithecid primates. The length of their second molars is approximately the same at a given body size. Primate species which eat significant proportions of leaves in their diets (species of *Indri* and *Alouatta* for example) tend to approximate this condition.

The generalization holds that cercopithecines tend to have more frugivorous diets than colobines but within each group there is considerable variation in the proportions of these foods taken. These differences show up clearly in the molar structure of different species. Folivorous species tend to have relatively higher cusps, longer shearing blades and larger crushing basins for a given tooth length than their frugivorous relatives. This is illustrated in Fig. 8 which compares a folivore, *Presbytis johni*, with a frugivore, *Cercocebus albigena*. On the basis of their molar structure it is hypothesized that several species of cercopithecines may take high proportions of leaves in their diets. *Cercopithecus lhoesti* illustrated in Fig. 8 is an excellent candidate for a folivorous cercopithecine.

ACKNOWLEDGEMENTS

I would like to express my gratitude to Dr Richard Thorington of the United States National Museum, Dr Sidney Anderson of the American Museum of Natural History and Dr P. Napier of the British Museum of Natural History for cooperation at their institutions. Many of the ideas developed in this chapter were incubated by Drs William Hylander and Matt Cartmill. Partial financial support was contributed by an N.S.F. Research Grant GS-43262.

REFERENCES

ALDRICH-BLAKE, F. P. (1966). Some aspects of blue monkey social organization. Presented at the 4th East African Acad. Symposium, Kampala.

ALDRICH-BLAKE, F. P. G., BUNN, T. K., DUNBAR, R. I. M. and HEADLEY, P. M. (1971). Observations on baboons, *Papio anubis*, in an arid region in Ethiopia. *Folia Primat.* **15**, 1–35.

ALTMANN, S. A. and ALTMANN, J. (1970). Baboon Ecology. *Biblio Primat.* **12y**, 1–220.

AMERASINGHE, F. P., VAN CUYLENBERG, B. W. B. and HLADIK, C. M. (1971). Comparative histology of the alimentary tract of Ceylon primates in correlation with the diet. *Ceylon J. Sci.: Biol. Sci.* **9**, 75–87.

ANSELL, W. (1964). Quoted from Hill, W. C. O. *Puku* **2**, 14–52.

BANKS, E. (1949). "Bornean Mammals." The Kuching Press, Kuching.

BATES, G. L. (1905). Notes on the mammals of the Southern Cameroons and the Benito. *Proc. zool. Soc. Lond.* 65–85.

BERNSTEIN, I. S. (1967). A field study of the pigtail monkey (*Macaca nemestrina*). *Primates* **8**, 217–228.

BERTRAND, M. (1969). The behavioral repertoire of the stumptail macaque. *Biblio Primat.* **11**, 1–273.

BLACKITH, R. E. and REYMENT, R. A. (1971). "Multivariate Morphometrics." Academic Press, New York and London.

BLANFORD, W. T. (1888). "The Fauna of British India, including Ceylon and Burma." Taylor and Francis, London.

Booth, A. H. (1956a) The Cercopithecidae of the Gold and Ivory Coasts: geographic and systematic observations. *Ann. Mag. nat. Hist.* **9**, 476–480.

Booth, A. H. (1956b) The distribution of primates in the Gold Coast. *J. W. Afr. Sci. Ass.* **2**, 122–133.

Booth, A. M. (1957). Observations on the natural history of the olive colobus monkey, *Procolobus verus* (Van Beneden). *Proc. zool. Soc. Lond.* **129**, 421–430.

Chalmers, N. R. (1968). The social behavior of free living mangabeys in Uganda. *Folia Primat.* **8**, 263–281.

Clutton-Brock, T. H. (1974). Primate social organization and ecology. *Nature, Lond.* **250**, 539–542.

Crompton, A. W. (1971). The origin of the tribosphenic molar. *In* "Early Mammals" (Kermack, D. M. and Kermack, K. A., eds.) *J. Linn. Soc.* (*Zool*) **50**, suppl. **1**, 65–87.

Crook, J. H. (1966). Gelada baboon head structure and movement —a comparative report. *Symp. zool. Soc. Lond.* **18**, 237–248.

Crook, J. H. and Aldrich-Blake, P. (1968). Ecological and behavioral contrasts between sympatric ground dwelling primates in Ethiopia. *Folia Primat* **8**, 192–227.

Cuvier, G. (1863). "The Animal Kingdom." Bohn, London.

Davis, D. D. (1962). Mammals of the lowland rainforest of north Borneo. *Bull. natn. Mus. St. Singapore* **31**, 1–129.

Deag, J. M. and Crook, J. H. (1971). Social behavior and "agonistic buffering" in the wild barbary macaque, *Macaca sylvanus*, L. *Folia Primat.* **15**, 183–200.

DeVore, I. and Hall K. R. L. (1965). Baboon ecology, *In* "Primate Behavior: Field Studies of Monkeys and Apes" (DeVore, I. ed.), pp. 20–52. Holt, Rinehart and Winston, New York.

DeVore, I. and Washburn, S. L. (1963). Baboon ecology and human evolution. *In* "African Ecology and Human Evolution" (Howell, F. C. and Bourliere, F. eds), pp. 335–367. Viking Fund Publications in Anthropology, No. 36, New York.

Dunbar, R. I. M. and Dunbar, E. P. (1974). Ecological relations and niche separation between sympatric terrestrial primates in Ethiopia. *Folia Primat.* **21**, 36–60.

Fooden, J. (1971). Report on primates collected in western Thailand, January–April 1967. *Fieldiana, Zool.*, **49**, (1), 95–118.

Forbes, H. O. (1894). "A Handbook of the Primates," Vols I and II. W. H. Allen, London.

Gartlan, J. S. and Brain, C. K. (1968). Ecology and social variability in *Cercopithecus aethiops* and *C. mitis*. *In* "Primate: Studies in Adaptation and Variability" (Jay, P. C., ed.), pp. 253–292. Holt, Rinehart and Winston, New York.

Gartlan, J. S. and Struhsaker, T. (1972). Polyspecific associations and niche separation of rainforest anthropoids in Cameroon, West Africa. *J. Zool. Lond.* **168**, 221–266.

Gautier, J.-P. (1966). L'ecologie et l'ethologie du talapoin (*Miopithecus talapoin talapoin*). *Rev. Biol. Gabon* **2**, 311–329.

Gautier-Hion, A. (1971). L'ecologie du talapoin du Gabon. *Terre et Vie*, **25**, 427–490.

Gautier, J.-P. and Gautier-Hion, A. (1969). Associations polyspecifiques chez les cercopitheques du Gabon. *Terre et Vie* **23**, 164–201.

Gould, S. J. (1966). "Allometry and size in ontogeny and phylogeny." *Biol. Rev.* **41**, 587–640.

GOULD, S. J. (1974). This view of life: The nonscience of human nature. *Nat. Hist.* **83** (4), 21–25.

HADDOW, A. J. (1952). Field and laboratory studies on an African monkey, *Cercopithecus ascanius schmidti* Matschie. *Proc. zool. Soc. Lond.*, **122**, 297–394.

HADDOW, A. J. (1956). The blue monkey group in Uganda. *Uganda Wildlife and Sport*, **1**, 22–26.

HADDOW, A. J., SMITHBURN, K. C., MAHAFEY, A. F. and BUGHER, J. C. (1947). Monkeys in relation to yellow fever in Bwanba Country, Uganda. *Trans. R. Soc. trop. Med. Hyg.* **40**, 677–700.

HADDOW, A. J., DICK, G. W. A., LUMSDEN, W. H. R. and SMITHBURN, K. C. (1951). Monkeys in relation to epidemiology of yellow fever in Uganda. *Trans. R. Soc. trop. Med. Hyg.* **45**, 189–224.

HALL, K. R. L. (1965). Ecology and behaviour of baboons, patas and vervet monkeys in Uganda. *In* "The Baboon in Medical Research" (Vagtborg, H., ed.), pp. 43–61. University of Texas Press, San Antonio.

HALL, K. R. L. (1966). Behaviour and ecology of the wild patas monkey, *Erythrocebus patas*, in Uganda. *J. Zool., Lond.*, **148**, 15–87.

HALL, K. R. L. and GARTLAN, J. S. (1965). Ecology and behaviour of the vervet monkey, *Cercopithecus aethiops*, Lolui Island, Lake Victoria. *Proc. zool. Soc. Lond.* **145**, 37–56.

HARRISON, J. L. (1954). The natural foods of some rats and other mammals. *Bull. Raffles Mus.* **25**, 157–165.

HICKSON, S. J. (1889). "A Naturalist in North Celebes." Murray, London.

HIIEMAE, K. M. and KAY, R. F. (1972). Trends in the evolution of primate mastication. *Nature, Lond.* **240**, 486–487.

HILL, W. C. O. (1966). "Primates: Cercopithecoidea," Vol. VI. Wiley-Inter-Science, New York.

HILL, W. C. O. (1970). "Primates: Cynopithecinae" (Second Part), Vol. VIII. Wiley-Interscience, New York.

HILL, W. C. O. (1974). "Primates: Cynopithecinae" (First Part), Vol. VII. Wiley-Interscience, New York.

HINGSTON, R. W. (1920). "A Naturalist In The Himalaya." Small, Maynard and Co., Boston.

HLADIK, C. M. and HLADIK, A. (1972). Disponsibilities alimentaire et domaines vitaux des primates a Ceylon. *Terre et Vie*, **2**, 149–215.

HORWICH, R. H. (1972). Home range and food habits of the nilgiri langur *Presbytis johni*. *J. Bombay nat. Hist. Soc.* **69**, (2), 255–267.

IZAWA, K. (1971). Japanese monkeys living in the Okoppe Basin of the Shimokita Peninsula: the first report of the winter follow-up survey after aerial spraying of herbicide. *Primates* **12**, 191–200.

IZAWA, K. (1972). Japanese monkeys living in the Okoppe Basin of the Shimokita Peninsula: the second report of the winter follow-up survey after the aerial spraying of herbicide. *Primates* **13**, 201–212.

JACKSON, G. and GARTLAN, J. S. (1965). The flora and fauna of Lolui Island, Lake Victoria, Uganda. *J. Ecol.* **53**(3), 573–598.

JEANNIN, A. (1935). "Les Mammiferes Sauvage du Cameroun." Lechevalier, Paris.

JERDAN, T. C. (1867). "The Mammals of India." Thomason College Press, Roorkee.

JONES, C. (1970) Stomach contents and gastro-intestinal relationships of monkeys collected at Rio Muni, West Africa. *Mammalia*, **34**, 107–117.

JONES, C. and SABATER-PI, J. (1968). Comparative ecology of *Cercocebus albigena* (Gray) and *Cercocebus torquatus* (Ker) in Rio Muni, West Africa. *Folia Primat* **9**, 99–113.

KANO, T. (1971). Distribution of the primates on the eastern shore of Lake Tanganyika. *Primates* **12**(3–4), 281–304.

KAWABE, M. and MANO, T. (1972). Ecology and behavior of the wild proboscus monkey, *Nasalis larvatus* (Wurmb), in Sabah, Malaysia. *Primates*, **13**(2), 213–228.

KAY, R. F. (1973). Mastication, molar tooth structure and diet in primates. Ph.D. Thesis, Yale University.

KAY, R. F. (1975a). Allometry and early hominids. *Science, N. Y.* **189**, 63.

KAY, R. F. (1975b) The functional adaptations of primate molar teeth. *Am. J. phys. Anthrop.* **43**, 195–216.

KAY, R. F. and HIIEMAE, K. M. (1974a). Jaw movement and tooth use in recent and fossil primates. *Am. J. phys. Anthrop.* **40**(2), 27–256.

KAY, R. F. and HIIEMAE, K. M. (1974b). Mastication in *Galago crassicaudatus*, a cinefluorographic and occlusal study. *In* "Prosimian Biology" (Martin, R. D. Doyle, G. A. and Walker, A. C., eds), 501–530. Duckworth, London.

KERN, J. A. (1964). Observations on the habits of the proboscis monkey, *Nasalis larvatus* (Wurmb), made in the Brunei Bay area, Borneo. *Zoologia* **49**, 183–192.

KLEIBER, M. (1961). "The Fire of Life". John Wiley and Sons, New York.

KUMMER, H. (1968). "Social organization of hamadryas baboons." *Biblio Primat.* **6**, 1–189.

KUMMER, H., and KURT, F. (1963). Social units of a free-living population of Hamadryas Baboons. *Folia Primat.* **1**, 4–19.

KURLAND, J. A. (1973). A natural history of Kra macaques (*Macaca fascicularis*, Raffles, 1821) at the Kutai Reserve, Kalimantan, Timur, Indonesia. *Primates*, **14** (2–3), 245–263.

LINDBURG, D. G. (1971). The rhesus monkey in north India: an ecological and behavioral study. *In* "Primate Behavior" (Rosenblum, L. A., ed.) Vol. 2. Academic Press, New York and London.

MACKENZIE, A. F. and JONES, T. S. (1952) The economic problems of the monkey population in Sierra Leone. *Proc. zool. Soc. Lond.* **122**, 541.

MAI BRANI, M. and MACLATCHY, A. (1949). "Faune de l'Equateur African Francais, Tome II, Mammiferes." Lechevalier, Paris.

MANDAL, A. K. (1964). The behavior of the rhesus monkeys (*Macaca mulatta* Zimmermann) in the Sundarbans. *J. Bengal nat. Hist. Soc.* **33**(1), 153–165.

MARINE, D., CYPRA, A. and HUNT, L. (1924). Influence of the Thyroid Gland on the increased heat production occurring during pregnancy and lactation. *J. metab. Res.* **5**, 277–291.

MCCANN, C. (1928). Notes on the common Indian langur (*Pithecus entellus*). *J. Bombay nat. Hist. Soc.* **33**, 192–194.

MCCANN, C. (1933). Notes on some Indian macaques. *J. Bombay nat. Hist. Soc.* **36**(4), 796–800.

MCCANN, C. (1934). Observations on some of the Indian langurs. *J. Bombay nat. Hist. Soc.* **36**, 618–628.

MEDWAY, L. (1970). The monkeys of Sundaland: ecology and systematics of the cercopithecids of a humid equatorial environment. *In* "Old World Monkeys" (Napier, J. R. and Napier, P. H., eds), pp. 513–554. Academic Press, New York and London.

MILLS, J. R. E. (1955). Ideal dental occlusion in primates. *Dent. Practnr., Bristol* **6**, 47–61.

MOHNOT, S. M. (1971). Ecology and behaviour of the human langur, *Presbytis entellus* (Primates: Cercopithecidae) invading fields, gardens and orchards around Jodhpur, Western India. *Trop. Ecol.* **12**(2), 237.

MUKHERJEE, A. K. (1969) A field study on the behavior of two roadside groups of rhesus macaque (*Macaca mulatta* Zimmermann) in northern Uttar Pradesh. *J. Bombay nat. Hist. Soc.* **66**(1), 47–56.

MUKHERJEE, A. K. and GUPTA, S. (1965). Habits of the rhesus macaque *Macaca mulatta* (Zimmermann) in the Sunderbans, 24—Parganas, west Bengal. *J. Bombay nat. Hist. Soc.* **62**(1), 145–146.

NAGEL, U. (1973). A comparison of anubis baboons, hamadryas baboons and their hybrids at a species border in Ethiopia. *Folia Primat.* **19**, 104–165.

NAPIER, J. R. and NAPIER, P. H. (1967). "A Handbook of Living Primates." Academic Press, New York and London.

NEVILLE, M. K. (1968). Ecology and activity of Himalyan foothills rhesus monkeys (*Macaca mulatta*). *Ecology* **49**, 110–123.

NISHIDA, T. (1968). Social groups of wild chimpanzees in the Mahali Mountains. *Primates* **9**, 167–224.

PILBEAM, D. and GOULD, S. J. (1974). Size and scaling in human evolution. *Science, N.Y.* **186**, 892–900.

POCOCK, R. I. (1939). "The Fauna of British India including Ceylon and Burma" Vol. I: Mammalia. Taylor and Francis, London.

POIRIER, F. E. (1970). "The nilgiri langur (*Presbytis johnii*) of south India." *In* "Primate Behavior" (Rosenblum, L. A., ed.), Vol. I, pp. 251–377. Academic Press, New York and London.

POURNELLE, G. H. (1959). Allen's Monkey. *Zoonooz* **32**(10).

PRATER, S. H. (1965). "The Book of Indian Animals," 2nd edition. Bombay Natural History Society, Bombay.

RIPLEY, S. (1970). Leaves and leaf-monkeys: the social organization of foraging in gray langurs (*Presbytis entellus thersites*). *In* "Old World Monkeys" Napier, J. R. and Napier, P. H., eds), pp. 481–509. Academic Press, New York and London.

ROMER, A. S. (1945). "Vertebrate Paleontology," 2nd edition. University of Chicago Press, Chicago.

ROWELL, T. E. (1964). The habitat of baboons in Uganda. *Proc. E. Afr. Acad.* **2**, 121–127.

ROWELL, T. E. (1966). Forest-living baboons in Uganda. *J. Zool., Lond.* **149**, 344–364.

RUMSEY, T. J. and WHITEN, A. (1972). Baby-care in Barbary apes. *Animals* **14**(12), 561–563.

SANDERSON, I. T. (1957) "The Monkey Kingdom." Hamish Hamilton, London.

SOUTHWICK, C. H., BEG, M. A. and SIDIGI, M. R. (1965). Rhesus monkeys in north India. *In* "Primate Behavior: Field Studies of Monkeys and Apes" (DeVore, I., ed.) pp. 111–159. Holt, Rinehart and Winston, New York.

STOTT, K. (1960). Stuhlmann's blue monkey in the Kayonsa Forest Uganda. *J. Mammal.* **41**, 400–401.

STOTT, K. and SELSOR, G. J. (1961). Observations of the maroon Leaf-monkey in north Borneo. *Mammalia* **25**, 184–189.

STRUHSAKER, T. (1967). Ecology of vervet monkeys (*Cercopithecus aethiops*) in the Masai, Amboseli Game Rserve, Kenya. *Ecology* **48**, 841–904.

STRUHSAKER, T. (1974). Of Monkeys and Men. *Animal Kingdom* **77**(2), 25–30.

SUZUKI, A. (1965). An ecological study of wild Japanese monkeys in snowy areas focused on their food habits. *Primates* **9**, 31–72.

SWINHOE, R. (1862). On the mammals of the island of Formosa (China). *Proc. zool. Soc. Lond.* 347–365.

SZALAY, F. S. (1969). Mixodectidae, Microsyopidae, and the insectivore-primate transition. *Bull. Am. Mus. nat. Hist.* **140**(4), 195–330.

SZALAY, F. S. (1972). Paleobiology of the earliest primates. *In* "The Functional and Evolutionary Biology of Primates" (Tuttle, R., ed.), pp. 3–35. Aldine and Atherton, Chicago.

TAPPEN, N. C. (1960). Problems of distribution and adaptation of the African monkeys. *Curr. Anthrop.* **1**(2), 91–120.

THORINGTON, R. W. and GROVES, C. P. (1970). An Annotated Classification of the Cercopithecoidea. *In* "Old World Monkeys" (Napier, J. R. and Napier, P. H., eds), pp. 620–648. Academic Press, New York and London.

VAN VALEN, L. (1966). Deltatheridia, a new order of mammals. *Bull. Am. Mus. nat. Hist.* **132**(1), 1–126.

WAHLSTEDT, W. C. and DAVIS, J. C. (1968). Fortran IV program for computation and display of principal components. *Kansas State Geol. Surv. Comput. Contrib.* **21**, University of Kansas, Lawrence.

WALLACE, A. R. (1869). "The Malay Archipelago." Macmillan, London.

WASHBURN, S. L. and DEVORE, I. (1961). The social life of baboons. *Scient. Am.* **204**, 62–71.

YOSHIBA, K. (1967). An ecological study of hanuman langurs *Presbytis entellus*. *Primates* **8**, 127–154.

YOSHIBA, K. (1968). Local and intertroop variability in ecology and social behavior of common Indian langurs. *In* "Primates: Studies in Adaptation and Variability" (Jay, P. C., ed.), pp. 217–242. Holt, Rinehart and Winston, New York.

21. The Relationship between Tooth Patterns and Jaw Movements in the Hominoidea

J. R. E. MILLS

Institute of Dental Surgery and University College London

It was shown many years ago by Butler (1952) that the movement of the lower teeth across the corresponding upper teeth leaves evidence behind in the form of wear facets, from which it is possible to reconstruct the path of movement of the lower jaw. I have used this technique (Mills, 1954, 1955, 1963, 1973) to investigate the pattern of jaw movement in representative groups of Primates. I concluded that chewing in the Hominoidea may be divided into two phases (Figs 1 and 2). The buccal phase commences when the teeth first come into contact (Fig. 2A), with the lower jaw displaced to the ipsilateral side, and continues, with the jaw moving upwards and medially, and rotating about the ipsilateral condyle, until the centric position is reached (Fig. 2B). It then passes smoothly into the lingual phase, as rotation transfers to the contralateral condyle (Fig. 2C). During this phase, the teeth are held in contact by contraction of the mandibular elevators, but, as the jaw continues to move medially, it also moves slightly downwards. This has recently been confirmed by Hiiemac and Kay (1973) and Kay and Hiiemae (1974).

An interesting feature is that, while facets used in the buccal phase of one side are in contact, those used in the lingual phase of the contralateral side are also in contact. That is, the buccal phase of the ipsilateral side is coincident with the lingual phase on the other side of the mouth. This is a condition sometimes called "balanced occlusion", and is found in all the higher primates, and in some, but not all, other groups. Its significance is not known, but it may be a mechanism to protect the mandibular joint from undue strain. It is difficult to visualize an animal chewing on both sides of the mouth simultaneously! These wear facets, produced by attrition, are highly polished and, under low-power magnification, resemble the cutting edge of an instrument such as a chisel. As I pointed out in a previous paper (Mills, 1955), these facets are covered with fine parallel scratch marks, which give an indication of the direction of jaw movement. The resemblance of these facets to the sharpened edge of a chisel is not coincidence; they in fact serve the same purpose, since chewing consists of a shearing action essentially between the edges of the facets. Every and Kühne (1971), and also Zingeser (1969), have

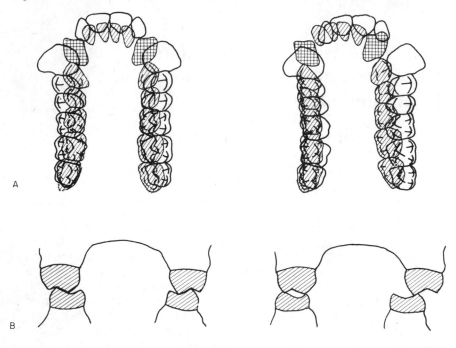

FIG. 1. (A) Upper and lower dentitions of *Gorilla* superimposed on the left in centric relationship, and on the right as the teeth first come into contact on the left side. The right side is consequently at the end of the lingual phase. (B) Coronal section of first molar of *Gorilla* through the tip of the hypoconid: left, in centric relation; right, at the commencement of the buccal phase on the left side.

suggested that these facets are produced, not during chewing, but during a sharpening activity which Every calls "thegosis". This seems not improbable. During chewing there is usually food between the teeth. Certainly at the end of a chewing cycle the molar teeth will come into contact, but this is surely the signal that the particular morsel has been comminuted, and that it is time to start a new cycle. One would expect chewing to have the effect of blunting the cutting edges, as use blunts a chisel. Zingeser (1969) has drawn attention to the marked wear facets on the large canines of certain monkeys; a similar

FIG. 2. The cheek teeth of *Gorilla*: (A) at the beginning of the buccal phase, (B) in centric relation, and (C) at the end of the lingual phase.

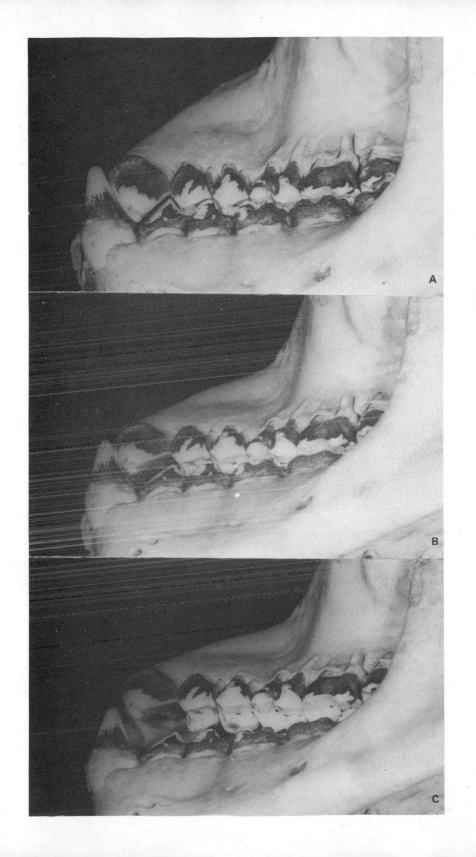

situation occurs in many groups of anthropoid primates, especially in the males. These facets produce fine, dagger-like cutting edges on the canines which have nothing to do with chewing. Nevertheless the facets are in the same plane and produced by the same jaw action as the smaller facets on the postcanine teeth. It may be that this balancing of the facets on the two sides of the mouth in the Hominoidea is further evidence of the existence of thegosis. That is to say, the balanced occlusion may, in some way, protect the weak joint during thegosis, when the teeth are in contact. It cannot do so in chewing, when food is between the teeth on one side only.

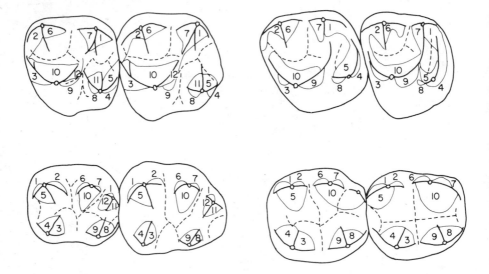

FIG. 3. "Map" of wear facets on first and second molars of *Gorilla* (left) and *Homo* (right) Homologous facets are numbered according to the method proposed by Butler (1973).

It has been shown (Mills, 1954) that the cusps and their associated ridges maintain a very constant relationship with opposing grooves during chewing, and moreover that this relationship does not vary greatly between genera. If the position of a cusp or ridge were to change, the opposing groove would also have to change. Wear facets therefore can be homologized from one genus to another over a wide range of animals, variations occurring only when cusps and ridges are lost, or new ones introduced.

The wear pattern in the Pongidae is easily explained. The large canines—larger in the male, but still interlocking in the female—prevent chewing along any but very narrow pathways. In man, the canine has become essentially a third incisor and has no affect on the path of jaw movement. Nevertheless, if we examine the teeth of a human skull (Fig. 3), and provided the dental occlusion is reasonably ideal, we find that the pattern of wear facets on the molar teeth is essentially similar to those on an ape such as, for example, the gorilla. Certain precautions are necessary in doing this. Modern man, in industrialized societies, has largely escaped the pressures of natural selection. This, together with a cooked and easily chewed diet, and with low cusps and ridges on the postcanine teeth, has allowed malocclusion to become the rule rather than the exception. For my purpose it is necessary to select a skull with a dental occlusion which is not too far removed from the ideal, and also in which wear of the teeth is not too far advanced, so that the wear facets have not merged into a continuous worn surface.

From an examination of these facets, it is possible to deduce the path of

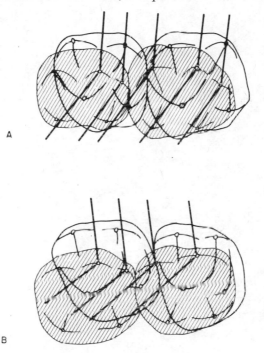

FIG. 4. Upper and lower first and second molars of (A) *Gorilla* and (B) *Homo* superimposed in centric relation. The heavy lines indicate the paths of the lower buccal cusps across the upper teeth.

molar cusps across the opposing teeth. Thus, during the buccal phase of occlusion, the hypoconid moves down the groove between the paracone and metacone, and into the centre of the trigon (Fig. 4). The protoconid similarly moves between the metacone of one upper molar and the paracone of the succeeding tooth, actually along a groove near the anterior edge of the more posterior molar. The path of the hypoconulid is of particular interest. It shears down a groove on the posterior side of the oblique crest of the upper tooth to the centric position, and then changes direction, following the oblique ridge, moving antero-lingually, and keeping just posterior to the

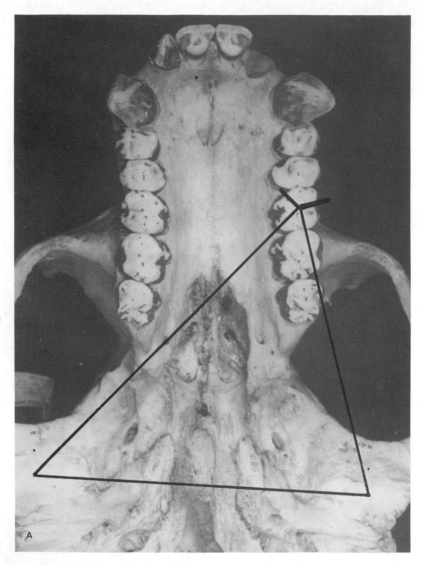

Fig. 5A. See facing page.

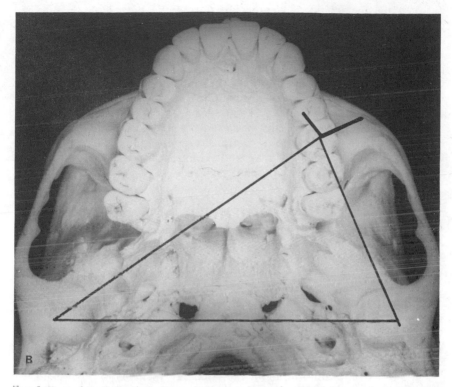

Fig. 5. Base of skull of (A) *Gorilla* and (B) *Homo*. The short thick lines in the centre of M^1 indicate the path of the hypoconid of M_1 in buccal and lingual phases.

ridge. The metaconid and entoconid duplicate this action on the lingual side of the tooth, shearing in grooves between the protocone and hypocone.

In the lingual phase, the path of the hypoconulid has already been described. In the more primitive primates, the hypoconid shears down a groove between the protocone and the paraconule. In Recent apes and man the paraconule is not recognizable, and essentially the lingual face of the hypoconid shears against the buccal face of the protocone. This rapidly wears away the enamel of these cusps, and exposes the dentine. The softer dentine wears more rapidly than the surrounding enamel, enabling the edges of the enamel to be used as a cutting edge, in a manner analogous to that seen in certain ruminants. Similarly the protoconid of the lower molar shears across the posterior part of the buccal surface of the hypocone of the adjacent upper tooth, duplicating the action of the hypoconid. The facet on the anterior part of the buccal surface of the hypocone (facet 11) is produced by the hypoconulid.

There is, of course, a reciprocal action by the cusps of the upper molars. I would mention particularly the protocone, which shears down the groove between the metaconid and entoconid during the buccal phase, into the centre of the talonid basin, and then along the groove between the hypoconid and hypoconulid in the lingual phase.

These relationships are, apart from cases of malocclusion, invariable. A cusp shearing down a groove must remain in this groove. If, in evolution, it were to transfer its relationship to a different groove, an intermediate stage would exist in which a cusp-to-cusp relationship would occur. Such a condition clearly could not exist.

Despite the similarity of the pattern of wear facets, and therefore of occlusal relations in function, there are certain essential differences between the masticatory apparatus of man and the apes, and the main purpose of this chapter is to probe these differences.

THE DRYOPITHECUS PATTERN

It is my contention that the main and principal difference between the masticatory apparatus of man and the apes lies in the shortening of the muzzle—the reduction of prognathism—which is the final stage of a typically primate development. Primates rely on sight rather than smell, and this is reflected during evolution in the prosimians, monkeys, apes and finally, man.

Shortening of the muzzle displaces the dentition backwards relative to a line joining the glenoid fossae or to that joining the mandibular condyles in the lower jaw. The effect of this is seen in Fig. 5.

Since the dentition comes closer to the bicondylar line, the joints are consequently placed more laterally relative to the dentition. If lateral chewing is due to alternate rotation about the condyles, then the lower molars will move lingually in the buccal phase and change direction more or less instantly at the centric position to an antero-lingual direction as rotation is transferred to the opposite condyle (Fig. 5A). With the more posterior displacement of the dentition in man, this change of direction will become much more marked (Fig. 5B).

If the dentition remained as in the gorilla, but the centre of rotation changed to the human condition, then, during the buccal phase the lower buccal cusps would be displaced from their appropriate groove, and would come into contact with the more anterior upper cusp, i.e. the hypoconid would strike the paracone and the protoconid the metacone. A simple modification corrects this. If a line is drawn through the long axis (bucco-lingually) of the molar teeth of any mammal, it usually passes close to the mandibular joint. This situation equally exists in man, because the buccal segments in fact diverge posteriorly, instead of being parallel, as in the apes. The cuspal relations in the buccal phase of occlusion are therefore maintained.

This fact does, however, have the effect of transferring the need for cuspal adjustment to those structures involved in the lingual phase. If man had the teeth of an ape, during the lingual phase the buccal cusps of the lower molars would follow the paths shown in Fig. 6, which shows the hominid direction of movement superimposed on the gorilla dentition. The hypoconid would ride laterally across the protocone of the upper molar, while the hypoconulid would slide up the posterior side of the oblique crest of the upper molar. The protoconid of the adjacent lower molar would have a very rough passage, passing across first the buccal hypocone crista, and then across the crista obliqua. To prevent this impossible situation, some cuspal reorganization is essential. A satisfactory result could be achieved by an anterior displacement

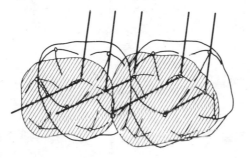

FIG. 6. Upper and lower first and second molars of *Gorilla* superimposed in centric relation. The thick lines show the paths which the lower buccal cusps would take if jaw movement were similar to that seen in *Homo*.

of protocone and hypocone. This does in fact occur in some primitive forms of man, as can be seen in Fig. 7, in the Australopithecine specimen which Broom *et al.* (1950) called *Plesianthropus transvaalensis*, and also in Neanderthal man. In recent man, however, the adaptations lie in the lower buccal cusps. The hypoconid and protoconid are displaced posteriorly. Thus, in Fig. 7C, while the first lower molar retains the *Dryopithecus* or Y5 pattern the second molar is of the " | 5" pattern, with the hypoconulid displaced to the extreme posterior end of the tooth.

As the jaws are shortened, with reducing prognathism, the length of lower molar necessary to accommodate this posteriorly displaced hypoconulid becomes an embarrassment, and the molars become of the "+4" pattern, as seen on M_2 of Fig. 7D, and on all the molars of Fig. 7E.

The hypoconulid having been eliminated, that part of the upper molar against which it sheared becomes superfluous. That is, only the more posterior part of the buccal face of the hypocone is functional and the facet in that area now covers the whole of the buccal face of the hypocone. The size of the hypocone is therefore reduced, again helping to shorten the tooth row. The effect on the third molars is variable. Not infrequently the hypoconulid is retained, even if absent on the second lower molar, and in this case it shears against the buccal face of the hypocone. If, as in Fig. 7E, it is eliminated here also, then there is a tendency also for the hypocone of M^3 to disappear.

Since the lower buccal cusps not only shear against the lingual part of the upper molar but also against the buccal part during the buccal phase, as the lower buccal cusps are displaced posteriorly, the appropriate grooves in the

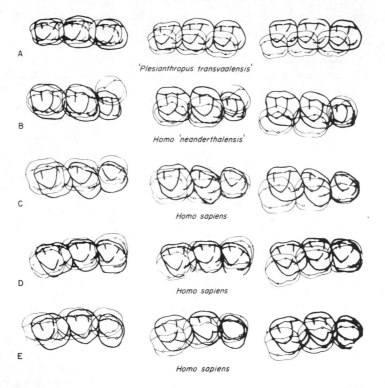

FIG. 7. Upper and lower molars of representative Hominoidea superimposed on the left at the beginning of the buccal phase; in the centre in centric relation; and on the right in the lingual phase of occlusion. A: after Broom; B: Le Moustier, after Gregory.

upper molars are similarly displaced. Clinically this is reflected by an increase in size of the paracone, and reduction of the metacone.

There are then, two differences in the molar patterns of man when compared with a typical pongid such as *Gorilla*. The lower buccal cusps are displaced backwards, so as to maintain their occlusal relationship with the upper lingual cusps in the lingual phase of occlusion. This brings about the change form the familiar "*Dryopithecus* pattern" to the +pattern. Secondly, the shortening of the tooth row is responsible for the reduction or elimination of the hypoconulid. This leaves part of the hypocone functionless, so that this cusp tends to be reduced in size. Both these differences are the result of a shortening of the muzzle.

THE PONGID CANINE

The Pongidae have enlarged, sectorial canines, the Hominoidea do not. There are doubtless many "reasons" for this. The development of the hands and of tools eliminated the need to use the canines as weapons or for tearing apart the food. Whatever the reason, man could not have evolved to his present form if he had kept his large canines. With large canines he could not have had reduced jaws, and therefore could not have had a large brain or binocular vision.

This can be seen by reference to Figs 1 and 8, which reiterate the point first made by Butler and Mills in 1959. In Fig. 1A the mandible is displaced to the left at the commencement of the buccal phase (on the left) and at the end of the lingual phase (on the right). On the left the lower canine passes smoothly through the diastema provided for it between I^2 and C^1. On the other side, the lower canine in the lingual phase passes across the lingual aspect of I^2. The height of the cusps causes the canine to move downwards slightly, and its tip essentially misses the upper tooth (although it does sometimes produce a small wear facet here).

Turning to Fig. 8, we see the corresponding situation in man. On the right

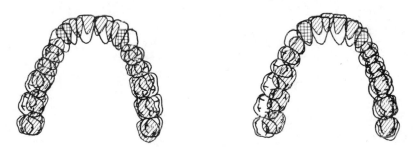

Fig. 8. Upper and lower dentition of *Homo sapiens* superimposed on the left in centric relation and on the right at the beginning of the buccal phase (to the right). The left side is therefore in the lingual phase. Note that the lower left canine (cross-hatched) moves along the line of the upper incisors.

side, during the buccal phase, the lower canine passes between I^2 and C^1. With small canines there is no need for a diastema to accommodate it, although such a diastema does occur in the milk dentition until the tip of the milk canine becomes worn. On the contralateral side the lower canine in its lingual phase moves along the incisal edge of the upper incisors. Since the lower canine is, in effect, a third incisor, this is a satisfactory working arrangement, but if it were the enlarged canine of even the female pongid, the lower canine would crash against the distal aspect of the upper second incisor and make lateral chewing movements impossible. Again this change in tooth relations in the lingual phase is the result of the shortening of the muzzle, and reduction of prognathism.

THE EMINENTIA ARTICULARIS

Figure 9 shows a coronal section through the first molars of three recent primates: *Lemur*, *Gorilla* and man. This section has been made through the tip of the hypoconid of the lower molar, so that on the upper molar it passes both through the deepest part of the groove between the paracone and metacone, and on the lingual side of the tooth, close to the tip of the proto-cone. In the case of *Lemur* the mandible is tapering, with its base lying well within the upper arch—a condition seen in the majority of mammals. The lower molars tend to lean buccally and the uppers lingually. In the case of *Gorilla* the mandibular base is somewhat rounded in the incisor region, and

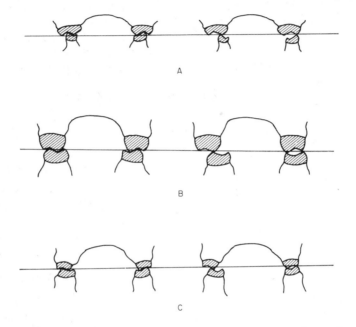

FIG. 9. Coronal sections through the tips of the hypoconids of lower first molars of (A) *Lemur*, (B) *Gorilla*, and (C) *Homo*. On the left, in centric relation; on the right, at commence-ment of buccal phase on the right side.

therefore in the molar region it is as wide as the maxillary base, so that both upper and lower molars are approximately upright. In *Homo* we again see the results of the increase in brain size and therefore of relative intercondylar width of the mandible, together with reduction of prognathism and therefore of jaw length. Because of these two factors the mandibular base is now wider than that of the maxilla. In order to occlude, the upper molars lean buccally and the lowers lingually.

Now, looking again at Fig. 9, a line can be noted which has been drawn joining the lowest points of the paracone–metacone grooves on each side of the mouth. On the left, the teeth are shown in centric relationship, and on the right, at the beginning of the chewing stroke on the right side of the mouth. On the right, therefore, the mandibular teeth are lower than on the left. In the case of *Lemur* the hypoconids on both sides of the mouth are touching the horizontal line. In the case of *Gorilla*, although the tip of the hypoconid on the right side is touching the horizontal line, that on the left side, occluding with the tip of the upper protocone, is below the line. In the case of man, despite the smaller teeth, the condition is exaggerated. That is, in lateral excursion of the mandible, the mandible tilts laterally towards the side in buccal occlusion. That this does, in fact, occur requires only a moment's reflection. During lateral movement the condyle on the contra-lateral side slides forwards down the eminentia articularis, and this action tilts the mandible. The eminentia is often stated to be a peculiarly human structure, but in fact a similar condition exists in *Gorilla*, where the contra-lateral condyle slides downwards as it moves forwards, on to the root of the zygoma. In *Lemur* this forward translation of the condylar head is horizontal. In *Galago* this area of the glenoid fossa actually slopes upwards, and this may account for the tilting of this animal's mandible in the opposite direction, observed by Kay and Hiiemae (1974).

The development of the eminentia articularis is man coincides with the development of the dentition. Lateral chewing would not be possible without the lateral tilting of the mandible and it seems reasonable to assume that the eminentia exists to provide this. This observation is not new—it was published previously (Mills, 1955), but it seemed worth repeating in the present context.

REFERENCES

BROOM, R., ROBINSON, J. T. and SCHEPERS, G. W. H. (1950). Sterkfontein Ape-Man –*Plesianthropus. Transv. Mus. Mem.* No. 4.

BUTLER, P. M. (1952). The milk-molars of Perissodactyla, with remarks on molar occlusion. *Proc. zool. Soc. Lond.* **121**, 777–817.

BUTLER, P. M. (1973). Molar wear facets in Early Tertiary North American Primates. *Symp. 4th Int. Cong. Primat.* 3, 1–27.

BUTLER, P. M. and MILLS, J. R. F. (1959). A contribution to the odontology of *Oreopithecus. Bull. br. Mus. nat. Hist. (Geol.)* 4, 1–26.

EVERY, R. G. and KÜHNE, W. G. (1971). Bimodal wear of mammalian teeth. *In* "Early mammals" (Kermack, D. M, and Kermack, K. A., eds). *J. Linn. Soc. (Zool)* Suppl. **1**, 23–28.

HIIEMAE, K. M. and KAY, R. F. (1973). Evolutionary trends in the dynamics of Primate mastication. *Symp. 4th Int. Cong. Primat.* 3, 28–64.

KAY, R. F. and HIIEMAE, K. M. (1974). Jaw movements and tooth use in recent and fossil Primates. *Am. J. phys. Anthrop.* **40**, 227–256.

MILLS, J. R. E. (1954). The dental occlusion of the Primates. M.Sc. thesis, University of Manchester.

MILLS, J. R. E. (1955). "Ideal dental occlusion in the Primates". *Dent. Practnr, Bristol* 6, 47–61.

MILLS, J. R. E. (1963). Occlusion and malocclusion in the teeth of Primates. *In* "Dental Anthropology" (Brothwell, D. R., ed.), pp. 29–52. Pergamon Press, London.

MILLS, J. R. E. (1973). Evolution of mastication in Primates. *Symp. 4th Int. Cong. Primat.* 3, 65–81.

ZINGESER, M. R. (1969). Cercopithecoid canine in tooth honing mechanisms. *Am. J. phys. Anthrop.* **31**, 205–213.

22. The Palate of *Pithecanthropus modjokertensis*

G. H. R. VON KOENIGSWALD

Senckenberg Museum, Frankfurt

Towards the close of the year 1938 our native collectors found in the Djetis Beds of Sangiran, Central Java, a fine heavily fossilized human palate, and a few months later other parts of the skull were discovered. Only the frontal bone was missing. In our catalogue of Javanese human fossils we called the find "*Pithecanthropus*-IV". Weidenreich's (1945: p. 96) opinion was, at the beginning, that this was only a male skull of *H. erectus*, but after his description of *Sinanthropus* skulls during the Second World War (I had been in Java as a prisoner of the Japanese, so we had no contact) he became aware of the differences, and proposed the name "*Pithecanthropus robustus*". This was not necessary, because from the same horizon in Eastern Java we had already the baby skull of *Pithecanthropus modjokertensis*, and it was evident that we had here for the first time an adult skull of the same type. The classical name of *Pithecanthropus* has been used here to indicate that this is a find from Java.

A few years ago our site in Eastern Java, near Modjokerto, could be dated by potassium/argon at $1 \cdot 9$ million $\pm$ 400 000 years. This means that this human type is more than 1 million years older than the classical *H. erectus*. The restored skull has a brain capacity of about 900 cm³, according to Holloway (1974); our own estimate, 750 cm³, had been too low.

Since the discovery in 1938, neither Java nor Africa has produced a similar complete specimen. But what formerly by some authors has been regarded as purely accidental has now, in the light of our absolute date (Jacob, 1972), developed phylogenetic meaning. While the details are discussed in a different paper, we want to underline the primitive character of this palate by some additional observations.

The general shape of the dental arcade is not parabolic, as is normally the

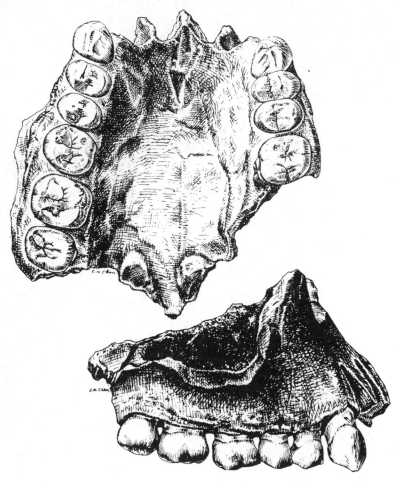

FIG. 1. Upper jaw of *Pithecanthropus modjokertensis* from the Lower Pleistocene Djetis Beds of Sangiran, Central Java. Actual size.

case in recent man and also in *Sinanthropus* (and most probably in *H. erectus*), but there are two slightly convergent straight tooth rows. In front of the canine is a marked diastema of 4 mm. A small fragment, with the canine still in place, shows that in this second specimen there also had been a diastema. In another specimen there is no simian gap. Our conclusion is that the male specimen still had a diastema, but that the females did not. The upper central incisors are strongly shovel shaped ($n = 2$), and the anterior upper premolar has three roots ($n = 2$). The canine is not worn down in one horizontal plane but, in spite of strong attrition, is still pointed. The second molar is strongly dominant over the first, a condition rarely observed in man but common in the anthropoids.

In fact, if the canine were enlarged then the maxilla could not be distinguished from that of an anthropoid. Only recently Krantz (1975) has mistaken our find for the dentition of a new species of orang-utan, which he called "*Pongo brevirostris*", but the entrance into the nose cavity is typically human, even with a well developed nasal spine. It is astonishing that the face had not been more prognathous. This provides a principal difference from the Australopithecinae, where the entrance into the nose is slanting and absolutely "chimpanzoid".

If this palate is accepted as the prototype of a human dentition of Lower Pleistocene age, a number of problems remain. As the dentition of *Pithecanthropus modjokertensis*, certainly a true member of the Hominoidea, is more primitive than in any known Australopithecinae, the only conclusion possible is that none of the latter can be regarded as a human ancestor. This conclusion has been reached before:

> In *Pithecanthropus*-IV this gap [the diastema] was unaccompanied by a simian overlapping of canines, and he was able to grind his food by moving his lower jaw from side to side in a true hominid fashion. The possession of this gap fails to make him an ape, but it also renders his descent from the kinds of Australopithecines found in South and East Africa unlikely (Coon, 1962: p. 380).

Another conclusion which can be drawn from the morphology of this dentition is that the canine has not been reduced in size by the pressure of the incisors dur to a reduction of a protruding face. The canine is of typical hominid dimensions, but the gap is still there. We might expect that man's Pliocene ancestor already had a similar dentition.

REFERENCES

COON, C. (1962). "The Origin of Races", pp. 1–724. Knopf, New York.
HOLLOWAY, R. L. (1974). The casts of fossil brains. *Scient. Am.* 7, 106–115.
JACOB, T. (1972). The absolute date of the Djetis Beds at Modjokerto. *Antiquity* 47.
KRANTZ, G. (1975). An explanation for the diastema of Javan erectus Skull IV. *In* "Paleoanthropology, Morphology and Palecology (Tuttle, R. H., ed.), pp. 361–372. Mouton, The Hague.
WEIDENREICH, F. (1945). Giant early man from Java and South China. *Anthrop. Pap. Am. Mus. nat. Hist* N.Y. **40**, 1, 1–134.

23. Mammalian Mastication: a review of the activity of the jaw muscles and the movements they produce in chewing

KAREN M. HIIEMAE

Unit of Anatomy in relation to Dentistry, Anatomy Department, Guy's Hospital Medical School, London

INTRODUCTION

There has been a great expansion of scientific interest in all aspects of mastication in mammals since the first of these conferences was held ten years ago. This is partly attributable to the development of new, and in some cases, very sophisticated techniques for the study of movements and muscle activity, but it is also due to a shift in the emphasis of evolutionary studies from the purely structural to functional and behavioural explanations for change. Not only are feeding and suckling important behaviours but their pattern of control may be analogous to that regulating other rhythmic and repetitive behaviours such as locomotion. By comparison with the limbs and their girdles, the jaw apparatus is a comparatively simple system with few joints and muscles (Fig. 1). It is, therefore, particularly useful for the investigation of the cause and effect relationships between the sensory input to, and motor output from, the central nervous system. This wide interest in the mechanisms of mastication has resulted in a rapidly growing literature, much of which is concerned with investigations into specific aspects of the more general problem of how mastication is controlled and how the actions of the various parts of the effector system are related.

Before 1965 there had been no experimental multidisciplinary study of oral behaviour in any single mammal which examined the action of the muscles, the pattern of movement and the mechanics of chewing (Fig. 1). Such studies have now been completed for the rat (Hiiemae, 1966, 1967, 1971a; Weijs, 1973a, b, 1975; Weijs and Dantuma, 1975), the little brown

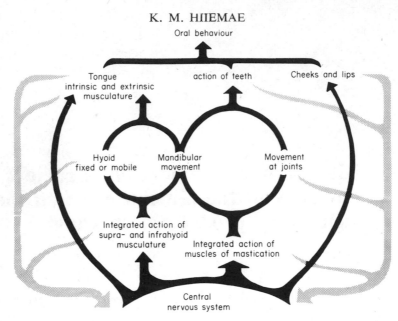

FIG. 1. The functional relationships between the various parts of the jaw apparatus. The solid arrows show the sequences of events producing oral activities such as biting or chewing. The shaded arrows indicate the sources of sensory feedback to the central nervous system. (The oral mucosa of the palate, an important part of the sensory system, has not been included.)

bat, *Myotis lucifugus* (Kallen and Gans, 1972), the miniature pig *Sus scrofa* (Herring and Scapino, 1973), and the pygmy goat, *Capra hircus* (de Vree and Gans, 1973; Gans and de Vree, 1974). Work on the American opossum, *Didelphis marsupialis*, is nearing completion (Hiiemae and Jenkins, 1969; Crompton and Hiiemae, 1969; Hiiemae and Crompton, 1971; Thexton and Hiiemae, 1975a, b; Crompton *et al.*, 1977). The pattern of masticatory movements in primitive mammals has recently been reviewed (Hiiemae, 1976). There is information available on the jaw movements of some primates, e.g. *Tupaia, Galago, Saimiri* and *Ateles* (Hiiemae and Kay, 1973; Kay and Hiiemae, 1974), and on the relationship between movements and muscle activity in the rhesus monkey, *Macaca mulatta* (Luschei and Goodwin, 1974). It is only recently that synchronous studies of jaw movement and muscle activity in man have been reported (Ahlgren, 1966 *et seq.*; Moller, 1966 *et seq.*) although there is a very large literature on both these as separate topics.

The mammals so far examined represent a spectrum of dietetic adaptations. It seems appropriate, therefore, to review the information now available in order to ascertain whether the differences in the anatomy of the jaw apparatus are reflected in the patterns of jaw movement or the activity of the muscles in chewing, or whether all mammals, including man, show fundamental similarities in their behaviour.

MOVEMENTS

Recent studies of jaw movements in mammals have, on the whole, been concerned less with the investigation of the pattern of jaw movement *per se* than with the correlations between movement and other phenomena such as muscle activity (Ahlgren, 1966 *et seq*; Kallan and Gans, 1972; Herring and Scapino, 1973; Gans and de Vree, 1974; Luschei and Goodwin, 1974; de Vree and Gans, 1974; Weijs and Dantuma, 1975; Crompton *et al.*, 1977), the force exerted on the food (Ahlgren and Öwall, 1970), the relationship between food consistency, particle size and movement pattern (Hiiemae and Thexton, 1975) and the nervous control of mastication (Goodwin and Luschei, 1974).

Serious examination of the occlusal relations between upper and lower teeth in chewing began after Butler's pioneering paper on the "Milk Molars of Perissodactyla" (1952) in which he developed a technique of wear facet analysis. This has been used in all subsequent studies and can be applied to fossil as well as to extant material without the difficulties inherent in the special clinical methods used in man for the study of molar occlusion during chewing (see Beyron, 1964). Attrition facets are produced by the contact or close approximation of upper and lower teeth and so record a very limited part of the whole range of jaw movement. The direction of the contact movement is along the axis of the subparallel striations, but other evidence is needed to confirm its actual direction. Although the shape, number and orientation of attrition wear facets in many vertebrates have been studied, Rensberger (1973) is alone in having considered the mechanical relationships between the food and the occlusal surface of the tooth. He evaluated the interactions between the dimensions of the food and its movement, tooth form, occlusal pressure and tooth wear by constructing a model for occlusion in some herbivorous mammals. This is a new and potentially valuable approach to the problem of the dynamics of the food as it is chewed, as well as to the larger problem of the evolution of tooth form.

A full account of the movements of the jaws in chewing requires a combination of experimental techniques and occlusal analysis (Hiiemae, 1967). However, the techniques used by some workers, especially those studying the relationship between movement and muscle activity, have often been so closely geared to the main, and usually neurophysiological, aims of their experiments that they have precluded the recording of some behavioural information.

Methods of Recording Jaw Movement. There are two main techniques for recording jaw movement: *continuous recording* which, at present, requires that some form of transducer system, usually a light source (Ahlgren and Öwall, 1970; Luschei and Goodwin, 1974), be attached to the jaws and gives a record of the continuous variation of jaw position with time; and *interrupted recording*, based on cinephotography or cinefluorography, which "samples" jaw position at regular intervals. Mandibular movements follow a complex path; this can be resolved into its components in the vertical, horizontal and transverse planes (vertical, antero–posterior and lateral movements). Interrupted recording methods such as cinefluorography can only provide a record of movement in two planes simultaneously unless a biplanar apparatus it used; so far this has not been reported. By using angled mirrors, cinephotographic recordings can be made which include movement in all three planes (Kallen and Gans, 1972). Continuous recording systems based on light sources pick up movement in three planes but record it in a maximum of two (Ahlgren and Öwall, 1970; Luschei and Goodwin, 1974). Other sensors, such as accelerometers (Gans and de Vree, 1974) or strain gauges record movement in only one plane.

Cranial flexion and extension are as intrinsic a part of masticatory movement as mandibular elevation and depression (Hiiemae, 1976). The importance of the cranial contribution to jaw movement varies between animals (see Kallen and Gans 1972; Herring and Scapino, 1973; Gans and de Vree, 1974) but any technique of recording or analysis which either inhibits or ignores the phenomenon must be treated cautiously. Analysis based on "a moving mandible", with the skull as a fixed reference point will contain a definite but variable distortion, i.e. the velocity and acceleration of the mandible in space will be exaggerated.

Jaw movement data is conventionally presented in the form of a "loop" showing the path through which a point on the lower jaw moves relative to a fixed reference point or plane on the upper, e.g. the incisal edges (Shepherd, 1960; Beyron, 1964), the intercuspal position (Ahlgren, 1966), the occlusal plane (Hiiemae and Kay, 1973; Herring and Scapino, 1973) or the tips of the upper canines (Kallen and Gans, 1972). Examples are shown in Fig. 4 but the "loop", although convenient, is an uninformative method of presenting jaw movement data since it condenses much information which has then to be reinterpreted. Unless clearly plotted by recording the position of a point in respect of the two included axes at regular, and stated, intervals of time (e.g. Beyron, 1964), loops give no information on the direction, time course or velocity of the movements involved, and can only show the change in relative position of the points between which the measurements were made. Unlike man, where the teeth make contact more or less simultaneously, many animals have an occlusal plane which is essentially flat in lateral view so the posterior teeth occlude ahead of those which are more anteriorly placed. No conclusions can therefore be drawn as to the relative position of teeth other than those used as the reference points.

Plots of jaw position against time can be obtained from both continuous and interrupted recordings, the former providing a trace of position against time in as many axes as sensors used. Velocity can be measured and acceleration, if required, can be calculated (Figs 2 and 3). Both interrupted and continuous recording techniques have other practical limitations. The analysis of interrupted recordings is laborious (Kallen and Gans, 1972) since the rate of sampling (the camera speed) must be fast enough to give enough observations (frames of film) for any movement to be fully reconstructed. In practice a camera speed of 60 f.p.s. has been found to be the minimum adequate for studies of Didelphis (Crompton and Hiiemae, 1970), which has a cycle time

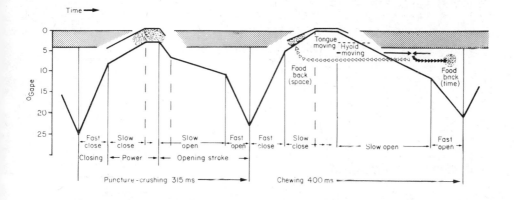

FIG. 2. A stylized gape/time plot of an "average" puncture-crushing cycle ($n = 18$) followed by a chewing cycle ($n = 24$). The horizontal axis is time (ms) and the vertical axis degrees gape, i.e. the angle between the upper and lower occlusal profiles seen in lateral projection. The shaded area between 0-4° gape indicates that cuspal interdigitation occurs within this range, full occlusion being 0° gape. The cycle profile therefore represents the changing relationship of upper and lower dentitions over time produced by both cranial and mandibular movement. Puncture-crushing is distinguished from chewing by the failure of the teeth to occlude, i.e. the dimensions of the food are such as to preclude tooth–tooth contact. In chewing, intercuspation and then full occlusion are achieved. In both types of cycle, there is a period in which no vertical movement can be observed but the lower jaw is moving medially and slightly forwards. There is a long "slow-open" stage in both cycles, shown here as discontinuous in puncture-crushing and continuous in chewing. The profile of this stage varies with the consistency and particle size of the food. As the mouth slowly opens, the hyoid bone is moved upwards and forwards (the duration of hyoid movement is shown by the length of the heavy arrows). The anterior part of the tongue is visibly protruded in the first part of slow opening (heavy arrow - - ➞) and then sharply retracted (heavy arrow ⚊ ⚊). This tongue movement "recycles" the untriturated part of the bite returning it to the postcanines (hollow-toothed arrow) during the fast opening stage (solid-toothed arrow).

in the range 300–400 ms. Inadequate camera speeds may result in distortion of the movement profile obtained. An engineering technique has been applied by Kallen and Gans (1972) to cinephotographic recordings of movement in the little brown bat. Polar coordinate plots showing the distribution of velocity, acceleration and time of dwell (=zero velocity and acceleration) for single "typical orbits" (an "orbit" is a chewing cycle), have been prepared. Whilst it is an elegant and spatially economical method of showing certain data, such plots leave the reader feeling subjected to presentational overkill.

Without exception, all the continuous recording techniques currently in use require some direct interference with the experimental subject which ranges from mild inconvenience (Taylor, 1969) to such gross interference with both posture and movement (Luschei and Goodwin, 1974) that it precludes the description "normal" for the behaviour recorded. Luschei and Goodwin (1974) fixed *Macaca mulatta* in a special restraining chair, immobi-

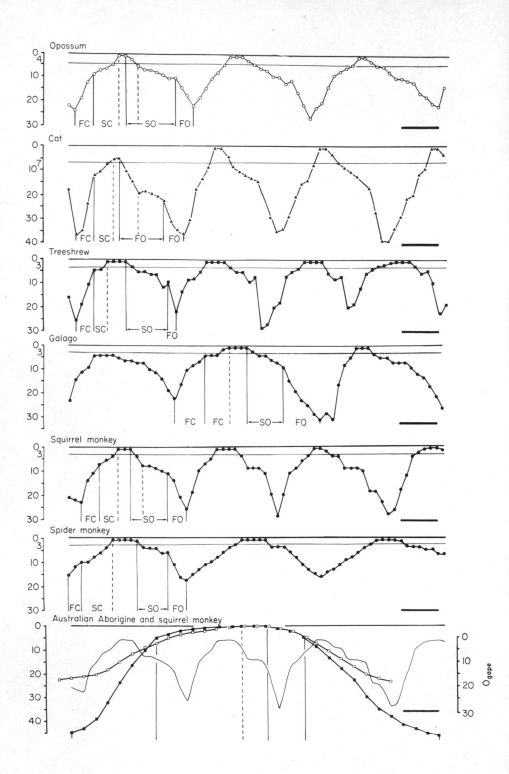

lized the cranium and attached a light source to the mandible with a surgically implanted coupling. This is an extreme example but all jaw movement transducers, including the accelerometer (Gans and de Vree, 1974) require anchorage to the lower jaw or preferably, to take account of cranial movement, to both skull and lower jaw. In man, head bands and a face bar are used and have been arranged so as to deliberately restrict the range of possible movement in some experiments (Ahlgren, 1967) All the methods for recording jaw movement so far available involve a significant diminution of resolution during the period in which the teeth are between initial cuspal interdigitation and full occlusion (and in the reverse direction); visibility is poor in photographic records and the slight movements occurring during this time may be missed by position transducers (Luschei and Goodwin, 1974).

Ideally, recordings of jaw movements in feeding would be made with the animal free in its natural habitat but this is patently impractical as a basis for detailed analysis. Some constraints, of which the laboratory environment is the most obvious, are unavoidable but these should at least be recognized and kept to the minimum consistent with standardizing recording conditions, analysis and measurement.

Terminology. Whatever the effect of the teeth on the food, the movements used to produce it are rhythmic and cyclical although both the rhythm and cycle profile can change with progression through the masticatory sequence (Hiiemae, 1976). The plethora of terms currently used to describe the masticatory cycle and its components is shown in Table I. The absence of any standardization either in the definition of the "start point" of a single cycle or even in the name given to it is due to the historical dichotomy between those studying mastication in man and those examining this behaviour from a neurophysiological or comparative anatomical standpoint. Some reconciliation is clearly needed. The term "chewing cycle" is well established in the literature, its retitling as a "masticatory orbit" by Kallen and Gans (1972) is unnecessary. It is even more confusing to describe a complete cycle as a "stroke" and a series of such strokes on one side of the mouth as a "cycle" (Herring and Scapino, 1973). But the real problems arise when the components of the chewing cycle are considered. Using the convenient convention that a single cycle begins at maximum gape it first involves a convergent movement of upper and lower teeth. This is completed at either the minimum vertical dimension (MVD) for that cycle or when the teeth reach "maximum

FIG. 3. Sample gape/time plots for the American opossum (*Didelphis*), the treeshrew (*Tupaia*), the cat (*Felis domesticus*), the squirrel monkey (*Saimiri*), the spider monkey (*Ateles*) and man. All are shown on the same time scale, each point on the plots represents the gape (or in the case of man, opening in mm from the horizontal plane of occlusion) in sequential single frames of cinefluorographs recorded at 60 f.p.s. (non-human mammals) and cinefilm taken at 30 f.p.s. (man). The time bar is 100 ms. The horizontal line at 4° (opossum), 7° (cat) and 3° (primates) is the level at which intercuspation first occurs. The plot for man has been obtained from two of Beyron's published "loops" (1964) and the contrast in the cycle time (see text) illustrated by the superimposition of the trace for the squirrel monkey.

TABLE I. To illustrate the major variants in the terminology used to describe or define the chewing cycle and its components. Where there are no specific definitions in the sources cited, the limits of each component have been derived from the texts. The arrows indicate the direction of movement of the lower jaw in the vertical plane.

Reference landmarks across the cycle (left to right): Maximum gape → Tooth–food–tooth contact / Centric occlusion → Loss of intercuspation → Maximum gape.

Source	Terminology across the chewing cycle
Atkinson and Shepherd (1961) / Hiiemae (1967 et seq.)	One chewing cycle
Kallen and Gans (1972)	One masticatory orbit (?)
Herring and Scapino (1973)	One masticatory stroke / One chewing stroke (?)
Beyron (1964) / Ahlgren (1966 et seq.)	One chewing cycle
Ahlgren (1966)	Closing phase — [Centric occlusion] — Opening phase
Herring and Scapino (1973)	Adduction (?) — Abduction
Ahlgren (1967)	Closing phase — Occlusal phase — Opening phase
Hiiemae (1967 et seq.)	Preparatory stroke — Power stroke — [Loss of intercuspation] — Recovery stroke
Mills (1955 et seq.)	Intercuspation / Occlusion (Buccal phase → Lingual phase); Phase I → Phase II
Hiiemae and Kay (1973)	Phase I — Phase II
Luschei and Goodwin (1974)	Rapid upwards — Slow upwards (?) — Isometric (?) — Recovery stroke
De Vree and Gans (personal communication)	Phase I — Phase II — Phase III

TABLE II. An attempt to reconcile the terminology used in movement, occlusal and electromyographic studies with the actual events occurring during or contributing to the completion of a single chewing cycle.

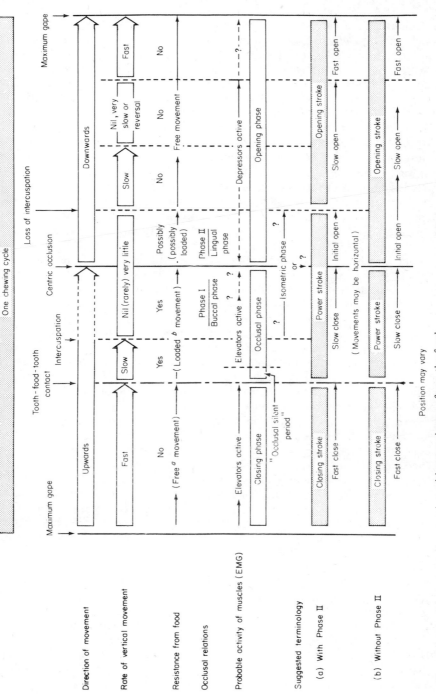

[a]Free movement is movement occurring without resistance from the food.
[b]Loaded movement is movement occurring with resistance from the food, i.e. work is being done in its trituration.

intercuspation" or centric occlusion (Table I). This closing movement is then followed by a return movement in which the teeth diverge to maximum gape at which point the convergent movements of the next cycle follow (Fig. 2). Whilst the direction of movement in the cycle is predominantly upwards or downwards (in respect of the lower jaw, but see Hiiemae 1976), the rate of such movement changes (Table II and Fig. 2) as the teeth come into contact with the food. All vertical movement may be suspended for a period in which the jaw moves transversely as the food is triturated. Three components or strokes in a single cycle can be distinguished (Fig. 2): a closing stroke (fast close) in which the teeth are converging and the lower jaw is moving rapidly upwards; a power stroke in which work, i.e. muscular effort, is being expended both in the trituration of the food and in moving the jaw, at least initially, slowly upwards (slow close); and an opening stroke in which the teeth are moved apart. [The author is dropping the terms "preparatory" and "recovery" (Hiiemae, 1967 et seq.) for "closing" and "opening strokes" respectively (see Hiiemae, 1976).]

There is, however, a problem in defining the beginning and the end of the power stroke since the term "occlusal phase" used by Ahlgren (1976) and others was defined as (that) "during which the teeth are in habitual occlusion (intercuspal position)". In the literature on human mastication there is no clear distinction between the point at which work to reduce the food can be regarded as beginning (tooth–food–tooth contact or tooth–tooth contact) or, alternatively, the former is assumed to occur within the intercuspal range of gape. It is obvious that the gape at which tooth–food–tooth contact occurs is variable and governed by the size of the food. It is equally obvious that the hardness or consistency of the food will determine, for any single cycle, the extent to which the teeth are finally approximated (MVD). Whilst it may be the case that most of the chewing effort of man is expended when the teeth are within intercuspal range (a function of our somewhat idiosyncratic dietary habits?), this is certainly not true of mammals in general and not even true of man in the early (puncture-crushing) phase of the masticatory sequence. Using the point of tooth–food–tooth contact to define the "start" of the power stroke is certainly consistent with the change in the rate of movement observed, possibly with the pattern of EMG activity in the elevators and, therefore, with the mechanics of chewing. A universally applicable and so wholly satisfactory definition for the "end point" of the power stroke is, in practice, much more difficult to achieve. In cycles where the MVD occurs outside the intercuspal range, that gape defines the end point in space but not necessarily in time. However, where the MVD coincides with centric occlusion, work in triturating the food, and in moving the lower jaw, may not have ceased (Table II). Occlusal studies (e.g. Mills, 1955 et seq., Kay and Hiiemae, 1974) have shown that after intercuspation in the power stroke, the teeth first move into centric occlusion ("buccal phase", Mills 1955; Phase I, Hiiemae and Kay, 1973) and then in many, but not all, mammals, including man, working contact is maintained as the teeth move out of centric occlusion and on towards the midline ("lingual phase" or Phase II; see Table II). The significance of Phase II varies between mammalian groups—it is certainly important in herbivores. In these circumstances the power stroke can be regarded as complete when tooth–food–tooth contact is lost and the opening movement begins. When the relationship between the EMG and the force produced by the elevator muscles is clearer, then a definition of the power stroke in terms of the EMG may be possible.

In the mammals so far examined for which gape/time plots are available there are two clearly defined stages in the opening stroke: an initial "slow opening" in which the gape slowly increases and may be held for some time, followed by a short "fast-open" stage in which there is rapid divergence of upper and lower teeth (Figs 2 and 3). Fast opening is complete at maximum gape. These terms and those discussed above in relation to the events occurring during a single chewing cycle are shown in Table III.

The Chewing Cycle

There is general agreement that, with the exception of man, the mammals so far studied have consistent chewing patterns both individually and specifically. Any variation in the chewing pattern is usually in the amplitude of movement and can be correlated with the consistency and particle size of the food (Hiiemae and Thexton, 1975; Hiiemae, 1976). In Australian aborigines and northern European populations (Beyron, 1964; Ahlgren, 1966) there is great individual variation in the movement profile.

The opossum (Crompton and Hiiemae, 1970), little brown bat (Kallen and Gans, 1972), treeshrew, bushbaby, squirrel and spider monkeys (Hiiemae and Kay, 1973), macaque (Luschei and Goodwin, 1974), cat (Hiiemae and Thexton, 1975), miniature pig (Herring and Scapino, 1973) and man (Atkinson and Shepherd, 1961, 1967; Ahlgren 1966) all have two distinct types of chewing cycle. One, "puncture-crushing" (Hiiemae and Crompton, 1971), occurs during the first stages of trituration: the teeth do not come into occlusion and may not even intercuspate, while the food is crushed rather than cut or ground (Fig. 2). This method of chewing has been called "inertial feeding" by Kallen and Gans (1972) and "chopping" (Ahlgren, 1966). Where hard foods or large volumes are "fed" into the side of the mouth as in the opossum and little brown bat, the bite is separated from the extra-oral mass in a series of puncture-crushing cycles; this is "ingestion by mastication" (Hiiemae and Crompton, 1971). In the cat, puncture-crushing appears to continue until the food is of a suitable consistency and particle size for chewing (Hiiemae and Thexton, 1975), the second type of chewing cycle. "A harmonious pattern is then developed" (Atkinson, 1960) as "regular mastication follows" (Luschei and Goodwin, 1974). Once pulped, the food is reduced by a rhythmic series of chewing cycles (sensu stricter) in which the teeth come progressively closer to and finally reach full occlusion (Fig. 2). Recent work (Hiiemae and Thexton, 1975; Hiiemae, 1976) has shown that whilst the general profile of all cycles is comparable, their duration and amplitude are highly variable even during the course of a single masticatory sequence (Fig. 3). There is, therefore, no "standard" chewing cycle, the

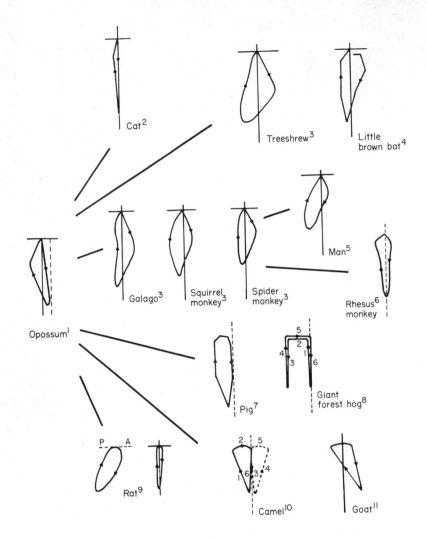

FIG. 4. The movements of the lower jaw in a "typical" chewing cycle in some mammals. The profiles are shown in frontal view with the working side on the right side of the jaws in all cases except the rat. Where crossed reference lines are shown, the horizontal line indicates the transverse plane of centric occlusion, the vertical is perpendicular to it at the point of centric occlusion. Where a single hatched vertical line is shown, this corresponds to the anatomical midline (centric relation). The profile for the rat is shown in both frontal and lateral view, the dotted line being the occlusal plane (A, Anterior; P, Posterior). Sources are as follows:

1. The American opossum (*Didelphis marsupialis*). From Crompton and Hiiemae (1970).
2. The cat (*Felis domesticus*). From work in progress (Hiiemae, in preparation).
3. The treeshrew (*Tupaia glis*), the bushbaby (*Galago crassicaudatus*); the squirrel monkey (*Saimiri scuireus*) and the spider monkey (*Ateles*). From Hiiemae and Kay (1973).
4. The little brown bat (*Myotis lucifugus*). From Kallen and Gans (1972, their Fig. 6).
5. Man, one specific case. From Ahlgren (1966).

closest approximation to it occurs in the later part of the sequence when a "steady state" lasting for several cycles may occur. Whether the food is actually cut, ground or a combination of the two depends on the form of the cheek teeth. Two variations of this pattern have so far been described. The miniature pig (Herring and Scapino, 1973) has a two-stage puncture-crushing system due to the hard particulate nature of its food which is first reduced in typical puncture-crushing cycles. These are followed by "chewing" cycles in which the teeth rarely come into occlusion. The rat (Hiiemae and Ardran, 1968; Weijs, 1975) and the rabbit (Ardran et al., 1958) rarely (the rat), if ever (the rabbit), puncture-crush their food, possibly due to the efficiency of their incisors in gnawing (cutting) it into a size suitable for chewing (Hiiemae, 1966). Puncture-crushing cycles have the same general movement profile as chewing cycles (sensu strictu) but with a greater vertical amplitude and reduced transverse component in the power stroke (Hiiemae and Crompton, 1971; Kallen and Gans, 1972; Herring and Scapino, 1973; Hiiemae and Kay, 1973; see Figs 2 and 3).

In most of the animals so far studied, chewing takes place on one side or the other of the mouth for a number of cycles and then active and balancing sides are reversed. Reversal may be at such regular intervals (five or six cycles in the bat) that Kallen and Gans (1972) concluded that it could be controlled by an "innate" mechanism. True bilateral chewing, as opposed to coincidental trituration on the balancing side (see Wictorin et al., 1971, on the position of the bolus in man), has been described in the rat (Hiiemae and Ardran, 1968; Weijs and Dantuma, 1975). It is only possible in those mammals such as rodents where the transverse width of the upper and lower jaws is the same (isognathy) or the lower jaw is the wider. The pig is isognathous and occasionally puncture-crushes bilaterally but the equally isognathous rabbit does not, due to the high "dorsal shield" on the tongue (Ardran et al., 1958). Primitive mammals such as Didelphis are sufficiently anisognathous for centric occlusion to be unilateral so that when the working side is moving through Phase 1 or is in centric occlusion, the balancing-side molars are out of contact. Chewing is, therefore, necessarily unilateral (Crompton and Hiiemae, 1970).

The Movement Profile in Chewing. The paths through which points on the

---

6. The rhesus monkey (*Macaca mulatta*). Drawn from Luschei and Goodwin (1974).

7. The miniature pig (*Sus scrofa*). Drawn from Fig. 11 (Cycle 1) of Herring and Scapino (1973).

8. The giant forest hog (*Hylochoerus meinhertzhageni*). From the text in Ewer (1958). Strokes 1, 2 and 3 have been separated from strokes 4, 5 and 6 for clarity. Ewer's description implies that the jaw returns along the "outward" path so that the "paired strokes" would overlap (but see text).

9. The rat (*Rattus norvegicus*). From Hiiemae and Ardran (1968) and Weijs (1975).

10. From the author's observation of specimens in the Zoological Society of London's collection. Cycles are alternating between right and left sides so that the normal sequence would be as shown. This pattern is found in cud-chewing and possibly in ordinary mastication. See Addendum.

11. The goat (*Capra hirvus*). From de Vree and Gans (1974).

lower jaw are moved during a single cycle as seen in frontal view in all mammals (for which data are available) are illustrated in Fig. 4. Given the form of the cheek teeth, the chewing cycle in *Didelphis* (Crompton and Hiiemae, 1970) may in fact correspond to that of primitive mammals. This is a view accepted by Kallen and Gans (1972).

The Closing Stroke. The closing movement brings the lower molars into alignment with the uppers in preparation for the power stroke. As is clear from Fig. 4 the degree of lateral excursion required depends on the position of maximum gape relative to the midline: this excursion is least in the cat and greatest in the goat. Maximum gape in man can occur to the balancing or active sides of the midline or coincident with it (Beyron, 1964; Ahlgren, 1966). There is some antero-posterior movement during the predominantly vertical closing stroke. This is greatest in the rodents, less marked in the pig, clearly discernible in the little brown bat and the primates examined by Hiiemae and Kay (1973), slight in the opossum and probably absent in the cat. This movement, which may involve an initial retraction followed by a slight protrusion, is partly due to the need to bring the cheek teeth into position for the antero-medially directed power stroke, but is also due to the anatomy of the squamo-dentary joint. The correlation between the movements of the mandibular condyle and disc on the articular fossa and the profile of the closing movement in man has been discussed by Griffin and Malor (1974). An upwards and backwards movement into tooth–food–tooth contact and thence into occlusion has not yet been observed in any primate although it may occur exceptionally in man. This makes the "orthal retraction" movement postulated on the basis of wear facet analysis by Gingerich (1972) for puncture-crushing in *Adapis* improbable. It is considered to be almost impossible on other criteria (see Kay and Hiiemae, 1974).

The Power Stroke. The closing stroke of the cycle merges smoothly into the power stroke. The "turn point" can be clearly distinguished in gape/time plots prepared from cinefluorographs as a change in velocity rather than as a sudden shift of direction (Fig. 2), although the latter does occur when the piece of food is extremely small and tooth–food–tooth and tooth–tooth contact occur almost simultaneously (Fig. 3, spider monkey). The general direction of the power stroke is, without exception, from buccal to lingual, upwards and variably forwards to centric occlusion (Fig. 4). There has been no observation of a retrusive power stroke in any experimental study to date. In fact recent work has tended to confirm the suggestion illustrated in Crompton and Hiiemae (1969, their Fig. 5) that the differences in the power stroke between a "primitive mammal" (opossum), a carnivore (the lynx) and a herbivore (the goat) are due to the length of the traverse from lateral to medial coupled with the steepness of the vertical movement in Phase I. The lower jaw of the active side is "rolled" about its long axis to bring the teeth through the first part of the power stroke and into centric occlusion in animals such as the opossum, little brown bat, tree-shrew and *Galago*, all with high-cusped molars and mobile mandibular symphyses. The protrusive component of the power stroke is greatest in the rodents and least, if it occurs at all, in the felid carnivores. In the latter the movement is almost completely vertical with a very slight transverse component (cat, Hiiemae and Thexton, 1975). The angulation of the first part of the power stroke (as seen from in front) has been shown, as might have been expected, to be related to the steepness of the "working" ridges on the occlusal surfaces of cheek teeth (Kay and Hiiemae, 1974, for primates; Beyron, 1964, for man). Beyron made the interesting observation that the verticality of the movement in the Australian aborigine decreased with age and related this to a reduction in the cuspal profiles of the cheek teeth with heavy wear. Phase I (the buccal phase on the active side) is completed at centric occlusion or in a closely comparable position if food is separating the occlusal surfaces of the molars. On the basis of the wear facets observed on mammalian molar teeth many authors have argued that the second part of the power stroke includes a slight downwards movement. Phase II as described by Kay and Hiiemae (1974) is an infero-medial movement from centric. No such movement could be detected in *Didelphis*, but Phase II facets have been related to the jaw movements seen in cinefluorographic recordings of jaw movements in some primates (Hiiemae and Kay, 1973) and have been deduced from wear facets in a wide range of mammals both living and extinct (see Mills, 1967; Butler, 1973). Examination of Beyron's frontal profiles of cycles in the aborigine suggests that they show a similar movement. It has been argued elsewhere (Kay and Hiiemae, 1973) that Phase II may have developed originally by the coincidental utilization of the opening movement required for the lower molar cusps to clear the uppers at the beginning of the opening stroke. With a shift from a predominantly shearing occlusion (*Didelphis*, *Tupaia* and *Myotis*) to a synchronous cutting and grinding mechanism (*Saimiri*, *Ateles* and *Homo*), Phase II has become nearly horizontal and a progressively more important component of the power stroke in the primates (see Chapter 20, this volume) and is an essential element in herbivores.

There is, however, a need to reconcile the data from occlusal (wear facet) analysis, movement recording and EMG studies in relation to the second part of the power stroke. Man (Shepherd, 1960; Ahlgren, 1966; Møller, 1966; Atkinson and Shepherd, 1967) and the macaque (Luschei and Goodwin, 1974) are described as having an "isometric phase" in the power stroke; the jaw is allegedly stationary in centric occlusion for a considerable period (about 100 ms in man, 75–100 ms in the macaque). This "stationary period" is followed by a rapid downwards acceleration into the opening stroke. Although the existence of an "isometric phase" in man has been denied by Fisch (1963, see Ahlgren, 1966), there is, in all the animals studied by the author including the cat, a period during the power stroke in which no vertical movement can be observed (Figs 2 and 3) in cinefluorographs. This does not necessarily mean that no such movement is occurring nor does it mean that there is no slight antero-medial movement. In short, there is, as yet, no unequivocal evidence to show whether all jaw movement ceases between Phase I and Phase II (but see Kay and Hiiemae, 1974) in which case conditions would be truly isometric, or whether the so-called "isometric phase" in fact covers part of Phase I, or Phase II or both (see Mathews, 1975; Hiiemae, 1976).

The pig, described by Herring and Scapino (1973) as an omnivore–herbivore, has closing and power strokes in its chewing cycle conforming to the general description given above but can have a "reverse power stroke since the lower teeth on one side may move either medially or laterally across the uppers on that side". If the pig does have a laterally directed power stroke, this will distinguish it from all other mammals examined. Herring and Scapino carefully point out in their discussion that Becht (1953) reported that the rodent *Myocastor* masticates with regular alternating transverse movements, and that Ewer (1958, 1970) has given a detailed verbal description of a complex cycle in the giant forest hog which has been reconstructed from her description (Fig. 4). It is, by comparison with all the other mammals shown, remarkably odd. If, however, the midline were shifted so that movements 2 and 5 crossed it, or approached it, then the pattern would be similar to that seen in the camel and each cycle, alternating between sides, would have a profile comparable to that seen in the pig. The movements of *Myocastor*, recorded with time-lapse cinephotography, almost certainly conform to a pattern of cycles on alternate sides. In view of the accumulating evidence, it seems reasonable to suggest that the power stroke of mammals has evolved from a simple antero-medially directed movement as seen in *Didelphis*, with an increase in the anteriorly directed component in the rodents, an increase in the vertical component in the carnivores, and in the transverse component in the herbivores. A slight exaggeration of one or two vectors would not involve a profound shift in the control of the pattern of muscle activity; a complete reversal, as in a laterally directed power stroke, almost certainly would.

The Opening Stroke. The antero-medial element in the power stroke means that the opening stroke begins with the jaw in a slightly forward position. In frontal view, the opening movement may either continue the medial direction of the power stroke towards the balancing side as in the goat; start with a further medial movement and then return to reach maximum gape in the mid-sagittal plane; cross the midline to a maximum gape on the active side *Tupaia, Myotis, Galago, Saimiri, Ateles, Macaca* and sometimes man); or be a simple downwards movement in the midline (*Didelphis*, the miniature pig, rat and rabbit) (Fig. 4). In lateral projection, the opening stroke is seen to incorporate a definite protrusion of the mandible (*Didelphis, Tupaia, Myotis, Galago, Saimiri* and *Ateles*) which occurs during the slow opening stage (Figs 2 and 3) while the vertical movement is slowed or suspended. Kallen and Gans (1972) give no indication of the vertical dimension (gape) at which this protrusion occurs in the bat. Opening is combined with mandibular protrusion in the rabbit (Ardran *et al.*, 1958) but there is a marked retrusion in the rat (Hiiemae, 1968; Weijs, 1975).

Despite the considerable anatomical differences in the jaw apparatus of the mammals so far studied *in vivo* and the limitations of occlusal analysis, there appears to be a consistent pattern in the profile of jaw movement, the most important aspect of which is the consistency in the upwards and medial direction of the first phase of the power stroke.

The Time Course of the Chewing Cycle. Amar (1914) said that the rate of mastication in mammals was correlated with the length and weight of the mandible. This cannot possibly be so. The data presented in Table III show that animals differing in weight by a factor of 3×10^3 (the little brown bat and the miniature pig) have a range of cycle times which overlap. It is clear from Table III that the duration of a single cycle is independent of total body weight or diet.

That there is variation in the percentage contribution of each of the major elevators (temporalis, masseter and medial pterygoid) to the total elevator muscle mass is well known (see Turnbull, 1970 for all data to that date) and can be broadly correlated with the animal's "dietetic group". It is reasonable to assume some relationship between the total elevator mass (as an index of the possible force generated in contraction), mandibular weight and "normal" resistance of the food. In practice, in those (few) cases for which figures are available, the possible elevator force greatly exceeds that exerted in normal chewing [80 kg as opposed to 5–15 kg in man (Anderson 1956)]. But it should be noted that chewing is not the only activity for which a powerful elevator force is needed· in some animals teeth are used as weapons and in the collection of food. Whether there is a point at which, in the larger mammals, some physical parameter, such as the inertia of the mandible, becomes significant in "slowing" the cycle is not yet known. The jaw of the zebu in which a single chewing cycle takes rather more than 1s (from Plate I of Becht, 1953) could be considered "heavy" in relation to body weight with its long body and comparatively reduced ramus. On the same criteria, the mandible of man could be considered light in relation to body weight, with its short body but wide ramus. Clearly further information in the cycle time in large mammals, on the biomechanics of the jaw apparatus, is needed (see Addendum).

All the evidence to date (Close, 1972) shows that all the mammalian striated skeletal muscles so far examined (but this does not include data on muscles from large mammals) have contraction times which fall within two specific ranges of, say, 8–30 ms and 50–100 ms. The jaw muscles have faster contraction times than most, *c.* 12 ms in the cat (Taylor *et al.*, 1973), ranging from 11–18 ms in *Didelphis* (Thexton and Hiiemae, 1975b) and 16 ms for the masseter in the macaque (Harrison and Corbin, 1942 cited by Matsunami and Kubota, 1972). The differences in cycle times shown in Table III are therefore unlikely to be due to the contractile behaviour of the muscle fibres.

Evidence is accumulating (Bremer, 1923; Dellow and Lund, 1971; Thexton, 1969, 1973, 1974) that the inherently rhythmic activity of chewing is due to an "oscillator" system which is probably located within the brain stem rather than in the higher centres of the CNS (see Matthews, 1975). On both behavioural and phylogenetic grounds it can be argued that if there is such an oscillator, it is likely to be present in all mammals and to have the same or closely similar characteristics throughout the class. Given this assumption and the evolutionary history of therian mammals, a "basic oscillator frequency" could be expected. This, as judged solely from the behavioural evidence in Table III could be in the range of 300–400 ms. In drawing such a conclusion, a distinction must be made between the intrinsic rhythm of an oscillator and the behavioural rhythm of successive chewing cycles. The former will be modified possibly by information from higher centres within the central nervous system and certainly by sensory feedback from the whole jaw apparatus (Fig. 1) and particularly the oral cavity. Moreover, chewing is a complex activity and a late arrival on the oral behavioural scene. The most fundamental rhythmic jaw activity in mammals is suckling, with its onto-genetic successor, lapping, both having their own faster rhythms (Thexton, 1969; Hiiemae and Crompton, 1971). Preliminary studies show that non-mammalian vertebrates also have rhythmic and cyclical jaw movements in feeding. It seems probable that if the mammals have evolved their own characteristic oscillator frequency, its intrinsic rhythm will be closer to that of suckling or lapping rather than that of chewing. In this context, it is worth noting that the mammalian (tribosphenic) molar evolved well after the first appearance of the mammals (Crompton 1971).

There is, however, a problem in considering the effect, if any, of the nature of the food on the cycle time. Not only is there no guarantee that food of a single type will have the same physical characteristics, in terms of consistency, "hardness" etc. on different occasions but, and probably more important, the condition of the food, once ingested, will not be uniform; the process of chewing is geared to changing it. The most efficient of contemporary grinding machines does not reduce material to a uniform particle size instantaneously —there is an interim period where some particles are small, some much larger. It follows that since teeth are unlikely to be as efficient as electrically driven steel blades, there will be times when larger particles have to be reduced and the cycle time will be affected, or a reversal from chewing to puncture crushing will occur (as has been recorded for *Ateles* by Hiiemae and Kay, 1973). Although there is considerable evidence that the size and consistency of the food ingested affects the pattern of chewing and the length of the masticatory sequence, it will not be possible to evaluate the actual relation-ship between the nature of the food, the manner in which it is reduced and the time taken for each cycle until controlled studies are completed for at least one mammal in which the type of food, its particle size and consistency at ingestion are all carefully regulated (see Hiiemae and Thexton, 1975).

Further, since there is no allometric relationship between increase in body size, and therefore in energy needs, and increase in molar size (Chapter 20, this volume), a greater food intake may require that more time overall be spent in mastication. The cycle time, given the evidence for non-human primates in Tables III and IV, does not increase with increase in body weight. Inevitably, given our present state of ignorance as to the factors controlling the total cycle time any suggestions as to why there is, apparently, little or no correlation between this time, body weight, jaw shape, muscle mass or diet (as inferred from molar pattern) beg almost as many questions

TABLE III. The total time, as the mean and standard deviation (where known) and, where possible, maxima and minima (in ms) for all mammals for which data are available. No distinction has been made between puncture-crushing and chewing cycles, although the minimum figures quoted are for the former (see text).

Animal	Source	Total Cycle Time	Minimum	Maximum	Body Weight
Little Brown Bat (*Myotis lucifugus*)	Kallen and Gans (1972)	250 average	143	333	c. 7 g
Treeshrew (*Tupaia glis*)	Hiiemae and Kay (1973)	238 ± 30 (n = 63)	221	289	c. 100–200 g
Rat (*Rattus notregicus*)	Weijs (1975)	192 ± 23 (n = 20)	140	250	c. 200 g
Squirrel Monkey (*Saimiri sciureus*)	Hiiemae and Kay (1973)	357 ± 63 (n = 67)	255	357	c. 350–750 g
Bushbaby (*Galago crassicaudatus*)	Hiiemae and Kay (1973)	314 ± 47 (n = 66)	255	408	c.
Rabbit (*Oryctolagus*)	Ardran et al. (1958)	158 ± 200 (on grass)		–	c. 1·5–2·0 kg
American Opossum (*Didelphis marsupialis*)	(work in progress)	390 ± 48 (n = 22)	255	493	c. 2–3 kg
Cat (*Felis domesticus*)	(work in progress)	308 ± 32 (n = 27)	250	366	c. 2–3 kg
Spider Monkey (*Ateles*)	Hiiemae and Kay (1973)	326 ± 100 (n = 66)	289	442	c. 5–7 kg
Rhesus Monkey (*Macaca mulatta*)	Luschei and Goodwin (1974)	317 + 30 (apple) 325 ± 20 (carrot) 360 ± 15 (biscuit)			c. 3–4 kg
Pygmy Goat (*Capra hircus*)	Gans and de Vree (1974)	333–500			c. 20 kg
Miniature Pig (*Sus scrofa*)	Herring and Scapino 1973	330 average	250	460	13 6–31 kg
Man (*Homo sapiens*)	Beyron (1964) Ahlgren (1966) Atkinson and Shepherd (1967)	858 ± 58[a] (meat) 580 (carrot) 770 (chewing gum) 880			(Australian aborigines) Scandinavian teenagers Australian whites

[a]Beyron quotes a figure of "just under one second" in the text of his paper, the value given has been calculated from his published movement profiles.

as they attempt to answer. However, this is an area in which there is currently very considerable interest (see Addendum).

Total cycle times (Table III) allow comparisons and provoke speculation but are not, in fact, very informative since they do not show how much time the animal spends in triturating the food or in free movement. An alternative method of comparing the chewing cycles of different mammals is to examine the duration of each stroke as a percentage of the total cycle time (Table IV). This has the advantage of eliminating the variation in total cycle time but requires that uniform criteria for determining when strokes begin and end are applied. There are, unfortunately, no data available on the time course of chewing in classic herbivores. The figures in the table have, with the sole exception of those for *Macaca* (obtained by measuring Luschei and Goodwin's (1974) published figures) been obtained from interrupted recordings, and the criteria used to determine the start and finish of each stroke are those outlined above (see section on Terminology). The data must, however, be

TABLE IV. The duration of the closing, power and opening strokes expressed as a percentage of the total cycle time (in ms). The "dietetic groups" are taken from Turnbull (1970). Sources are as follows:
[1] measured directly from gape/time plots based on sequential single frame tracings (Hiiemae, work in progress);
[2] based on frame counts only (Hiiemae and Kay, 1973);
[3] from measurements of published continuous recordings (Luschei and Goodwin, 1974): (a) is the power stroke inclusive of the "isometric phase", (b) is the power stroke exclusive of the "isometric phase" which has been calculated as part of the opening stroke (see text);
[4] Kay (Chapter 20, this volume);
[5] based on gape/time plots derived from measurements of Beyron's (1964) displacement loops;
[6] from the minimum and maximum figures given by Herring and Scapino (1973);
[7] from data kindly supplied by Dr W. A. Weijs.

	Total Cycle Time (ms)	Closing Stroke	Power Stroke	Power and Closing	Opening Stroke	Phase II Present	Dietetic Group
		(As a percentage of the Total Cycle Time)					
Opossum[1] (n = 17) (Didelphis marsupialis)	392 ± 50	18·0 ± 4·6	22 ± 4·2	40	60 ± 5·3	No	"Generalized group"
Cat (n = 27) (Felis domesticus)	308 ± 32	21·4 ± 5·6	23·4 ± 5·6	45	55·5 ± 5·2	No	"Carnivore shear"
Treeshrew[2] (n = 63) (Tupaia glis)	238 ± 30	31·1 ± 4·6	24·5 ± 5·9	56	44·8 ± 6·0	Yes	"Generalized (insectivore)"
Bushbaby[2] (n = 66) (Galago crassicaudatus)	314 ± 47	29·2 ± 1·5	24·2 ± 6·2	53	45·56 ± 5·1	Yes	"Generalized (primate)"
Squirrel Monkey[2] (n = 67) (Saimiri scireus)	357 ± 63	26·2 ± 8·7	33·2 ± 5·0	59	38·3 ± 1·3	Yes	"Generalized (primate)"
Spider Monkey[2] (n = 66) (Ateles)	326 ± 100	32·2 ± 1·4	28·3 ± 5·4	60	39·0 ± 5·9	Yes	"Generalized (primate)"
Rhesus Monkey[3] (n = 19) (Macaca mulatta)	388·5 ± 36	21·5 ± 3·8	a) 56·87 ± 6·7 b) 38·6 ± 7·5	78 60	22·2 ± 3·8 40·21 ± 4·6	Yes[4]	"Generalized (primate)"
Man[5] (n = 9) (Homo sapiens)	857·6 ± 59	28·3 ± 4·8	28·33 ± 3·8	57	43·22 ± 4·4	Yes	"Generalized (primate)"
Miniature Pig[6] (Sus scrofa)	(a) 250 (min) (b) 460 (max)	33 27 } 30	17 36 } 26·5	56	50 36 } 43	Unlikely	"Ungulate-grinding"
Rat[7] (Rattus norvegicus)	192 ± 23	37·0	28·0	65	35	Yes	"Rodent-gnawing"

treated with some reservations: the "turnpoints" for the strokes of the cycle in the rat are difficult to determine accurately (Weijs, personal communication) and only maximum and minimum figures based on an unknown size of sample are available for the pig. Further, the figures for the rhesus monkey differ so much from those for other primates that they must be viewed with suspicion. In the absence of any other time course data on this animal, the author can only suggest that Luschei and Goodwin (1974) have, by excluding all possibility of cranial movement, obtained a record of a modified pattern of mandibular movement. There is some similarity between their profiles and those obtained for lower jaw movement in the opossum when plotted against extra-cranial reference planes (see Fig. 8 in Hiiemae, 1976). Both show a relative reduction in length of the fast-closing and fast-opening stages and an exaggeration of the time spent near occlusion in the power stroke and slow-opening stage. If this inference is correct, then the time course data for *Macaca* will necessarily be distorted by comparison with that obtained from conventional gape/time plots. For this reason the "isometric" period of Luschei and Goodwin's profiles has been included in the opening stroke (case b, Table IV).

There is both absolutely (in ms) and relatively in the percentages shown in Table IV a reciprocal relationship between the duration of the closing and power strokes; as one lengthens the other shortens, but the total time for both appears to fall within fairly narrow limits. This finding is to be expected as the length of the free movement (closing stroke) and the loaded movement (power stroke) are related to particle size, tooth–food–tooth contact marking the transition from one to the other. However, gape/time plots for the masticatory sequence show that in puncture-crushing, the working movement does not continue until a particular degree of closure is achieved but ceases after a fairly short period of time. Its duration therefore appears a function of the time elapsed, or, rather, the muscular effort expended. As might be expected, the gape at which tooth–food–tooth contact occurs diminishes as the food is reduced until, in chewing, it can reach a steady level.

In terms of the percentage time spent in the three strokes of the cycle, the animals cited in Table IV fall into two groups: those with a short power stroke, no Phase II and an aggregate percentage for closing and power strokes of less than 50% of total cycle time (opossum and cat), and those with a relatively longer power stroke, Phase II and an aggregate percentage for closing and power strokes in excess of 50% of total cycle time (primates, pig and rat). The pig is an unexpected member of the second group; the similarity between it and the primates lends support to Herring and Scapino's (1973) remark that it seems to be an omnivore incompletely adapted to a herbivorous grinding habit!

The percentage duration of the power stroke in the opossum, cat, treeshrew and *Galago* is shorter than in the remaining animals (the minimum figure for the pig almost certainly refers to puncture-crushing). All four have a predominantly shearing occlusion (Crompton and Hiiemae, 1970; Kay and Hiiemae, 1973) although both *Tupaia* and *Galago* have a short, grinding

Phase II. The elongation of the power stroke in the monkeys and man could be attributed to the second phase with its longer transverse movement.

In the first study of mastication in *Didelphis* (Hiiemae and Crompton, 1971) the opening stroke was observed to occur in two stages: an initial opening to about 7° gape followed after a pause, or a period of further slow opening, by a fast downwards movement from about 11° gape (Hiiemae, 1976). This pattern of opening movement has also been observed in some primates (Hiiemae and Kay, 1973) and in the cat (Hiiemae and Thexton, 1975). Fast opening starts at about 15° gape in the cat, at a level well clear of the intercuspal range in *Tupaia*, *Galago* and *Saimiri* and just within it in *Ateles* (Fig. 3). In the last three the slow-opening period is associated with a marked protrusion of the mandible.

During slow opening, the food in the mouth is recycled by the tongue in preparation for the next power stroke. The position of the bite and the direction of movement of the anterior part of the tongue in successive cycles have now been plotted both for the opossum (Fig. 2) and for the cat: the bite is "collected" by the tongue at the end of the power stroke and, as the jaw is slowly opened, is carried forwards on it. Visible protrusion of the anterior part of the tongue continues for most of slow opening and is followed by an abrupt reversal of direction just before the fast-opening movement begins. The bite is then moved backwards and reaches the posterior cheek teeth during the rapid downstroke (Fig. 2). It has recently been shown (Crompton et al., 1975; Crompton et al., 1977) that slow opening in the jaw movement cycle corresponds to the stage of the hyoid cycle in which marked upwards and forwards movement of the hyoid is occurring. Fast opening of the jaws does not begin until the hyoid has completed its movement and the base of the tongue has been both elevated and protruded. On present evidence, the profile of hyoid movement appears consistent throughout the stages of the masticatory sequence, the profile of jaw movement in slow opening is not. In both the opossum and the cat, slow opening can be discontinuous, i.e. involve an intiial opening movement to beyond the intercuspal range followed by a period of as long as 100 ms in which movement is slowed, suspended or even transitorily reversed (Fig. 3, opossum and cat, first cycle) or involve a steady slow opening (Fig. 3, opossum and cat, last cycle). The discontinuous form of slow opening is seen in puncture-crushing and the earlier stages of chewing when the animals are feeding on hard food. Steady slow opening is associated with soft food or with the later stages of a sequence on hard food. This suggests a relationship between the pattern of slow opening, tooth form and both the consistency and particle size of the food. The opossum, tree-shrew and cat have high-cusped cheek teeth which are so aligned that on closing the mouth the posterior teeth occlude ahead of those more anteriorly placed, giving a scissor-like action. This forces the food, especially a large bite, forwards and medially. At the same time fully triturated material is guided into the channels between the palatal rugae (Crompton and Hiiemae, 1970) and then collected on the dorsum of the tongue. For a large bite to "clear" the cusps of the anterior postcanines, the mouth must be opened fairly widely. It can then be "collected" by the tongue and repositioned in readiness for the next cycle. As chewing proceeds, the need for a distinct initial opening movement to clear the bite will be progressively reduced. As, by comparison with the more primitive mammals, the spider monkey and man have both low-cusped teeth and a curved occlusal plane, all the cheek teeth can occlude more or less simultaneously; even a large bite is not driven forwards in the power stroke. Further, the well developed cheeks of the anthropoids assist the tongue in controlling the position of the bite. The activities of the "slow-opening" stage can therefore begin within or much closer to the intercuspal range of gape. It is possible that the long "isometric" phase described in the rhesus monkey and in man includes a period functionally equivalent to the distinct slow opening of other mammals in which elevation and protraction of the hyoid is occurring. Confirmation of this suggestion will wait on the result of suitable experiments using a good human analogue in which simultaneous recordings of jaw, hyoid movement and food position can be made. It is, however, clear that there is a complete integration of jaw and hyoid movement (Fig. 1) during mastication and other oral activities, to the extent that the movement of one during any part of the cycle can be predicted from that of the other (Crompton et al., 1977).

MUSCLES

The elevators of the lower jaw in mammals are the temporalis, masseter* and medial pterygoid. It has been argued that in primitive mammals, temporalis was the largest of the elevator muscles and the masseter and pterygoids were of approximately the same size and smaller (Adams, 1919; Crompton, 1963a, b; Barghusen, 1968). In the opossum, which has been used as an experimental analogue for early mammals (Crompton and Hiiemae, 1969 et seq.), the separation of temporalis and the deeper part of masseter is so incomplete as to justify their being regarded on anatomical grounds as a single muscle mass (Hiiemae and Jenkins, 1969). In contrast to the large bulk of the elevator muscles, the depressors of the jaw are very small. Although the lower fibres of the lateral pterygoid are considered to act as a mandibular depressor and as the initiators of jaw opening in man (Moyers, 1950), the digastric, which connects the symphyseal region to the para-occipital area of the cranial base with, usually, an intermediate connection to the hyoid (du Châine, 1919) is classically regarded as the major jaw opening muscle. In practice, at least in Didelphis, jaw opening depends on a combination of mandibular depression through the combined activities of digastric, particu-

*No attempt is made in this review to reconcile either the names given or the homologies assigned to the various muscle blocks in the elevator musculature. The terms temporalis and masseter are used simply to indicate large blocks of muscle whose location can be recognized. The numbers of parts into which these muscle masses are anatomically separable, or physiologically divisible, vary greatly between the genera described and the authors describing them. The scale of the problem is implied by Turnbull (1970), although his use of both a standard nomenclature and a convention for its application to some extent masks the true position.

larly the anterior belly, geniohyoid and the inferior fibres of genioglossus, coupled with the sternohyoid and omohyoid and elevation of the cranium, presumably by the action of the nuchal and cervical musculature (see Hiiemae, 1976, for movements; Crompton *et al.*, 1977, for muscles).

The disproportion in bulk between the large elevator and small depressor musculature is explained by the nature of jaw movement in feeding: the jaws are closed against resistance, opening (with the possible exception of Phase II) is a free movement with gravity as a synergist. However, the working relationships between the various parts of the elevator mass during the closing and power strokes of the cycle are not yet clear and without this information it is difficult to explain the differential evolution of the various parts of this mass as mammals have specialized for herbivorous or carnivorous diets. Such attempts as have been made (notably Turnbull, 1970; but also Arendsen de Wolff-Exalto, 1951a, b; Becht, 1953; Crompton and Hiiemae, 1969, for extant mammals in general; Scapino, 1973, for the equid lineage) have either described the differences in the proportions of the major elevators or their constituent parts in each "dietetic group" (Turnbull, 1970) or have produced "mechanical reconstructions" of varying complexity. With two exceptions (Hiiemae, 1971b; Weijs and Dantuma, 1975) all such reconstructions have involved a number of, usually unstated, assumptions of which the two most important are: first, that all the elevator muscles contract maximally with the jaw in centric occlusion (or its equivalent); and second, that this is the critical functional position of the jaws. Both are ill-founded. It is inherently unlikely, and evidence has recently been obtained to substantiate this view (Thexton and Hiiemae, 1975b), that all the elevator muscles are maximally effective in a position corresponding to that at which the major muscular effort in mastication, i.e. the power stroke, is actually complete. Experiments have shown that these muscles are most efficient, as measured by the twitch tension they produce, over different, but overlapping, ranges of gape in the opossum. Temporalis is most effective at the wider range of gapes associated with the beginning of the closing stroke, followed by masseter in the middle range and medial pterygoid when the teeth are approaching occlusion. Masseter in the rat is also most efficient with the mouth slightly opened (Nordstrom and Yemm, 1974). This does not mean that these muscles do not contract outside their optimum range nor that they cannot contract simultaneously—indeed they do—but that when considering their mechanics in a single mammal or, more important, in the context of evolutionary change, due weight must be given to the likelihood that the proportions and internal architecture of each muscle or part thereof, have developed in relation to that muscle's optimum functional range within the envelope of motion rather than to its potential for force production in centric occlusion.

It is difficult to ascertain whether the second assumption, that centric occlusion is the critical jaw position, has arisen from a genuine, if mistaken, belief that this epitomizes its normal working arrangements or, and this is more likely, from a static approach to what is essentially a dynamic problem.

The difficulties of considering the dynamics of even the simplest bone–muscle–joint system have been amply demonstrated by Stern (1974). However, the moments of the muscles were shown to change with jaw movement by Hiiemae (1971b) who considered this aspect of their mechanics at the three turnpoints between the strokes of the cycle in the rat. This approach has been refined by Weijs and Dantuma (1975) who have achieved a synthesis of EMG and mechanical data by considering the conditions operative in eight positions of the jaw during a statistically standardized chewing cycle, again in the rat. In practice, as the jaw moves, the line of action of each muscle changes, as does its moment and the force it produces in relation to the occlusal plane. Since the mechanics of each muscle at any moment of time are a function of its immediately preceding behaviour, it is as yet impossible, in view of the number of variables, to achieve a dynamic analysis.

The behaviour of the jaw muscles, like that of all mammalian skeletal muscles, depends on both extrinsic and intrinsic factors. The former are the intracranial connections of the motor nerves and, most important, give the actual pattern of firing through the nerves to the motor units within the muscle. These extrinsic factors combine to form the "output" side of the control system regulating jaw muscle activity and thence jaw movement (Fig. 1). The sensory receptors, their nerves and intracranial connections form the "input" side. There is an extensive and growing literature on the control of mastication but since this is largely concerned with studies of various aspects of the relationship between controlled sensory input and specific components of the motor output rather than with normal behaviour, it is considered to be outside the scope of this review (see Kawamura, 1974). The intrinsic factors governing the actual contractile behaviour of a muscle are: its architecture; the way the fibres are arranged in pennate, multipennate or parallel systems (Gans and Bock, 1965); the size and distribution of the motor units within it; and lastly, the contractile characteristics of the fibres themselves (Close, 1972; see Taylor et al., 1973 for data on cat; Thexton and Hiiemae, 1975b, for data on Didelphis). There is some irony in the fact that the most useful and widely applied technique for the study of muscles in vivo, electromyography (EMG), provides a record of the impact of the extrinsic factors on the muscle over time and no information whatsoever on the effect of that impact in terms of how the muscle itself behaves or on the mechanical consequences of that behaviour.

Electromyography of the Jaw Muscles

An electromyogram (EMG) is a record of the electrical state of a muscle over time. It cannot show whether the muscle is contracting isotonically, isometrically or changing from one condition to the other. Since it is the velocity and direction of movement produced by a muscle contracting isotonically or the tension generated by one contracting isometrically that is of major interest in the study of movement in vivo, considerable effort has been expended in attempts to correlate the EMG with either one or the other.

Correlations have been based on the "integrated EMG". This term is very loosely used. It usually means that the investigator has rectified and filtered the raw signal to give a wave-form, the deviations of which from the baseline can be taken as a measure of the electrical activity in the muscle (see *inter alia* Møller, 1966, 1974; Ahlgren, 1967; Ahlgren and Öwall, 1970). To obtain a true integration, the area enclosed by the raw wave-form has to be accurately calculated. Only under the most stringent and rigidly controlled laboratory conditions has a relationship between the genuinely integrated EMG and the performance of a muscle been proved for the force produced in isometric contraction (Inman *et al.*, 1952; Lippold, 1952; Thexton *et al.*, 1973) and the velocity of movement in isotonic contraction (Bigland and Lippold, 1954; Close *et al.*, 1960).

The EMG obtained from a muscle is greatly affected by the instrumentation used. The properties of the various types of electrodes and of the components of recording systems have been discussed by Møller (1966). All the studies of non-human mammals have used the fine wire indwelling electrodes developed by Basmaijan and Stecko (1962). It is, however, important to recognize that when recording simultaneously from a number of electrodes in different muscle blocks, the timing of activity as shown by the different electrodes can be compared, but the performance (force or work) as signalled by one single electrode cannot be compared with that from any other. The amplitude of the raw traces or the peaks in filtered or integrated traces only record the changing levels of activity within the fields of each electrode.

Despite this limitation, the EMG of the jaw muscles can be used both as an index of the pattern of motor activity in studies on jaw movement control and on the effects of stimulating peripheral receptors (e.g. Taylor and Davey, 1968; Hannam *et al.*, 1970; Munro and Basmaijan, 1971; Matsunami and Kubota, 1972; Goodwin and Luschei, 1974; Kawamura, 1974). It can also be used to examine the activity of the muscles in relation to jaw movements (Moyers, 1950, Carlsöo, 1952, 1956a, b, 1958; Ahlgren, 1966, 1967; Møller, 1966, 1974). The application of EMG techniques in studies of mastication in mammals other than man (Kallen and Gans, 1972; Herring and Scapino, 1973; de Vree and Gans, 1974; Thexton and Hiiemae, 1975a; Weijs and Dantuma, 1975; Crompton *et al.*, 1977) is very recent and can be attributed, at least in part, to the technical difficulties involved in synchronizing jaw movement and EMG recordings. Only man can be instructed to eat to order, or in time to a metronome (Ahlgren, 1967)!

Muscle Activity in the Chewing Cycle

The pattern of EMG activity in the jaw muscles during a masticatory sequence changes as the food is reduced (Thexton and Hiiemae, 1975a) and differs between various types of food (Ahlgren, 1967; Luschei and Goodwin, 1974; Møller, 1974; de Vree and Gans, 1974). The details of this pattern change from cycle to cycle in a single chewing sequence recorded from one animal chewing one type of food (Hiiemae, 1976; Thexton and Hiiemae, 1975a). Given the differences in the properties of the recording systems used, reliable comparisons can only be made between the records obtained in different studies in the light of the methodology used. Any discussion of the pattern of EMG activity in the jaw musculature of mammals must, therefore, be based on generalizations.

Data has been presented in the form of a visually derived "average" pattern of EMG activity in relation to a "standard" cycle (Kallen and Gans, 1972; Herring and Scapino, 1973) or as a statistical model in relation to time Møller, 1974) or a standardized cycle (Weijs and Dantuma, 1975). Even where differences have been noted in relation to diet, these have not been quantified.

The classical work of Sherrington (1906) in the early part of this century described the reciprocal innervation of antagonistic muscle systems throughout the body. Carlsöo (1956a, b), based on his EMG studies of chewing in man, advanced the concept of "reciprocity" between the elevators and depressors of the jaw. As the mouth is opened, the activity of the elevators is inhibited and the depressors activated. During closing, the activity of the elevators gradually increases and that of the depressors diminishes. Mammalian studies have shown that instead of clear alternation of elevator and depressor activity associated with closing and opening movements, there is in fact a considerable degree of overlap (Fig. 5 A, B).

In describing the EMG of the muscles, a distinction has to be drawn between the beginning and end of all activity in a given muscle during a single cycle and the period in which peak activity occurs. This difference is clearly shown by Møller (1974, his Fig. 9) where the duration of activity is represented as a bar and the period of "strong activity" within that time plotted from a statistical analysis of the level of activity in a series of cycles. Within any period of activity, the amplitude of the EMG can fluctuate so that sudden shifts between high and low level activity or between either and electrical silence can be recorded. In the following necessarily very generalized account, the correlations suggested between the activity of the muscles and the occlusal relations of the teeth have been deduced from the available data, but not always by the authors cited.

The Closing and Power Strokes. The last stage of opening and the first part of closing involves some lateral movement in all mammals (Fig. 4). This is followed by a free closing movement to tooth–food–tooth contact. Some activity in the medial pterygoid is observed at or close to maximum gape in all the mammals except the pig. In man this muscle is the first to be activated, 10–40 ms ahead of the remainder (Møller, 1974). Activity in the temporalis and masseter follows, reaching maximum levels as the teeth come into contact with the food at the beginning of the power stroke (Fig. 5, A and B). The variations on this general pattern, as seen for example in the pig, where the "m. zygomaticomandibularis" fires first, may not so much reflect a difference in the pattern of motor outflow from the central nervous system, but the relative development (and labelling) of various parts of the musculature; the fibres of the zygomaticomandibularis in the pig are homologous with the outermost fibres of the middle temporalis or "external adductor" in the opossum (Hiiemae and Jenkins, 1969).

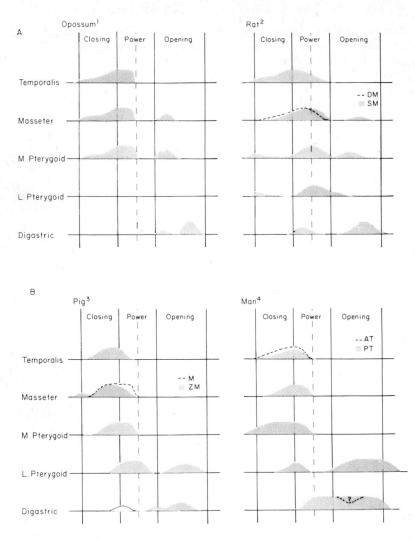

FIG. 5. To illustrate the "average" pattern of EMG activity in the major muscles of mastication. The lengths of the cycle have been standardized using the data in Table IV so that, taking the total cycle time as 100%, then the closing and power strokes are each shown as 30% and the opening stroke as 40% of total time. The midway point of the power stroke has been arbitrarily defined as "centric occlusion". (The same convention has been used in Fig. 6.) The pattern of EMG activity in chewing is not constant, neither in its timing nor in the level of activity in each muscle (Thexton and Hiiemae, 1975). The figures are, therefore, only a guide as to when the muscles are active and at what level. The data for the opossum (Thexton and Hiiemae, 1975; Crompton et al., 1977) and for pig (Herring and Scapino, 1973) are based on visual impression, that for the rat (Weijs and Dantuma, 1975) and man (Møller, 1974) on a statistical analysis.

A. Both the opossum and rat have mobile mandibular symphyses and show activity in the masseter and medial pterygoid as well as in the digastric during "slow opening". The

One feature of the EMG pattern, so far reported only in man, is less clear and therefore somewhat controversial. According to Ahlgren (1967) and Ahlgren and Öwall (1970), all elevator activity is cut off abruptly for about 30 ms at the beginning of the occlusal phase (= power stroke, Ahlgren, 1967), and there is then a second short burst lasting through Phase I. This abrupt cut-off or "occlusal silent period" would provide an extremely useful marker for this critical point in the upward movements of chewing if it was a constant feature of the EMG and correlated with tooth–food–tooth contact. Møller (1966, 1974) has not recorded such a cut-off in his careful and exhaustive studies. Griffin and Munro (1969) reported a silent period of about 13 ms following tooth contact in the somewhat artificial situation of the "open–close–clench" cycle in man. Other workers have reported a similar phenomenon with a duration ranging from 5–50 ms (see Hannam et al., 1970). Ahlgren (1967) was unable to correlate the silent period with either tooth–food–tooth contact or tooth–tooth contact during normal chewing but such a correlation has been reported by Hannam et al. (1970), there being a 12 ms delay after tooth–tooth contact. With the evidence available it is impossible to say whether the silent period is a normal feature of the human EMG in chewing or whether it only occurs when the jaws are moved in a predetermined manner (Griffin and Munro, 1969) or are deliberately tapped (Hannam et al., 1970).

Although the major electrical activity of the elevators ceases abruptly during the power stroke when the teeth are close to or have reached centric occlusion, there follows a period (related to time to reach peak tension and the subsequent decay time of the active muscle fibres) in which force continues to be produced. This force persists for up to 100 ms in man (Ahlgren and Öwall, 1970) and will sustain the power stroke for that period. The extended EMG activity in the rat (Weijs and Dantuma, 1975) can be correlated with the elongation of Phase II in that animal. Kallen and Gans (1972) found that the medial pterygoid on the working side in the bat was active throughout the power stroke and into the opening stroke (Fig. 6).

A second burst of activity in the elevator muscles, particularly the deep and superficial masseter and medial pterygoid, is seen in the early part of the opening stroke in the opossum (Thexton and Hiiemae, 1975b). At this time the anterior and posterior suprahyoid muscles are acting to raise the hyoid, and the activity of the elevator muscles serves to control the movement of the lower jaw which would otherwise be depressed by the hyoid muscles (Crompton et al., 1977).

---

secondary burst of activity in the superficial masseter of the rat is due to the pars reflexa of that muscle, described by Weijs (1973).

SM = superficial masseter; DM = deep masseter (all parts combined).

B. The pig and man have immobile mandibular symphyses. The burst of activity in the digastric of the pig during the early part of the power stroke is not a constant feature. The dip in the activity level for this muscle in man indicates the reduction or cut-off in activity that sometimes occurs.

M = masseter; ZM = zygomaticomandibularis; PT = posterior temporalis; AT = anterior temporalis.

The Opening Stroke. The two depressor muscles, lateral pterygoid and digastric, can be identified in EMGs by their characteristic pattern of activity. Møller (1966) describes the former in man as having two main bursts: the first, "primary activity", begins as the teeth move into Phase II and continues throughout the opening movement, ceasing at maximum gape. There is then a secondary burst of activity synchronous with the main activity of the elevators in closing (Fig. 5B). This pattern has been observed in the rat and the pig but not in the bat (Fig. 6). Kallen and Gans (1972) found that

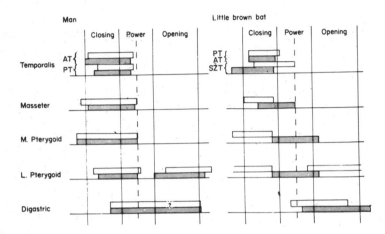

FIG. 6. The firing order and duration (but not amplitude) of electrical activity in the jaw muscles of right (stippled) and left sides during a chewing cycle when the active side is on the right. The data for man is taken from Møller (1974) and is used to represent the general mammalian pattern in broad outline (see Fig. 5) and for the little brown bat from Kallen and Gans (1972). Asynchrony on the onset of firing is shown in all the muscles of man except the medial pterygoid and the digastric. In the former, there is marked asynchrony in the timing and level of peak activity within the active period. Kallen and Gans (1972) recorded alternation in the activity of the medial and lateral pterygoids between active and balancing sides. This has not been reported in any other mammal.

AT = anterior temporalis; PT = posterior temporalis; SZT = suprazygomatic part of the temporalis.

the lateral pterygoid of the working side fired during the power stroke and in the early stages of opening. The contralateral muscle fired during the later stages of opening and the first part of the closing stroke (Fig. 6). There is no clear evidence of "double-bursting" in the lateral pterygoid in the macaque (Luschei and Goodwin, 1974). However, the results obtained by McNamara (1973) also in the rhesus monkey show an interesting difference between the activity in the superior and inferior heads. The superior head fired in synchrony with the elevators (particularly masseter) during closing but the inferior head fired in synchrony with the suprahyoids during opening. Kawamura *et al.* (1968) found that the very small lateral pterygoid in the cat showed EMG activity both prior to the actual opening movement and also in the first stages of closing. They attribute the first burst of activity to the bulk of the fibres, which insert into the capsule and disc of the joint, and the latter to the more inferior fibres attaching to the condylar neck. These observations suggest that the two functions of this muscle, the stabilization of condylar position during jaw closure against resistance and the rotation of the condyle during jaw opening, have become progressively localized so that in the primates, the upper head subserves one function, and the lower head the other.

The pattern of activity in digastric is so characteristic that it has been used by a number of authors, including Thexton and Hiiemae (1975) as a reference muscle. Digastric activity begins early in the power stroke or even in the later stages of closing, either coincident with peak activity in the anterior temporalis (man, Møller, 1974) or immediately on cessation of activity in that muscle (opossum). Activity then continues throughout the power stroke reaching a peak during fast opening. In the opossum, rat and pig, there is evidence of a drop in activity at the end of the power stroke and a second peak during opening. No digastric activity coincident with that of the elevators was reported by Kallen and Gans (1972) in the little brown bat (Fig. 6).

Asynchrony in the EMG Record

All the EMG studies to date have shown some asynchrony in either the time of onset of activity or the timing of peak activity between the muscles of the active and balancing sides (Møller, 1974). In man, time dispersal between the active and balancing side muscles is most marked in those muscles known or considered to contribute to the production of transverse mandibular movement. Differences in activity levels are greatest in those muscles considered to be responsible for the comminution of the bite, such as the masseter (Møller, 1974). Herring and Scapino (1973) used this difference in activity level as diagnostic of the active or "dominant" side, since they could not determine this from their movement records. In no study, other than that one of Kallen and Gans (1972) on *Myotis*, has alternation of activity as between "working side" and "balancing side" muscles been found. These authors recorded some asynchrony in the onset of activity in the various parts of the temporalis, a distinct lag between the balancing and working sides in the masseter and a clear alternation in activity between working and balancing sides in the medial and lateral pterygoids (Fig. 6). The timing of the two bursts, one from each muscle, in the bat, corresponds to the timing of each of the bursts from both muscles in the other mammals studied. The bat is therefore either atypical of mammals in general or the "second burst" level of activity in *Myotis* was such as to be "cut out" by the properties of the recording apparatus. The first alternative is difficult to accept given the degree of variation in the anatomy of the jaw apparatus of the other mammals studied and the similarity of the EMG pattern. The second alternative is the likelier. Møller (1966) has pointed out that since the EMG actually recorded is dependent on the apparatus used, pen recorders, such as that employed by Kallen and Gans, could result in their not observing the true signal.

The figures published by Luschei and Goodwin (1974) show no elevator activity in the early stages of closing. EMG activity first appears at a point which, based on the change in the velocity of closing movement, could be regarded as marking the point of tooth–food–tooth contact. Ahlgren (1966) found that the elevators appeared inactive in the first part of the closing stroke, particularly when his subjects were chewing gum. He did, however, find (1967) that when the rate of chewing (mandibular lowering and elevation) was increased, then action potentials appeared at the beginning of the closing stroke. Møller (1966, 1974) found no such lag, nor has it been reported in mammals other than man. It is, however, possible that the initial upwards movement of the closing stroke is produced in certain circumstances by the recoil of the elastic components of the elevator muscles stretched during the preceding opening (Clemmensen, 1963).

The Pattern of Muscle Activity in Mammals

It is clear that the pattern of EMG activity in the major jaw muscles is broadly similar in all the mammals so far studied despite the difference in their profile of movement (cf. Figs. 4 and 5 A, B) and in the structure of the jaw apparatus. This is an interesting commentary on the observation based on the extensive data available for man, that the EMG pattern is essentially the same even where the associated movement path is very different (Ahlgren, 1966; Møller, 1966), and its corollary, that movements are difficult to predict from the EMG record. The uniformity of the firing pattern might have been expected since there is a "basic mammalian jaw apparatus" (possibly exemplified by *Didelphis*) and since the jaws are approximated and move apart in a regular rhythm in chewing. A central control system will, presumably, be "programmed" for the alternating pattern of muscle activity required to produce a cyclical movement.

The overall similarity in the general EMG pattern suggests that the pattern of firing in the motor neurones initiated in the central nervous system must also be similar (Fig. 1). If this is so, then the differences in the profile of mandibular movement (Fig. 4) must be due either to the mechanical properties of the fibres, or to the anatomy and internal architecture of the muscles or, more likely, to both.

The Actions of the Muscles

It is possible to describe the action of a muscle on the classical principle that it will tend, on contraction, to approximate its origin and insertion. Whilst this implies something about the arrangement of the muscle, it says very little about its pattern of interaction with the other muscles in a given system and its consequent contribution to the movements or mechanics of normal behaviour. The movements of the lower jaw are produced by a pattern of muscle activity based on combinations of muscles forming couples. These may include muscles of the same side or of both sides which may fire asynchronously or synchronously but with peak activity at different times or at different levels.

The movements of the closing stroke are directed upwards and laterally (Fig. 3) turning medially just before or on tooth–food–tooth contact. The lateral movement is produced by a couple formed by the posterior temporalis of the working side (including the suprazygomatic fibres where these are separately identified) and the contralateral lateral pterygoid. The upwards movement of the jaw during free closing is produced by the anterior temporalis in man (Møller, 1974) and, given the EMG picture seen in Figs 5A, B and 6, this may well be true of other mammals. As the closing stroke begins, the two other elevators, masseter and medial pterygoid, which are more or less symmetrically placed on the inner and outer sides of the ramus of the jaw come into action and provide the main force for the comminution of the food. The conspicuous difference in the activity levels between these muscles on the working and balancing sides reported by Møller (1974) for man, and Herring and Scapino (1973) for the pig (and indicated in the preliminary results for the opossum) supports this view. The balancing-side masseter and medial pterygoid will, according to Møller (1974), stabilize the jaw, an action requiring less force and therefore fewer active motor units.

The power stroke is antero-medial in direction. The anterior component is exaggerated in rodents and the medial is emphasized in herbivores (Fig. 4). Although the posterior temporalis of the balancing side and the lateral pterygoid of the working side are active during the stroke, acting as a couple rotating the jaw medially on the active side, the medial and forwards vectors of both masseter and medial pterygoid will assist this movement. The exaggeration of the anterior movement in the rodents may be attributable to the action of the nearly horizontal superficial masseter in these animals. Similarly the enlargement of the masseteric complex and the medial pterygoid in the herbivores must be related to the increase in the medial excursion of the power stroke. In this context it is interesting to note that Møller found a very marked asynchrony in the activity of the masseters in individuals with a very large medial movement in the closing and power strokes of chewing: the balancing side muscle fired first with short-lived low level activity; the working-side muscle then showed a large peak of activity as the jaw moved medially.

The pattern of activity in the opening stroke shows the greatest variation. Whilst the digastric is a "mandibular depressor" its activity is very closely correlated with that of the remainder of the hyoid musculature and the effect of their combined activity is to produce movement of both the lower jaw and the hyoid (Crompton et al., 1975; Crompton et al., 1977).

The variation in the form of the chewing cycle shown in Fig. 4 can, therefore, be attributed to slight shifts in the balance between pairs of muscles. This may be due to an adaptive response tending to enhance one or other of their vectors by alterations in their mass or the orientation of their fibres. Quantification of these modifications based on detailed studies of mastication in a wide range of mammals will provide the essential basis for the evaluation of their adaptive advantages in the groups concerned.

Mammalian Mastication

Mammals apparently conform to a basic pattern of masticatory behaviour. The teeth of mammals are very different. Even without the evidence presented and reviewed in this chapter, the first conclusion should not, on reflection, be surprising. The second statement implies that were the teeth the only parts of the jaw apparatus available for study, no such conclusion would be drawn.

This chapter has discussed aspects of behaviour; how the various components of the jaw apparatus are known, or assumed, to function. The variations in the shapes and proportions of those components have had only the briefest mention and then only in relation to particular features which can be associated with modifications of the basic behavioural pattern. There are, however, substantial differences in the form of the teeth, the detailed anatomy of the muscles and in the overall proportions of the jaw apparatus in the mammals. How can these differences be reconciled with the concept of a fundamental masticatory pattern?

It can be argued that the "basic mammalian pattern" was definitely established with the appearance of the squamo-dentary joint and the development of the patterns of muscular activity required to control the position of a freely moving lower jaw. Further, that this "basic pattern" was very flexible; a simple cycle such as that found in *Didelphis*, with a path of antero-medial and upwards movement in the power stroke brought the then comparatively simple teeth into occlusion and allowed the development of tribosphenic molars capable of piercing, cutting, crushing and later grinding food of a wide variety of size and consistency. The adaptations resulting from the opening up of wider adaptive zones which led to the mammalian radiation in the Paleocene could have involved the progressive optimization of capacities already present in the system and their later fixation with changes in tooth form or muscle proportions. It is suggestive that the greatest variation in the parts of the jaw apparatus in the Mammalia is in the shape of the teeth. Although there are considerable variations in the detailed architecture of muscles and bones there is much less variation in the overall plan of both.

The answer to the question posed above cannot yet be given, but the reality may prove to be that although structure limits behaviour in the short term, behaviour provides the context in which structural change takes place over the longer term.

Summary

Oral behaviour such as biting, chewing or speaking, depends on a complex series of interrelated actions in the jaw apparatus. The integrated actions of the jaw muscles, in response to a cranial outflow down the motor nerves, produces mandibular movement which in turn leads to relative movement between upper and lower teeth. At the same time, the muscles of the hyoid apparatus control the position of that bone, and with the other extrinsic and the intrinsic muscles of the tongue, regulate the shape and position of that organ. There is a continuing sensory feedback from the periphery modulating these activities. In the last decade there has been a great expansion of interest in all aspects of oral behaviour but particularly in the activities of the parts of the jaw apparatus during mastication and in the mechanisms by which these activities and oral behaviour in general are controlled. Chewing is based on the repetition of a cyclical movement produced by the interplay of "elevator" and "depressor" muscles. These movements, and the activity patterns of the muscles in mammals have been reviewed and areas of future experimental interest have been outlined.

ACKNOWLEDGEMENTS

The experimental work on *Didelphis* referred to in this chapter has been supported by U.S.P.H.S. Grants Nos DE-02648 and 03219 and was carried out with Dr A. Thexton and Professor A. W. Crompton at the Museum of Comparative Zoology, Harvard University, Cambridge, Massachusetts.

I should particularly like to thank the many people, but especially Dr W. A. Weijs, who have been kind enough to make available unpublished data or their manuscripts in advance of publication in order that this review should be as complete as possible. In addition, I should like to thank Dr A. Thexton, Professor J. W. Osborn, Mr A. Sita-Lumsden and my husband, Mr R. W. Holmwood, for reading the manuscript and for their helpful comments; Mrs. P. Elson, who typed the manuscript; and Messrs S. P. A. Kariyawasam, M. Lyons and S. Metcalfe, who have also helped in its preparation.

REFERENCES

ADAMS, L. A. (1919). A memoir on the phylogeny of the jaw muscles in recent and fossil vertebrates. *Ann. N. Y. Acad. Sci.* **28**, 51–166.

AHLGREN, J. (1966). Mechanism of mastication. *Acta odont. scand.* **24**, suppl. 44, 5–109.

AHLGREN, J. (1967) Kinesiology of the mandible. An EMG study. *Acta odont. scand.* **25**, 593–611.

AHLGREN, J. and ÖWALL, B. (1970). Muscular activity and chewing force. A polygraphic study of human mandibular movements. *Archs oral Biol.* **15**, 271–280.

AMAR, J. (1914). "Le Moteur Human or The Scientific Foundation of Labour and Industry" (Doolittle Brown, ed.). George Routledge and Sons, London (1920).

ANDERSON, D. J. (1956). Measurement of stress in mastication. *J. dent. Res.* **35**: I, 664–670; II, 671–673.

ARDRAN, G. M., KEMP, F. H. and RIDE, W. D. L. (1958). A radiographic analysis of mastication and swallowing in the domestic rabbit *Oryctolagus caniculus* L. *Proc. zool. Soc. Lond.* **130**, 257–274.

ARENDSEN DE WOLFF-EXALTO, E. (1951a) On differences in the lower jaw of animalivorous and herbivorous mammals I. *Prov. K. med. Akad. Wet. Ser. C.* **54**, 237–246.

ARENDSEN DE WOLFF EXALTO, E. (1951b). On differences in the lower jaw of animalivorous and herbivorous mammals II. *Proc. K. ned. Akad. Wet. Ser. C.* **54**, 405–410.

ATKINSON, H. F. and SHEPHERD, R. W. (1961). Temporomandibular joint disturbances and the associated masticatory patterns. *Aust. dent. J.* **6**, 219–222.

ATKINSON, H. F. and SHEPHERD, R. W. (1967). Masticatory movement and tooth form. *Aust. dent. J.* **12**, 49–53.

BARGHUSEN, H. R. (1968). The lower jaw of cynodonts (Reptilia, Therapsida) and the evolutionary origin of mammal-like adductor jaw musculature. *Postilla* **116**, 1–49.

BASMAIJAN, J. V. and STECKO, G. (1962). A new bipolar electrode for electromyography. *J. appl. Physiol.* **17**, 849.

BECHT, G. (1953). Comparative biologic-anatomical researches on mastication in some mammals I and II. *Proc. ned. Akad. Wet. Ser. C.* **56**, 508–527.

BEYRON, H. (1964). Occlusal relations and mastication in Australian aborigines. *Acta odont. scand.* **22**, 597–678.

BIGLAND, B. and LIPPOLD, O. C. J. (1954). The relation between force, velocity and integrated electrical activity in human muscle. *J. Physiol.* **123**, 214–224.

BREMER, F. (1923). Physiologie nerveuse de la mastication chez le chat et le lapin. *Archs int. Physiol.* **21**, 309–352.

BUTLER, P. M. (1952). The milk-molars of Perissodactyla, with remarks on molar occlusion. *Proc. zool. Soc. Lond.* **121**: IV, 777–817.

BUTLER, P. M. (1973). Molar wear facets of Early Tertiary North American primates. *Symp. 4th int. Cong. Primat.* **3**, 1–27.

CARLSÖO, S. (1952). Nervous co-ordination and mechanical function of the mandibular elevators. *Acta odont. scand.* **10**, Suppl. 11.

CARLSÖO, S. (1956a). An electromyographic study of the activity of certain suprahyoid muscles (mainly the anterior belly of digastric muscle) and of the reciprocal innervation of the elevator and depressor musculature of the mandible. *Acta Anat.* **26**, 81–93.

CARLSÖO, S. (1956b). An electromyographic study of the activity and an anatomic analysis of the mechanics of the lateral pterygoid muscle. *Acta Anat.* **26**, 339–348.

CARLSÖO, S. (1958). Motor units and action potentials in the masticatory muscles. *Acta morph. neerl.-scand.* **2**, 13–19.

DU CHÂINE, T. (1914–1919). Le digastrique (abaisseur de la mandible des mammifères). *J. Anat. Physiol., Paris*, **80**, 248–319; 393–417.

CLEMMENSON, S. M. (1963). "Some Neurophysiological Foundations of Therapeutic Exercises". Munksgaard, Copenhagen.

CLOSE, R. I. (1972). Dynamic properties of mammalian skeletal muscles. *Physiol. Rev.* **52**, 129–197.

CLOSE, J. R., NICKEL, E. D. and TODD, F. N. (1960). Motor-unit action-potential counts. Their significance in isometric and isotonic contractions. *J. Bone Jt Surg.* **42**-A, 1207–1222.

CROMPTON, A. W. (1963a). On the lower jaw of *Diarthrognathus* and the origin of the mammalian jaw. *Proc. zool. Soc. Lond.* **140**, 697–753.

CROMPTON, A. W. (1963b). The evolution of the mammalian jaw. *Evolution* **17**, 431–439.

CROMPTON, A. W. (1971). The origin of the tribosphenic molar. *In* "Early Mammals" (Kermack, D. M. and Kermack, K. A., eds), pp. 65–87. Academic Press, London and New York.

CROMPTON, A. W. and HIIEMAE, K. M. (1969). How mammalian molar teeth work. *Discovery* (*Yale Peabody Museum*) **5**, (1) 23–34.

CROMPTON, A. W. and HIIEMAE, K. M. (1970). Molar occlusion and mandibular movements during occlusion in the American opossum, *Didelphis marsupialis*. *J. Linn. Soc. (Zool)* **49**, 21–47.

CROMPTON, A. W., COOK, P., HIIEMAE, K. and THEXTON, A. J. (1975) Movements of the hyoid apparatus during chewing. *Nature, Lond.* **258**, 69–70.

CROMPTON, A. W., THEXTON, A. J., PARKER, P. and HIIEMAE, K. (1977). The activity of the hyoid and jaw muscles during the chewing of soft food in the American opossum. *In* "The Biology of Marsupials. II. Biology and Environment" (Gilmore, D. and Robinson, B eds), pp. 287–305. Macmillan, London.

DELLOW, P. and LUND, J. (1971). Evidence for the central timing of rhythmical mastication. *J. Physiol., Lond.* **215**, 1–13.

EWER, R. F. (1958). Adaptive features in the skulls of African Suidae. *Proc. zool. Soc.Lond.* **131**, 135–155.

EWER, R. F. (1970). The head of the forest hog, *Hylochoerus meinhertzhageni* *E. Afr. Wildlife J.* **8**, 43–52.

GANS, C. and BOCK, W. J. (1965). The functional significance of muscle architecture— a theoretical analysis. *Ergebn. Anat. Entw Gesch* **38**, 115–142.

GANS, C. and DE VREE, F. (1974). Correlation of accelerometers with electromyograph in the mastication of pygmy goats (*Capra hircus*) *Anat. Rec.* **306**, 1974 (Abstract).

GINGERICH, P. (1972). Molar occlusion and jaw mechanics of the Eocene primate *Adapis*. *Am. J. phys. Anthrop.* **36**, 359–368.

GOODWIN, G. M. and LUSCHEI, E. S. (1974). Effects of destroying spindle afferents from jaw muscles on mastication in monkeys. *J. Neurophysiol.* **37**, 967–981.

GRIFFIN, C. J. and MALOR, R. (1974). An analysis of mandibular movement. *Front. oral Physiol.* **1**, 159–198.

GRIFFIN, C. J. and MUNRO, R. R. (1939). Electromyography of the jaw closing muscles in the open–close–clench cycle in man. *Archs oral Biol.* **14**, 141–149.

HANNAM, A. G., MATTHEWS, B. and YEMM, R. (1970). Receptors involved in the response of the masseter muscle to tooth contact in man. *Archs oral Biol.* **15**, 17–24.

HERRING, S. W. and SCAPINO, R. P. (1973). Physiology of feeding in miniature pigs. *J. Morph.* **141**, 427 460.

HIIEMAE, K. (1966). The Development, Structure and Function of the Temporomandibular Joint in Rat. Ph.D. Thesis, University of London.

HIIEMAE, K. M. (1967). Masticatory function in the mammals. *J. dent. Res.* **46**, 883–893.

HIIEMAE, K. M. (1971a). The structure and function of the jaw muscles of the rat. II. Their fibre type and composition. *J. Linn. Soc. (Zool)* **50**, 101–109.

HIIEMAE, K. M. (1971b). The structure and function of the jaw muscles of the rat. III. The mechanics of the muscles. *J. Linn. Soc. (Zool)* **50**, 111–132.

HIIEMAE, K. M. (1976). Masticatory movements in primitive mammals. *In* "Mastication" (Anderson, D. J., and Matthews, B. eds), pp. 105–118. Wright and Sons, Bristol.

HIIEMAE, K. M. and ARDRAN, G. M. (1968). A Cineradiographic Study of Feeding in *Rattus Norvegicus*. *J. Zool., Lond.* **154**, 139–154.

HIIEMAE, K. M. and CROMPTON, A. W. (1971). A cinefluorographic study of feeding in the American opossum, *Didelphis marsupialis*. *In* "Dental Morphology and Evolution". (Dahlberg, A. A. ed.) pp. 299–334. University of Chicago Press.

HIIEMAE, K. M. and JENKINS, F. A. (1969). The anatomy and internal architecture of the muscles of mastication in the American opossum, *Didelphis marsupialis*. *Postilla* **140**, 1–49.

HIIEMAE, K. M. and KAY, R. F. (1973). Evolutionary trends in the dynamics of primate mastication. *In* "Craniofacial Biology of Primates" (Zingeser, M. R., ed.). Karger, Basle. *Symp. 4th Int. Cong. Primat.* **3**, 28–64.

HIIEMAS, K. M. and THEXTON, A. J. (1975). Consistency and bite size as regulations of mastication in cats. *J. dent. Res.* **54**, (special issue A), 194 (Abstract).

INMAN, V. T. RALSTON, H. J., SAUNDERS, T. B. DE C. M., FEINSTEIN, B. and WRIGHT, E. W. (1952). Relation of human electromyogram to muscular tension. *Electroenceph. clin. Neurophysiol.* **4**, 187–194.

KALLEN, F. C. and GANS, C. (1972). Mastication in the little brown bat (*Myotis lucifugus*). *J. Morph.* **136**, 385–420.

KAWAMURA, Y. (1974). Neurogenesis of Mastication. *Front. oral Physiol.* **1**, 77–120.

KAWAMURA, Y., KATO, I., and MYOSHI, K. (1968). Functional anatomy of the lateral pterygoid muscle in the cat. *J. dent. Res.* **47**, 1142–1148.

KAY, R. F. and HIIEMAE, K. M. (1974). Jaw movement and tooth use in Recent fossil primates. *Am. J. Phys. Anthrop.* **40**, 227–256.

LIPPOLD, O. C. J. (1952). The relation between integrated action potentials in a human muscle and its isometric tension. *J. Physiol, Lond.* **117**, 492–499.

LUSCHEI, E. S. and GOODWIN, G. M. (1974). Patterns of mandibular movement and jaw muscle activity during mastication in the monkey. *J. Neurophysiol.* **37**, 954–966.

MATSUNAMI, K. and KUBOTA, K. (1972). Muscle afferents of trigeminal mesencephalic tract nucleus and mastication in chronic monkeys. *Jap. J. Physiol.* **22**, 545–555.

MATTHEWS, B. (1975). Mastication. *In* "Applied Physiology of the Mouth" (Lavelle, C. L. B., ed.), pp. 199–242. Wright and Sons, Bristol.

MCNAMARA, J. A. (1973). The independent functions of the two heads of the lateral pterygoid Muscle. *Am. J. Anat.* **138**, 197–206.

MILLS, J. R. E. (1955). Ideal dental occlusion in the Primates. *Dent. Practnr, Bristol.* **6**, 47–61.

MILLS, J. R. E. (1967). A comparison of lateral jaw movements in some mammals from wear facets on the teeth. *Archs oral Biol.* **12**, 645–661.

MØLLER, E. (1966). The chewing apparatus: an electromyograph study of the action of the muscles of mastication and its correlation to facial morphology. *Acta physiol. scand.* **69**, Suppl. 280.

MØLLER, E. (1974). Action of the muscles of mastication. *Front. oral Physiol.* **1**, 121–158.

MOYERS, R. E. (1950). An electromyographic analysis of certain muscles involved in temporomandibular movements. *Am. J. Orthod.* **36**, 481–515.

MUNRO, R. R. and BASMAIJAN, J. V. (1971). The jaw opening reflex in man. *Electromyography*, **2**, 191–206.

NORDSTROM, S. H. and YEMM, R. (1974). The relationship between jaw positions and isometric active tension produced by direct stimulation of the rat masseter muscle. *Archs oral Biol.* **19**, 353–359.

RENSBERGER, J. M. (1973). An occlusion model for mastication and dental wear in herbivorous mammals. *J. Paleont.* **47**, 515–528.

SCAPINO, R. P. (1973). Adaptive radiation of mammalian jaws. *In* "Morphology of the Maxillo–Mandibular Apparatus" (Schumacher, G. H., ed.), pp. 33–39, YEB. George Thieme, Leipzig.

SHEPHERD, R. W. (1960). A further report on mandibular movement. *Aust. dent. J.* **5** (6) 337–342.

SHERRINGTON, C. S. (1906). "The Integrative Action of the Nervous System". Scribner, New York.

STERN, S. (1974). Computer modelling of gross muscle dynamics. *J. Biomech.* **7**, 411–428.

TAYLOR, A. (1969). A technique for recording normal jaw movements in conscious cats. *Med. Biol. Eng.* **7**, 89.

TAYLOR, A. and DAVEY, M. R. (1968). Behaviour of jaw muscle stretch receptors during active and passive movements in the cat. *Nature, Lond.* **220**, 301–302.

TAYLOR, A., CODY, F. W. J. and BOSLEY, M. A. (1973). Histochemical and mechanical properties of the jaw muscles of the cat. *Expl Neurol.* **38**, 99–109.

THEXTON, A. J. (1969). Reflex control of jaw movement in the cat. Ph.D. Thesis, University of London.

THEXTON, A. J. (1973). Some aspects of neurophysiology of dental interest. 1. Theories of oral function. *J. Dent.* **2**, 49–54.

THEXTON, A. J. (1974). Oral reflexes and neural oscillators. *J. Dent.* **2**, 141–137.

THEXTON, A. J., STEINER, T. J. and WEBER, W. V. (1973). The electromyogram as a measure of reflex response in experimental animals. *J. appl. Physiol,* **35**, 762–369.

THEXTON, A. J. and HIIEMAE, K. M. (1975a). Masticatory electromyographic activity as a function of food consistency. *J. dent. Res.* **54** (special issue A,) 193.

THEXTON, A. J. and HIIEMAE, K. M. (1975b). The twitch tension characteristics of opossum jaw musculature. *Archs oral Biol.* **20**, 743–748.

TURNBULL, W. D. (1970). Mammalian Masticatory Apporatus. *Field. Geol.* **18**, (2) 153–356.

DE VREE, F. and GANS, C. (1973). Masticatory responses of pygmy goats (*Capra hircus*) to different foods. *Am Zool.* **13**, 1342–1343 (Abstract).

WEIJS, W. A. (1973a). Functional morphology of the masticatory apparatus of the albino rat. *Acta morph. neerl.-scand.* **11**, 321–340.

WEIJS, W. A. (1937b). Morphology of the muscles of mastication in the albino rat, *Rattus norvegicus* (*Berkenhout, 1769*). *Acta morph. neerl.-scand.* **11**, 321–340.

WEIJS, W. A. (1975). Mandibular movements of the albino rat during feeding. *J. Morph.* **154**, 107–124.

WEIJS, W. A. and DANTUMA, R. (1975). Electromyography and mechanics of mastication in the albino rat. *J. Morph.* **146**, 1–34.

WICTORIN, L. B., HEDEGARD, B. and LUNDBERG, M. (1971). Cineradiographic studies of bolus position during chewing. *J. Prosth. Dent.* **26**, 235–246.

ADDENDUM

Since this review was submitted M. Fillery, C. N. Kay, S. H. Perry and the author have been examining patterns of chewing and rumination in herbivores. This work is still in progress but the following points should be noted in relation to the main text.

(a) In all the herbivores so far examined (including the horse, cow, sheep, goat, camel, llama and giraffe) the lower jaw on the active side moves from lateral to medial during the power stroke. It also moves upwards as noted by Hendrichs (1965). The general direction of movement in the chewing cycle of herbivores is therefore the same as in other mammals.

(b) The camel, llama and guanaco chew alternately on right and left sides as illustrated for the camel in Fig. 4. The actual profile of the loop when plotted from cinefilm is shallower in the vertical plane and wider in the transverse so there is no abrupt transition from opening to closing strokes as shown in the figure. The lower jaw moves downwards and towards the balancing side in the opening stroke and into the upwards movement of the closing stroke from a long laterally directed near horizontal sweep through maximum gape.

(c) The duration of a chewing cycle in "initial mastication" (when the food is first chewed after ingestion) is, in some cases markedly, different from the length of a cycle in rumination. The duration of chewing cycles is also affected by the consistency of the food. This has been documented for initial mastication in a range of animals (Hendrichs, 1965).

(d) The duration of the chewing cycle is affected by the weight (size) of the animal and is related to its age. Hendrichs gives figures of chewing frequency (numbers of cycles min^{-1}) for a wide range of herbivores and shows that in animals of very similar weight the cycle frequency can be very different and, conversely, that animals with weights ranging from 50–500 kg can have very similar cycle frequencies. There is, therefore, no direct relationship, at least in herbivores, between body weight and the duration of the chewing cycle.

(e) Cinefilm taken in the present study showed that ewes ruminate significantly more slowly (either in terms of cycle frequency or cycle time) than do their lambs. Although Hendrichs (1965) was able to monitor some of the animals used in his study for long periods, and give data for cycle frequency as against increasing body weight, he offers no further comment. The relationship between increase in cycle time and increasing age is currently being investigated.

REFERENCE

HENDRICHS, H. (1965). Vergleichende Untersuchung des Wiederkauverhalten. *Biol. Zbl.* **84**, 651–751.

24. Another Look at Dental Specialization in the Extinct Sabre-toothed Marsupial, *Thylacosmilus*, compared with its Placental Counterparts

WILLIAM D. TURNBULL

Department of Geology, Field Museum of Natural History, Chicago, Illinois, U.S.A.

The striking similarities of the highly specialized canine teeth of marsupial and placental sabre-toothed forms have caught the imagination of both scientists and the public. They constitute a prime example of parallelism, well known now for 40 years, since my predecessor discovered and described *Thylacosmilus* (Riggs, 1933, 1934). Placental sabre-toothed cats have been known for a much longer time, of course (Warren, 1853; Hatcher, 1895; Matthew, 1901, 1910; Barbour and Cook, 1915; Schaub, 1925; Merriam and Stock, 1932; to name but a few). Most of these and a number of other workers have attempted to analyse the way or ways in which the sabre teeth were used (Brandes, 1900; Weber, 1904; Scott and Jepsen, 1936; Marinelli, 1938; Bohlin, 1941; Simpson, 1941; Kurtén, 1968; Miller, 1969). The parallelism is indeed remarkable as Fig. 1 shows, but it has overshadowed some very real differences which exist and which deserve attention.

I will show that *Thylacosmilus* was in many ways more highly specialized for the sabre-toothed niche than any of the machairodontines such as *Dinobastis*, *Smilodon* or even *Barbourofelis* due to the following features of its sabre teeth:

(a) they were relatively larger and more slender and they apparently eliminated the need for functional incisors;

(b) they were far more securely anchored in the skull;

(c) they were hypsodont and self-sharpening perhaps through wear and

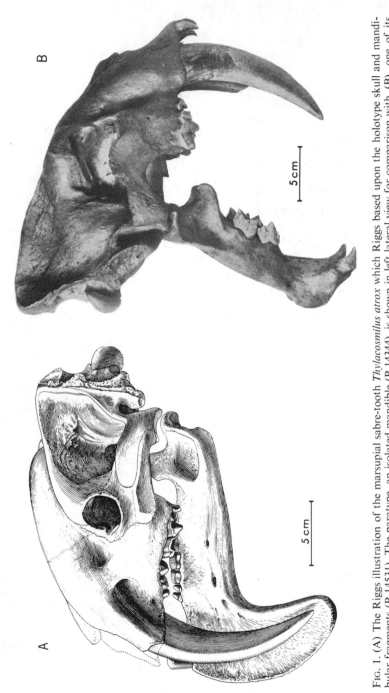

FIG. 1. (A) The Riggs illustration of the marsupial sabre-tooth *Thylacosmilus atrox* which Riggs based upon the holotype skull and mandibular fragments (P 14531). The paratype, an isolated mandible (P 14344), is shown in left lateral view for comparison with (B), one of its placental counterparts. (B) The skull and jaws of the placental machairodont, *Smilodon californicus* Bovard (taken from Stock, 1953) shown in right lateral view. The parallel development of the sabres and occipital cresting are strikingly apparent.

certainly by thegosed occlusion with the lower canine tooth which served the sharpening function (Every and Kühne, 1970);

(d) they were protected by a more highly developed symphyseal flange; and

(e) they were powered by the force of a lunge, as, of course, were the placental counterparts. They accomplished this with the additional capability of more forceful downward and backward head movements judging by the remarkably developed head and neck flexing musculature (Riggs, 1934; Turnbull, 1976). These were far more powerful movements than those which their placental counterparts were capable of.

The remainder of what I have to say will be an attempt to document these points, and I will attempt to illustrate both the differences that I wish to emphasize as well as to reiterate the similarities which have tended to obscure them.

THE SABRE TEETH AND THE REST OF THE DENTITION

In both marsupial and placental sabre-toothed forms the primary specialization beyond that of the immediate ancestral (borhyaenid or felid) condition of each is the parallel, extreme development of the upper canine teeth. Whatever the sabre-toothed forms did with their sabres, it was an act largely superimposed over the normal masticatory functions of their immediate non-sabre-toothed ancestors, to judge by the close similarity of the cheek teeth in ancestral and specialized forms in both stocks. But there were differences suggested by the extent to which the sabre teeth appear to have supplanted functions of, or needs for, other parts of the dentition. In *Thylacosmilus* this aspect appears to have been carried to a greater degree than in the placental sabre-toothed cats, for the cheek teeth are relatively reduced in size, although they still retain advanced shearing specializations. The incisors have been abandoned completely, while in the machairodontines (*Smilodon* and *Barbourofelis*), the carnassials show both size increase and a greater specialization, although some of the other cheek teeth have become reduced and the incisors have remained standard (Merriam and Stock, 1932; Schultz *et al.*, 1970).

Let us look at the marsupials in some detail. Figure 2 compares the cheek teeth of *Thylacosmilus* with those of other marsupials: the closely related borhyaenid stock (*Cladosictis* and *Borhyaena*), two other carnivorously specialized modern forms (*Thylacinus* and *Sarcophilus*) and a modern form representative of the morphotype for all marsupials, the omnivorous *Didelphis*. Note the progressive trend of marsupial carnivores away from broad upper molars with sizeable protocones (*Didelphis*) where shear surfaces are concentrated along deep interdental embrasures, towards narrower upper molars with reduced protocones and with shear concentrated in a more linear manner along parastyle–paracone, metacone–metastyle crests, to the extreme condition represented by *Thylacosmilus*. A functionally similar trend is expressed in the lower cheek teeth by a progressive dominance and lesser angulation of the trigonid crests in the same sequence of forms.

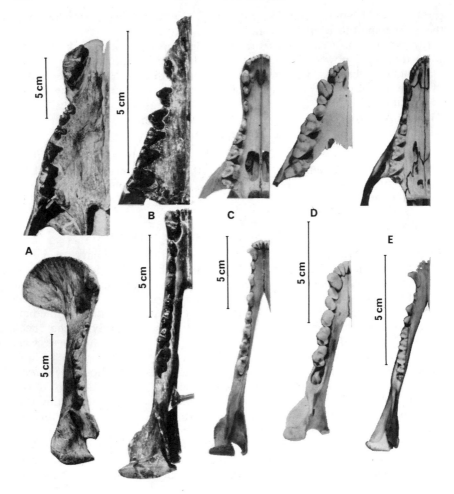

Fɪɢ. 2. Upper and lower dentitions of *Thylacosmilus atrox*, P 14531 and P 14344 (A) are compared with those of a series of other marsupials: two borhyaenids (B), *Cladosictis lustrata*, P 13255, (above) and *Borhyaena tuberata*, P 13253, representative of the ancestral stock; two modern carnivorously specialized forms, (C) *Thylacinus cynocephalus*, FMNH 81522, and (D) *Sarcophilus harrisi*, FMNH 57801; and a modern form approximately representative of the ancestral morphotype of all marsupials (E), the omnivorously specialized *Didelphis marsupialis virginianus*, FMNH 41088. Not to scale.

The relative size of the sabres is slightly greater for *Thylacosmilus* than for *Smilodon* or even *Barbourofelis*, and their cross-sections are different, indicating that they had been specializing in somewhat different directions. In all of them the section is oval and the antero-posterior diameter is greatest, but in dirk-toothed machairodontines it is either oval (but comparatively thick transversely and narrow antero-posteriorly—*Smilodon*) or it has some degree of constriction medially and laterally (*Barbourofelis*). Conversely, in scimitar-toothed machairodontines it is very thin transversely and broad antero-posteriorly and has sharp anterior and posterior edges (*Dinobastis, Homotherium*) as Kurtén (1968) has shown. In *Thylacosmilus* the section is rather triangular as Riggs noted with the medial side quite flat and the lateral side ridged so that two nearly equal lateral faces extend for the full length of the tooth (Fig. 3).

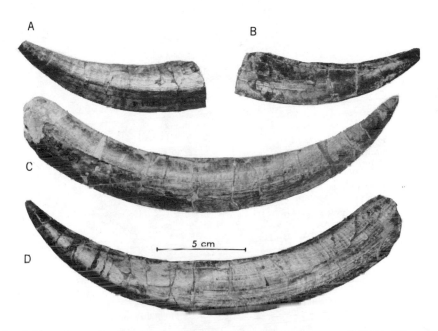

FIG. 3. The sabre teeth of the holotype specimen of *Thylacosmilus atrox*, P 14531. (A) and (B): lateral and medial sides of the broken off right canine tooth. (C) and (D): lateral and medial sides of the removed left canine. The longitudinal faceting of the lateral side of the tusk is well illustrated by (A), and the "thread" of enamel referred to by Riggs is apparent in (B), while (C) and (D) demonstrate the unrooted, hyposdont condition.

ANCHORAGE TO SKULL

Here we have perhaps one of the most telling bits of evidence for concluding that in spite of overall similarities between *Thylacosmilus* and the sabre-toothed cats, the former had reached a stage of specialization that appears to be far more advanced. Riggs (1934) has noted the condition well, and commented on it, although apparently not forcefully enough to drive the point home. In *Thylacosmilus* more than half of the tooth is contained within an alveolus which is so expanded backwards as to crowd between the orbits and to encroach upon the roof of the braincase for half the distance between the orbits and the occiput (Fig. 4). Riggs' comparison was with *Eusmilus*, but

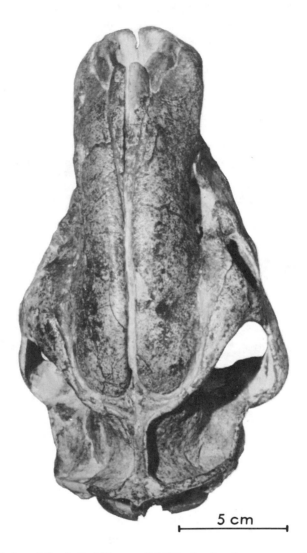

FIG. 4. Dorsal view of the skull of *T. atrox*, P 14531, showing the very expanded maxillary bones into which the canine sabres are implanted.

Smilodon or *Barbourofelis* would serve as well; in them the canine alveolus is extensive, but usually it does not extend beyond the antero-medial edge of the orbit, and it never reaches the back of it. Hence the sabres of *Thylacosmilus* must have been much more securely anchored, which I regard as a higher degree of specialization.

HYPSODONTY AND SELF-SHARPENING

In this area we not only have evidence for the most extreme specialization in *Thylacosmilus*, but that which suggests a fundamentally different sort of use of the canine tusks than other sabre tooths employed. It is surprising in a way that it hasn't been widely noted before,* and we probably have Riggs (1934, p. 17) to blame for this, for he states categorically that:

The enamel coating extends throughout the entire length of the tooth.

He makes no mention of loss anywhere through wear. In the following paragraph he continues:

The enamel coating of the upper canine teeth is very thin. In general it is restricted to the lateral surface, though in the tooth of the larger specimen a thread of enamel extends halfway down the exposed mesial surface. At no point is the enamel more than one fifth millimeter in thickness. It is minutely striated in the transverse direction, giving rise to minute denticulations, barely visible to the naked eye where the enamel is exposed at the cutting edge.

Finally in the next paragraph after describing the cross-sections of various positions along the tusk he states:

There is much less evidence of wear on the canines of this animal than upon the corresponding teeth of *Smilodon*.

This last statement is quite incorrect. Careful examination shows that he is probably correct in stating that enamel extended throughout the length of the tooth, for in an unworn or little-worn tooth it doubtless did, but certainly thegosis and probably wear breaches the enamel soon after the tooth becomes functional. Figure 3 shows the mesial aspects of the broken canine (A and B) and the unrooted, removed complete tooth (C and D). The advanced state of hypsodonty is readily seen in the complete tooth, where there is no evidence of an end to growth or a closing-off of the pulp by a constriction. Such is never the case in mature machairodonts where tusks each have distinct crown and root, and the root closes off early in life (Fig. 5).

Riggs was also correct in his statement that the enamel is nowhere very thick; he gave 0·2 mm as the maximum. I have found a maximum of about 0·25 mm on both of the lateral facets. Close to the front and back edges of the tooth on the lateral side the enamel band abruptly diminishes in thickness to a lamina no more than about 1/20th the thickness of that covering the lateral side. This very thin layer extends around the medial surface. It has

---

*It has in fact been noted twice to my knowledge. First by Dalzel who happened to visit when I was preparing my restoration of the masticatory musculature of *Thylacosmilus*, and saw the sabre teeth in my laboratory. She immediately grasped the significance of the truncated enamel banding as evidencing thegosis. Second by Kühne (1973) as an aside in his expanded report of the paper he presented originally in 1971 in Brussels, in which he dealt with serrated edges of teeth (pp. 300–301 in his paper). I did not attend the Brussels meeting, and only became aware of Kühne's comments a few weeks after the Cambridge meeting when his reprint arrived. His is a remarkably perceptive comment and I refer to it again in more detail.

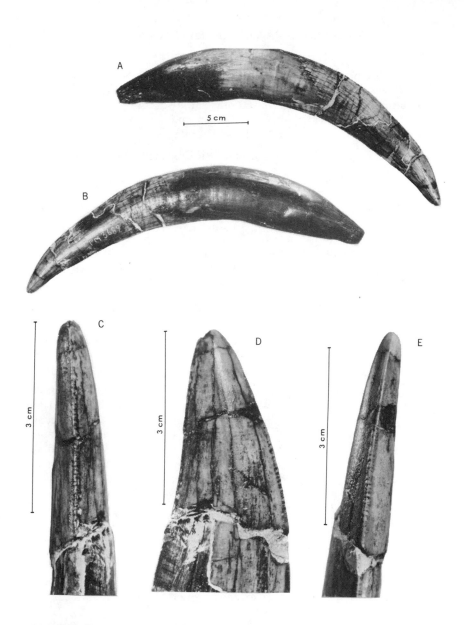

FIG. 5. (A) and (B): Medial and lateral (lingual and buccal) views of a left upper canine tooth of *Smilodon californicus*, PM 3689, with its distinct crown and nearly closed, tapered root. Note the contrast with hypsodont condition of the canine of *Thylacosmilus* in Fig. 3. (C), (D) and (E): Closer views of the enamel beading along the anterior and posterior crests seen in posterior, lateral and anterior views.

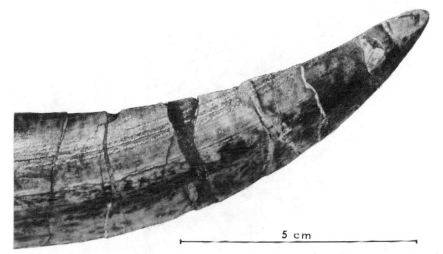

FIG. 6. Close-up view of the lateral side of the distal third of the left upper canine of *Thylacosmilus atrox* showing more detail than is visible in Fig. 3C. Note the many near-parallel longitudinal bandings in the enamel and the way that these are truncated by the thegosed posterior edge (top edge as shown).

minor thickenings (and thinnings) which cause it to be longitudinally marked by fine parallel striae (as Fig. 3B and D shows), the coarsest of which may be beaded. Such a thin veneer of enamel is easily worn away, and only an occasional one of the thickened bands (Fig. 3B; Riggs' thread of enamel) persists for very long on the worn part of the tooth.

The distal one-third of the lateral side of the left canine beautifully illustrates the phenomenon of thegosis tooth sharpening.* Here and all along the lateral

*As indicated earlier, in a paper which I received after I gave this one, Kühne (1973) has commented on and correctly and astutely deduced the true condition for *Thylacosmilus*. Following a paragraph in which he points out that sharpness and hypsodonty go hand in hand and "are only explicable under Thegosis", he further gleans from the one clue that Riggs (1934) gave (but the significance of which eluded him—see the above quotes) that here the serrations differed from those of the usual long-lived, beaded enamel thickenings. In *Thylacosmilus* the serrations are formed by, and constantly renewed through thegosed wear of a broad and minutely crenulated enamel surface. Kühne's reasoning is sound as my reporting here shows, and in this context most of his second paragraph is deserving of repetition:

> Behind the cutting edge, dentine is exposed. If anything, the description reveals a corrugation of the enamel, which, when cut longitudinally, leads to a serrated edge. RIGGS: "There is much less evidence of wear on the canines of that animal than upon the corresponding tooth of *Smilodon*." What Riggs really wanted to convey is that the nonsharpened upper canine of the sabre-tooth tiger shows abrasion, while on the same tooth of *Thylacosmilus*, which is subjected to Thegosis, abrasion marks are deleted. The lower canine of *Thylacosmilus* is described as follows: . . . "it is a strong tooth, oval in cross-section. . . . It has an antero-posterior diameter of 11 mm and a transverse diameter of 6 mm at the root. The crown . . . is worn and blunted leaving no trace of enamel". This arrangement of the upper and lower canine of *Thylacosmilus* only makes sense if the lower canine acts as a whetstone for the lingual Thegosis-facet of the upper canine since the permanently sharpened posterior cutting edge of this tooth is permanently serrated due to the transverse striation viz. corrugation of the enamel.

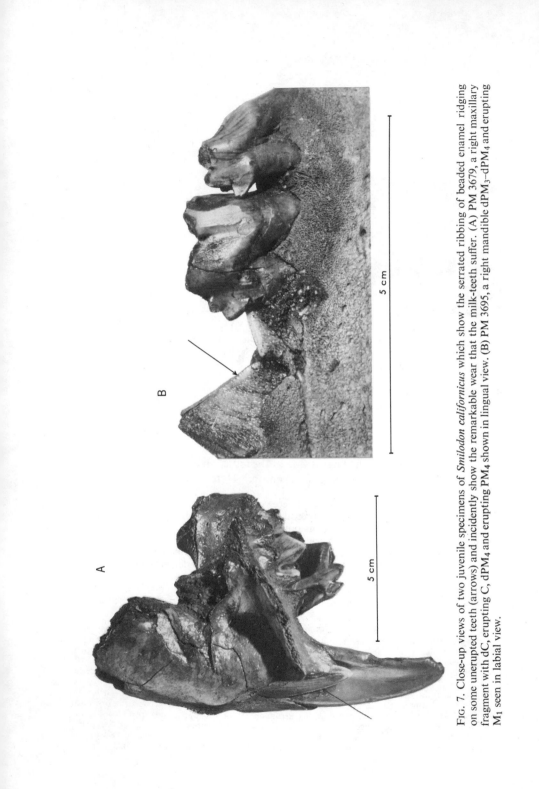

Fig. 7. Close-up views of two juvenile specimens of *Smilodon californicus* which show the serrated ribbing of beaded enamel ridging on some unerupted teeth (arrows) and incidently show the remarkable wear that the milk-teeth suffer. (A) PM 3679, a right maxillary fragment with dC, erupting C, dPM$_4$ and erupting PM$_4$ shown in lingual view. (B) PM 3695, a right mandible dPM$_3$–dPM$_4$ and erupting M$_1$ seen in labial view.

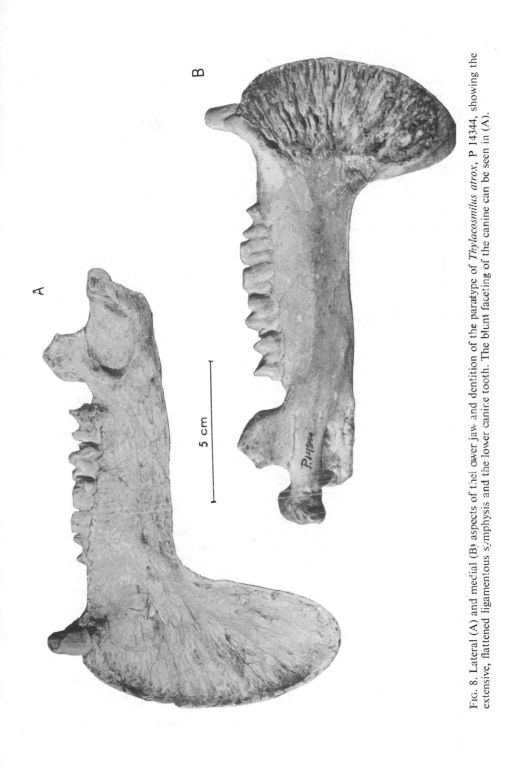

FIG. 8. Lateral (A) and medial (B) aspects of the lower jaw and dentition of the paratype of *Thylacosmilus atrox*, P 14344, showing the extensive, flattened ligamentous symphysis and the lower canine tooth. The blunt faceting of the canine can be seen in (A).

5 cm

surface the enamel bears (Fig. 3C, and in a closeup view, Fig. 6) nearly parallel, minute transverse grooves and ridges, with occasionally some anastomosing of the grooves and ridges (Riggs' minute striae which are too small to show at this scale). A much coarser longitudinal, irregular thickening and thinning which shows as fine bands or striae is also present. These striae are readily seen to be truncated at a low angle as a result of combined thegosis (tooth-sharpening) and wear phenomena, along the posterior cutting edge of the tooth (top as shown in Fig. 6) where the truncated portion cuts across nearly all of the distal third of the tooth.

In the machairodonts no such thing happens; instead the anterior and posterior edges of the blade are reinforced rather symmetrically by a fine serrated enamel band designed to persist by virtue of its hardness and thus to maintain the cutting edge. Fig. 5 (C, D and E) shows three aspects of a specimen of an adult individual of *Smilodon* in which the serrations have been somewhat reduced by wear. However, nowhere except at the very tip of the tooth has the enamel been breached. In a juvenile specimen (Fig. 7A) this serrated ribbing is clearly seen (arrow) on an unerupted canine tooth lying mesial to the worn deciduous canine. Note also in Fig. 7A the extent of wear on the deciduous cheek teeth which even extends on to the mesial root of dPM[4]. In the lower dentition (another individual, Fig. 7B) a similar serration marks the crest of the unerupted M_1 (see also Fig. 3 of Mawby, 1965) and comparable wear is also evident from facets on the milk teeth. These are examples of the usual (standard) sort of tooth crest serrations.

Evidence suggesting that the lower canine of *Thylacosmilus* served as the hone to sharpen the sabre is to be found, not on the jaw of the type which lacks the tooth, but on another specimen, the paratype, where this tooth bears two blunted facets, the posterior oblique one of which appears to have been generated by the thegosis act (Fig. 8A).

SYMPHYSEAL FLANGE

In *Thylacosmilus* the symphyseal flange is greatly expanded and meets its counterpart through a broad ligamentous band covering virtually all of its medial surface. None of the placental sabre-toothed forms have developed as broad and complete a symphyseal flange as has *Thylacosmilus* (Fig. 8A and B), and there is wide variation to the extent of development of the flange in machairodontines. *Barbourofelis* comes the closest to *Thylacosmilus* in this regard; its flange is more massively built (i.e. thicker) but less extensive. Some of the earlier (Oligocene) genera such as *Eusmilus* and *Hoplophoneus* possessed distinct, but nowhere nearly as developed a flange, and some other machairodonts, such as *Dinictis* and *Nimravus*, lacked a flange. *Smilodon* varies in this regard; the earlier forms had a slightly better developed flange than the later ones. There does not seem to be any tendency for the dirk-toothed machairodonts to have a better developed flange than the scimitar-toothed ones, or vice versa.

Apparently the sabre-toothed way of life is served about equally well whether or not the symphyseal flange is there to give a scabbard-like protection for the tusks. With maximum expansion of the flange as in *Barbourofelis* and *Thylacosmilus* it would seem that the limits must have been reached, for with a wide open gape, exaggerated as it must have been to free the upper canines, it must be close to, if not already at the point of, encroaching on the neck in a damaging way.

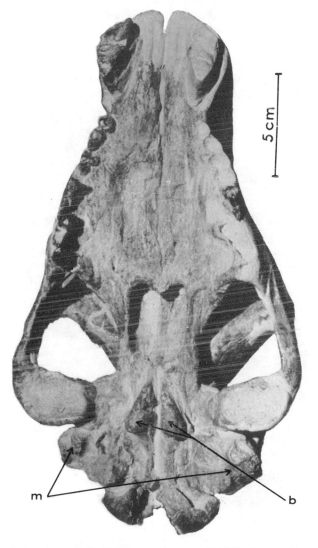

FIG. 9. Ventral view of the skull of *Thylacosmilus atrox*, P 14531, showing the very expanded basilar (basisphenoid) tubercles and mastoids (arrows b and m). These hyper-developed muscle attachment areas serve the powerful head and neck flexors.

Some (Schultz *et al.*, 1970) have argued that *Thylacosmilus* used its sabres differently from the machairodontines because it had diverging tusks and that therefore it could not have stabbed using both, for such a stroke would force the teeth apart. From my examination of the only slightly distorted skull, I have concluded that they were not diverging to any very great extent, and the symphyseal flange, which presumably bore a thick, fibrous, connective tissue pad, does not indicate much flare either. The notion comes I think from Riggs' figure of the skull which I believe exaggerates the amount of divergence and hence is somewhat erroneous.

HEAD AND NECK FLEXING

All sabre-toothed forms apparently combined a lunging attack with a stabbing thrust which was then embellished with varying degrees of slashing.

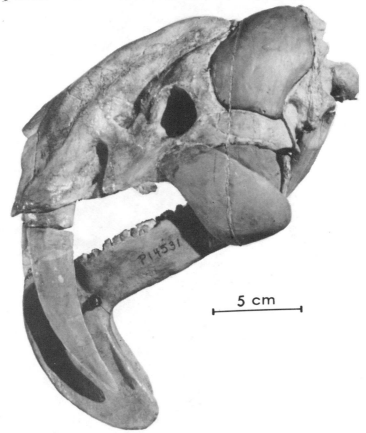

FIG. 10. A cast of the skull and jaws of *Thylacosmilus atrox* on to which the masticatory musculature has been restored. As reported elsewhere, the jaw-closing musculature appears to have been quite comparable with that of most carnivores, which indicates that it probably was not involved in the use of the sabres.

Simpson (1941) has analysed the action most thoroughly, and Kurtén (1968 and elsewhere) distinguished those that mostly stab as the dirk-toothed forms, and those that stab and then mostly slash as the scimitar-toothed forms. *Thylacosmilus* has the most extreme development of the head and neck-flexing musculature judging by the basilar (basisphenoid) tubercles (Fig. 9; see Riggs, 1934; Turnbull, 1976) and the drawn-out mastoids (Turnbull and Segall, unpublished). The former represent an attachment for an extremely hyper-developed *M. rectus capitis ventralis major*, for no other form has developed such large, prominent attachment bosses. To me this indicates a most specialized stabber–slasher. With its thin, sharpened blades alone, *Thylacosmilus* is equipped for slashing in much the same way as are the scimitar-toothed forms, and with the thegosed self-sharpening feature added to this, I am forced to conclude that it was also at least as specialized a slasher as any scimitar-toothed form, probably considerably more so.

The jaw closing musculature itself is in no way remarkable being neither of unusual proportions nor form judging from my restoration attempts (Fig. 10; Turnbull, 1976) and I see no sign of its being reduced in mass, as has been suggested for the machairodonts (because of the reduced coronoid process, I suspect). Figure 10 shows the cast of the skull and jaws onto which the masticatory muscles have been restored. Such restorations are based primarily upon individual muscle scars. Then beginning with the deepest muscle masses, the restoration is carried out to the superficial-most layers to afford an in-depth and somewhat self-correcting procedure. If I am reasonably correct in this restoration and the muscle proportions are as standard as I believe them to be, the use of the sabres in no way involved the masticatory musculature. This then reinforces the notion that head and neck flexion and the lunge itself are all that is required for use of the sabres.

CONCLUSIONS

Every point stressed suggests a greater degree of specialization for one or more of the aspects of the sabre-toothed way of life for *Thylacosmilus* than for its placental counterparts. It apparently became so proficient at both stabbing and slashing that it in effect combined the dirk- and scimitar-toothed specialities and in so doing it was able to abandon its incisors and their related functions.

Hence it is not only remarkably parallel to the placental sabre-toothed forms, but has its own unique specialized variant of that way of life.

REFERENCES

BARBOUR, E. H. and COOK, H. J. (1915). A new sabre-toothed cat from Nebraska. *Nebraska Geol. Surv.* 4(17), 235–239.

BOHLIN, B. (1941). Food habits of the machairodonts, with special regard to *Smilodon*. *Bull. Geol. Inst. Upsala*, **28**, 156–174.

BRANDES, G. (1900). Über eine Ursache des Aussterbens einiger diluvialer Säugethiere. *Corr. blatt Dt. Ges. Anthrop.* **31**, 103–107.

EVERY, R. G. and KÜHNE, W. G. (1970). Funktion und form der Säugerzahne. *Z. Säugetierk* **35**(4), 247–252.

HATCHER, J. B. (1895). Discovery in the Oligocene of South Dakota of *Eusmilus*, a genus of sabre-toothed cats new to North America. *Am. Nat.* 1091–1093.

KÜHNE, W. G. (1973). The evolution of a synorgan, nineteen stages concerning teeth and dentition from the Pelycosaur to the mammalian condition. *Bull. Group Int. Rech. Sc. Stomat.* **16**, 293–325.

KURTÉN, B. (1968). "Pleistocene Mammals of Europe", pp. i–viii and 1–317. Weidenfeld and Nicolson, London and Aldine, Chicago.

MARINELLI, W. (1938). Der Schadel von *Smilodon*, nach der Funktion des Kieferapparates analysiert. *Paleobiologica* **6**, 246–272.

MATTHEW, W. D. (1901). Fossil mammals of the Tertiary of northeastern Colorado. *Mem. Am. Mus. nat. Hist.* **1**, 355–446.

MATTHEW, W. D. (1910). The phylogeny of the Felidae. *Bull. Am. Mus. Nat. Hist.* **28**(26), 289–316.

MAWBY, J. E. (1965). Machairodonts from the Late Cenozoic of the panhandle of Texas. *J. Mammal.* **46**(4), 573–587.

MERRIAM, J. C. and STOCK, C. (1932). The Felidae of Rancho La Brea. *Carnegie Inst. Washington* **422**, i–xvi, 1–231.

MILLER, G. J. (1969). A new hypothesis to explain the method of food ingestion used by *Smilodon californicus* Bovard. TEBIWA. *J Idaho State Univ. Mus.* **12**(1), 9–19.

RIGGS, E. S. (1933). Preliminary description of a new Marsupial saber-tooth from the Pliocene of Argentina. *Geol. Ser. Field Mus. nat. Hist.* **6**: 61–66.

RIGGS, E. S. (1934). A new Marsupial saber-tooth from the Pliocene of Argentina and its relationships to other South American predaceous Marsupials. *Trans. Am. Phil. Soc. N.S.* **24**(1), 1–32.

SCHAUB, S. (1925). Über die Osteologie von *Machaerodus cultridens* Cuvier. *Ecol. Geol. Helvet.* **19**, 255–266.

SCOTT, W. B. and JEPSEN, G. L. (1936). The mammalian fauna of the White River Oligocene—Part I. Insectivora and Carnivora. *Trans. Am. Phil. Soc. N.S.* **27**(1), 1–153.

SCHULTZ, C. B., SCHULTZ, M. R. and MARTIN, L. D. (1970). A new tribe of sabertoothed cats (Barbourofelini) from the Pliocene of North America. *Bull. Univ. Nebraska State Mus.* **9**(1), 1–31.

SIMPSON, G. G. (1941). The function of saber-like canines in carnivorous mammals. *Am. Mus. Novit.* **1130**, 1–12.

STOCK, C. (1953). "Ranchro La Brea. A Record of Pliestocene Life in California" (5th edition), Sci. Ser. No. 15, pp. 1–81. Los Angeles County Museum.

TURNBULL, W. D. (1976). Restoration of masticatory musculature of *Thylacossmilus*. *In*. "Athlon: Essays on Paleontology in Honour of Loris Shano Russell" (Churcher, C. S. ed.), pp. 169–185, Figs 1–5. Royal Ontario Museum, Life Sciences, Miscel. Publ.

TURNBULL, W. D. and SEGALL, W. (unpublished). The ear region of *Thylacosmilus* and the influence of the dentition upon it.

WARREN, J. C. (1853). Remarks on *Felis smylodon*. *Proc. Boston Soc. nat. Hist.* **4**, 256–258.

WEBER, M. (1904). *Die Säugetiere*. Gustav Fischer, Jena. i–xi, 1–866.

25. Scanning Electron Microscopy of Wear and Occlusal Events in Some Small Herbivores

JOHN M. RENSBERGER

Department of Geological Sciences, University of Washington, Seattle, U.S.A.

INTRODUCTION

The characteristics of occlusal wear in mammals are probably consequences of multiple factors operating during the small interval of the chewing stroke. These factors potentially include all of the events which collectively may be termed the occlusal process. What is known about several of the components of the occlusal process which most closely bear upon the interpretation of wear is reviewed below.

Evidence concerning the occlusal processes of mastication has been derived from several sources of observations: mapping of wear facets and striation directions; cinefluorography of masticatory movements; and the relationships of specialized non-random cusp and crest patterns to occlusal motion and shapes of worn surfaces. Butler (1952a, b) showed that a complex series of wear facets were homologous throughout the Perissodactyla, and Mills (1955, 1963, 1966) extended these homologies to the primates and the insectivores. Wear facet analyses have also shown that there are two directions or phases (buccal or Phase I and lingual or Phase II) to the power stroke in insectivores and primates (Mills, 1955, 1963, 1967) and this sequence has been further documented by Butler (1973). Cinefluorographic studies of jaw movements led to the observation that two types of power strokes, vertical puncture-crushing and dorso-medioanterior movement, are used by *Didelphis* (Crompton and Hiiemae, 1970; Hiiemae and Crompton, 1971), in which food is first punctured by a series of vertical movements not involving tooth–tooth contact and subsequently subdivided by translatory movements producing facets. Gingerich (1973) observed facets indicating two types of jaw motion in the Jurassic mammal *Docodon* and concluded that one of these may involve a primitive and different sort of puncturing during contact between pointed cusps.

Opposing curvature of enamel crests in the upper and lower dentitions of many mammals suggests phyletic selection for occlusal configurations limiting the area of tooth–tooth contact and thereby maximizing occlusal pressure at contacts (Rensberger, 1973; Kay and Hiiemae, 1974). That the curvature is most often concave in the direction of relative motion also implies a function involving a control over the movement of food (Rensberger, 1973).

It has been shown that thickening of enamel on one side of a tooth and thinning or loss on another is related to the direction of relative motion and configuration of the occlusal crests in fossorial geomyoid rodents (Rensberger, in press). In these forms the loss occurs either where the enamel crest is oriented parallel to the direction of motion, and cutting efficiency is lowest, or where the crest is parallel to and rests conformably against a crest of an adjacent tooth. The loss of marginal enamel in geomyoids provides for the attainment of uniform contact and uniformly high pressures across the occlusal surface. Loss in areas of lower cutting efficiency eliminates elevations which otherwise result from differential rates of food abrasion, and thereby contributes to the maintenance of the occlusal surface at an optimum angle with respect to the direction of masticatory force. Loss of compliant enamel involves the same advantage and emphasizes the importance of enamel crest length (as opposed to crest thickness) in food subdivision, and the importance of crest thickness in controlling occlusal elevation. The absolute thickening of enamel occurs where food and detritus becomes most concentrated and is seemingly a response to intensive food and detrital abrasion. Computer simulation of a basic set of quantitative postulates relating occlusal surface topography, pressure, wear and food movement reproduce these findings and further suggest that a change in occlusal pattern documented by a phyletic series of fossils of *Entoptychus* would have been advantageous only under conditions of increased food abrasion.

Every and Kühne (1971) noted the presence of two patterns of wear in mammalian enamel. In one type, the enamel is curved in many planes, striae trend in diverse directions, and the enamel is raised in rounded relief above recessed dentine. In the other type (called facets by most workers), the enamel is curved (at most) in only one plane, the striae are strictly parallel and enamel is worn flush with the dentine. Every and Kühne concluded that the second type of surface is produced by a sharpening process (thegosis) which is not a consequence of mastication, and that the first is caused by mastication. They believed that mastication of food causes the second type of surface to be quickly obliterated so that non-masticatory strokes are necessary in order to restore the edges of the surfaces. Rensberger (1973, pp. 520–522 and Fig. 5) has interpreted these patterns as being due entirely to the normal process of mastication, in which opposing crests accomplish food subdivision as they meet along leading edges, and food is thereby normally excluded from contact with the interiors of the occlusal facets where enamel–enamel wear maintains the flat surface. Additional evidence for this interpretation is that the facets are normally striated, and that chips of enamel, being of the same hardness as the surface, would not produce striae; the striae would require ingestion of a harder grit as part of or as an accessory to food (Gingerich, 1973).

It is becoming increasingly apparent that the occlusal processes of food subdivision and dental wear differ not only among taxa, but even within the apparatus of a single individual. The extent to which the type of food, the quantity of food, occlusal pressure and detritus vary among mammalian taxa may be recorded in the fine details of the worn surface, just as the trail of a detrital particle is preserved. The present study is an attempt to recognize and interpret differences in the microscopic morphology of wear in some small Recent herbivores with differing diets and cheek teeth.

MATERIALS AND METHODS

A series of rodent taxa with differing molar morphologies and diets were chosen for examination in the belief that, with such prominent differences, some range in the characteristics of wear might be apparent. Rodents were selected because of the variety of both tooth forms and diets. The small size of most of the rodent taxa facilitated study because the teeth of most of them easily fit within the limited space of the microscope stage. With large herbivores the study would have required either subdividing teeth or making replicas. Only one specimen, that of *Hydrochoerus*, the largest living rodent, required replication.

The scanning electron microscope (SEM) employed was a Japan Electron Optical Laboratory model JSM V3. Magnifications up to 10 000 diameters were obtained using specimens coated with 100 Å of gold within a vacuum evaporator. The replicated specimen was cast using an epoxy resin poured in a Silastic rubber-moulding compound. Some circular pits $0 \cdot 1$–$0 \cdot 5$ μm in diameter, and not observed in the other specimens, were present on the replica along with a few larger bubbles. In other features the replica resembled the original specimens examined.

The following specimens were examined by SEM: *Sciurus griseus*, University of Washington (UWZ) 20638, left M^2, King County, Washington; *Aplodontia rufa*, UWZ 20502, left M^2, western Washington; *Peromyscus maniculatus*, UWZ 17539, left M^1, Grant County, Washington; *Peromyscus maniculatus*, UWZ 12585, left M^1, Kittitas County, Washington; *Microtus townsendi*, UWZ 26499, left M^1, right M^1, Seattle, Washington; *Microtus townsendi* (unnumbered), left M^2; *Lagurus curtatus* (unnumbered), left M^1, Deschutes County, Oregon; *Hydrochoerus* sp., UWZ 22397, right M_2, Woodland Park Zoo, Seattle, Washington. In addition, numerous other individuals of each taxon (except *Hydrochoerus*) were examined under light microscopy to verify constancy of such gross characteristics of wear as convex enamel, facets and major features of relief.

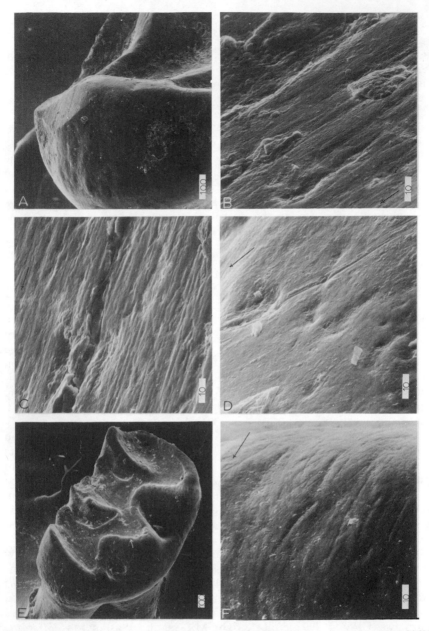

FIG. 1. SEM micrographs of worn occlusal enamel. (A) *Sciurus griseus*, UWZ 20638, postero-lingual view of protocone, left M². (B) Same, protoconid II facet (i.e. facet caused by contact with protoconid during Phase II of the power stroke) on protocone. (C) Same, metaconid I facet on protocone. (D) Same, hypoconid "facet" of metaloph between areas of Phase I and Phase II facets. (E) *Peromyscus maniculatus*, UWZ 17539, antero-lingual, occlusal view of left M¹; anterior towards lower left, lingual towards lower right. White arrow points to area of (F). (F) Same, anterior enamel of protocone (area of arrow). Scale lengths (long dimensions of white rectangles): A—100 μm; B, C and D—10 μm; E—100 μm; F—10 μm. Black arrows denote motions of opposing surfaces.

Morphology of Worn Molar Enamel

The descriptions in this section are organized by taxon. In the following section the different features of wear and their possible causes are discussed in sequence. Finally, under "Systems of Wear" the functional interrelationships of the features are interpreted as contributions to the overall wear in each taxon.

Sciurus. Figure 1(A–D) of a left M^2 is viewed in each case from a position postero–lingual to the protocone. The four illuminated crests extending diagonally towards the upper right from the protocone in Fig. 1A are, from left to right, the anterior cingulum, the protoloph (leading to the paracone), the metaloph (leading to the metacone) and the posterior cingulum. Two flat surfaces of wear, or facets, are visible on the left and lingual sides of the most elevated part of the protocone. The anterior and more horizontal of these facets (almost parallel to the viewer in Fig. 1A) was produced by contact with the protoconid during Phase II* of the power stroke. This facet is well developed in rodents, in which a prominent anterior cingulum occludes with a portion of the protoconid surface, but is apparently not present in most other mammalian genera. Butler (1973, his Fig. 12) illustrated it for both *Paramys* and *Phalanger*, but did not describe it. It is important in the rodents because, together with the other recipient of the protoconid, the posterior cingulum of the adjacent anterior tooth, it provides a major component of the Phase II contacts. The more steeply inclined of the two facets was produced by contact with the metaconid during Phase I. This is homologous to the facet in primates designated 3 by Butler (1973, his Figs 4, 7 and 10) and 5 by Kay and Hiiemae (1974, their Figs 4, 5 and 6).

The metaconid I facet is dominated by striae, as seen under high magnification (Fig. 1C). The widths of the striae range from about 10 μm down to 1 μm or less. Many of the small grooves extend for more than 20 μm and some are recognizable over 50 μm. The tops of the ridges separating the grooves are usually smooth, whereas the lower elevations appear more irregular at this magnification, especially the bottoms of the large, shallow pits. Some of the pits bear a few fine striae. Almost all of the grooves are parallel to one another, and, from consideration of the occlusal relationships, parallel to the direction of the power stroke. The surface is a true facet, for it is nearly flat in the direction of occlusal motion although slightly concave in the transverse direction.

The protoconid II facet (Fig. 1B) is also dominated by striae, but there

---

*Phase II is equivalent to the lingual phase of Mills, whose earlier studies of wear facets [1955, 1963, 1967] showed the existence of two directions of jaw motion, which he termed buccal and lingual; the corresponding names Phase I and II for the initial and final directions of motion (p. 228 in Kay and Hiiemae, 1974) seem less confusing in the present context because Phase I facets occur on both buccal and lingual cusps, and also because the numerals I and II become a convenient shorthand in the labelling of facets.

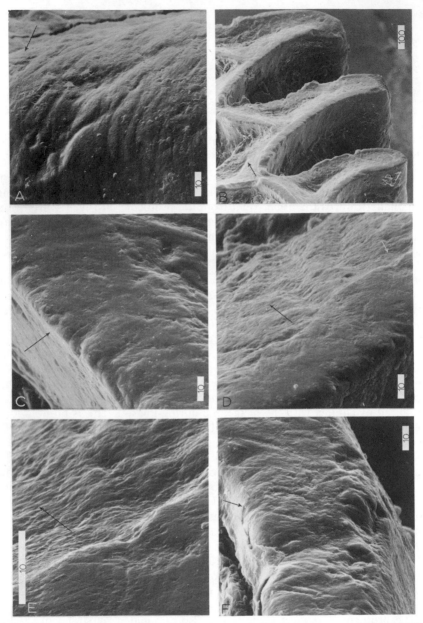

FIG. 2. SEM micrographs of worn occlusal enamel. (A) *Peromyscus maniculatus*, UWZ 12585, left M[1], anterior enamel of protocone (see Fig. 1E). (B) *Lagurus curtatus*, left M[1], posterior occlusal view; anterior towards top. (C) Same, but anterior towards right; posterior enamel of central loph of (B); enamel crest is on upstroke side of dentinal platform (upper right). (D) A different location on crest of (C); anterior towards upper left; lighter area (upper left half of micrograph) is dentine. (E) An enlargement of area of white arrow in (D). (F) *Microtus townsendi*, labial occlusal view, left M[2], anterior enamel; anterior towards right. Scales: A—10 μm; B—100 μm; C, D, E and F—10 μm. Black arrows denote motions of opposing surfaces.

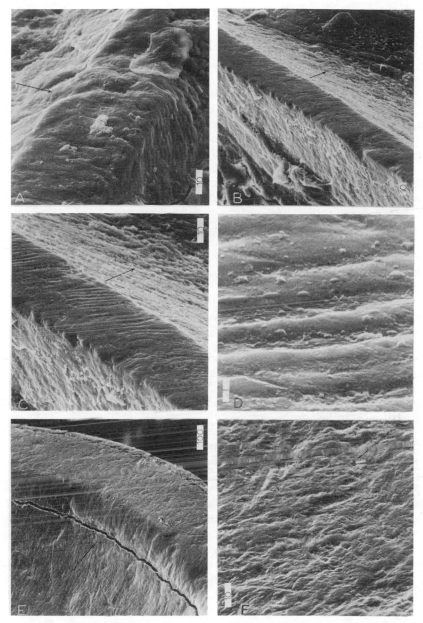

FIG. 3. SEM micrographs of worn occlusal enamel. (A) *Lagurus curtatus*, antero-labial occlusal view, left M¹, anterior enamel; anterior towards right. (B) *Microtus townsendi*, UWZ 26499, postero-labial occlusal view, left M¹, enamel on upstroke side of dentinal platform (upper right). (C) Enlarged view of crest in (B). (D) Enlarged view of enamel furrows on top of the flat crest in (C). (E) *Aplodontia rufa*, UWZ 20502, antero-lingual occlusal view, left M², lingual enamel crest in region of protocone; anterior towards right; dentine in lower left, below crack; cementum is thin lamina in upper right. (F) Same, enlarged view of flat enamel surface. Scales: A, B and C—10 μm; D—1 μm; E—100 μm; F—10 μm. Black arrows depict motions of opposing surfaces.

are fewer medium-sized (2–3 μm) grooves. The relatively smooth areas are marked by very fine striae of 0·5 μm diameter or less. Wide, shallow pits are present, and the bottoms of these are irregularly rough.

The hypoconid facet in the central region of the metaloph (Fig. 1D) is smooth compared to the other facets. A moderate number of pits are present, but these frequently lack elongate axes in the direction of relative motion, which is approximately aligned with the one prominent groove. The margins and bottoms of the pits are smoother than those of the other facets, although these areas have more texture than the elevated regions. Some variation in the fineness of the polish of the higher regions is evident; most of it bears a visible texture, but in a few areas there is no perceptible fine relief, even at $\times$ 10 000 magnification. The surface as a whole is not as flat as the other two facets.

The facets, metaconid I and protoconid II, among those of the other taxa examined in this study, are most suggestive of the flat, striated surface of a Phase I facet in *Galago*, a primate illustrated by Kay and Hiiemae (1974, their Fig. 17B). These facets differ, however, in the greater degree of parallelism of the striae, the absence of a set of diagonal grooves produced by balancing-side occlusion and less irregularity of the crests which separate the striae.

Peromyscus. The area illustrated (Figs 1F and 2A) in this cricetine is the enamel on the posterior side of the antero-lingual inflexion. This position lies on the antero-lingual side of the protocone (Fig. 1E), receives wear during the late phase of the masticatory stroke and thus is analogous to the protoconid II facet in *Sciurus*.

This, as well as other surfaces in *Peromyscus*, differ from those of *Sciurus* in the absence of facets, except in young individuals. Instead, the enamel edges, exposed as a result of loss of the enamel capping the cusps, are prominently convex (Figs 1F and 2A). The surfaces are covered by striae of widths ranging from 3 or 4 μm down to 0·5 μm or smaller (Figs 1F and 2A). The grooves in the individual of Fig. 1F are less consistently parallel than are those in *Sciurus*, indicating occlusal motion in slightly different directions, but the variation in direction is not as great as in *Galago*. In the other individual of *Peromyscus* (Fig. 2A) the directions of the striae are more consistent than in that of Fig. 1F. A conspicuous difference between the wear surfaces of *Peromyscus* and the striated facets of *Sciurus* and *Galago* is the dominantly smooth character of the entire surface—even in the bottoms of the grooves (Figs 1F and 2A) and within chipped areas (Fig. 2A).

Microtus and Lagurus. The nature of enamel wear in these taxa varies with position, depending upon whether it is on the "upstroke" or the "downstroke" side of the dentinal platform (i.e. in front of or behind the dentine, with respect to direction of relative motion of the opposing lower dentition). Furthermore, wear on the downstroke enamel depends upon whether or not it is near the transverse centre of an enamel crest.

Upstroke enamel crests (Figs 2C, D, E and 3B, C) are characterized by deep, wedge-shaped fissures along the leading edge and wide shallow cavities near the trailing (downstroke) edge. The depths as well as the prominences of the leading fissures are polished, whereas the depths of pits elsewhere are frequently rough, unlike those in *Peromyscus*. Most of the surface of the crest is dominated by polish. Only minor irregularities, consisting of pits or poorly defined striae, neither of which are abundant, are present. The surface is dominantly smooth, more so than the surfaces of any of the other taxa investigated in this study. Unlike those in *Peromyscus*, these surfaces are essentially flat, and those in different regions of the tooth lie in the same plane.

In both *Microtus* and *Lagurus* the crests on the downstroke side of the dentinal platform are similar to those on the upstroke side at positions near the labial or lingual margins of the teeth. But near the transverse centres of the crests, especially at the centres of the anterior bends (Fig. 2B), the surfaces are coarsely gouged and chipped, striae of widths 2–3 μm are common, wedge-shaped fissures at the leading edge may extend entirely across the enamel, and the cavities of the trailing edge are often larger and more steeply inclined than those away from the centres of the crests (Figs 2B and 3A).

An unexpected pattern of grooves is present on the occlusal enamel surface in one of the three arvicolines examined (Fig 3B, C, D). Unlike the random sizes and diameters of the striae observed in other taxa, these grooves are not only parallel but also of approximately uniform diameter and spacing, like a fabric. They appear to occur on the downstroke three-fifths of the enamel, where the surface is slightly depressed. The intervening and higher areas are smoothly polished, but bear in a few places a faint trace of the fabric-like grooves (Fig. 3C). The fabric pattern is present, though less prominent, in the shallow pits of the trailing edge. The surfaces of the ridges separating the grooves are polished (Fig. 3D) and where these are faintly detectable on slight elevations (Fig. 3C), they appear to be polished vestiges of a pattern which was more prominent at one time. They are not present on the vertical side of the enamel in this specimen. One large depressed area (Fig. 3C, near right end of enamel) lacks them. The enamel is otherwise worn in a fashion like that of the other arvicolines, with polished wedge-shaped fissures on the leading edge, broader, shallower pits near the trailing edge and few striae marking the polished surfaces. *Lagurus* (Fig. 3A) bears possibly related structures on the vertical face of the enamel.

Aplodontia. Much of the contacting facet on the antero-lingual enamel of M^2 is flat (Fig. 3E) but irregularly pitted (Fig. 3F). This is the region of the protocone although there would be, of course, no vestige of a cusp in such a hypsodont tooth, except in an unworn state. The direction of relative motion (lower left to upper right in the micrographs) is not evident in Fig. 3F, for the pattern of pits is almost lacking in directional orientation. There are a few grooves running parallel to the direction of the power stroke, and some in oblique directions. However, many of the ridges, although short and quite

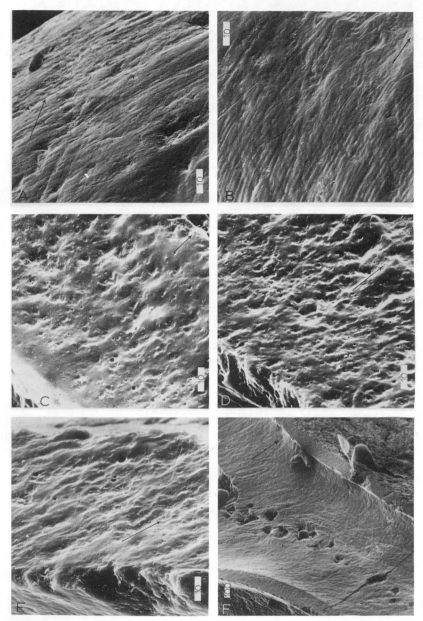

FIG. 4. SEM micrographs of worn occlusal enamel. (A) *Aplodontia rufa*, UWZ 20502, labial occlusal view, left M², lingual enamel posterior to area of Fig. 3 (E and F); anterior towards right. (B) Same specimen; enamel of Fig. 3E, between dentine and edge of occlusal facet; upper right corner joins lower left corner of Fig. 3F. (C) Cast of *Hydrochoerus* sp., UWZ 22397, antero-lingual view, right M₂, enamel crest of downstroke side of dentinal platform; same crest as in upper right of Fig. 4F. (D) Same specimen; enamel crest on upstroke side of dentinal platform (lower left of Fig. 4F). (E) As (D), but different location along crest.

irregular in elevation, show a slight elongation in the direction of the power stroke. The leading edge of the enamel and the adjacent dentine (below the prominent crack) exhibit many striae in the vertical plane of the power stroke (Fig. 3E) and a few oblique to that plane. The leading edge bears a few wedge-shaped fissures, and is more heavily rounded than in the arvicolines. The trailing edge lacks shallow pits and is covered lingually by a relatively thin lamina of cementum.

The convex surface of the enamel along the leading edge bears in places a set of fabric-like furrows (Fig. 4B) in the vertical plane of the power stroke and similar to those observed in *Microtus*. The pattern fades away near the edge of the occlusal facet.

The occlusal surface near the antero-posterior centre of the lingual enamel is more elevated than other parts in this region, and is dominated by grooves of varying diameters (Fig. 4A). This surface most closely resembles those of *Sciurus* among the taxa examined. The direction of the grooves is not parallel to those of the more anterior part of the lingual enamel in *Aplodontia* (described above), nor the more posterior, and are probably not produced by the power stroke. The apex of the metastylid of the lower molar could briefly contact this surface, but this would produce grooves parallel to the direction of the power stroke. Manipulation of the skull and mandible indicates that these grooves may be produced by contact of this more elevated region with the lower tooth during extension or retraction of the mandible during gnawing motions using the incisors.

Hydrochoerus. The edge of the enamel crest is sharply angular in this taxon, and like that of the arvicolines, frequently bears wedge-shaped fissures (Fig. 4E). The surfaces of these fissures are rough when occurring on enamel upstroke of the dentinal platform. The edge of the enamel on the downstroke side of the dentine is heavily polished (Fig. 4C) but is not as convex as the edge of the downstroke enamel in *Aplodontia*. The downstroke edge of the enamel on either side of the dentinal platform exhibits shallow pits, as in the arvicolines. The occlusal facet of the enamel crest is flat over the entire tooth, but is quite heavily pitted and locally may contain irregular striae up to 10 μm in diameter. The striae are short and usually pitted themselves. The smaller, circular pits are almost certainly artefacts of the moulding process; they are only present in this taxon, and this was the only instance in which the original specimen had to be replicated. The bottoms of many of the irregular pits are rough, whereas the margins and intervening surfaces are polished.

(F) Same specimen, showing dentinal platform, upstroke enamel (lower left) downstroke enamel (upper right) and cementum (extreme upper right); several prominent bubbles are artefacts of casting process. Scales: A, B, C, D and E—10 μm; F—100 μm. Black arrows depict motions of opposing surfaces, except in (B), where an occlusal surface is not seen (arrow there is aligned with direction of movement of food near the surface).

Features of Wear

Below is a classification of distinctive surface characteristics, most of which were observed in more than one individual.

Facets (*Contact Wear*). The name facet is here applied to:

(a) flat or nearly flat surfaces of wear, or
(b) rotational surfaces which are flat in only one direction.

Both flat and rotational facets exhibit distinct angular margins where they are bounded either by other facets in different planes, or by non-planar surfaces. The flatness of facets indicates repeated contact or near contact between opposing tooth surfaces during occlusion (p. 520 in Rensberger, 1973). Where the contact is maintained for a considerable interval of the power stroke, it is usually of the second type because a change in direction of motion is involved.

Convex Wear. Convex enamel surfaces are usually distinguishable from rotational facets by the absence of a distinct angular boundary. They are produced by wear from food masses between surfaces which do not normally contact one another. *Peromyscus* is the only taxon examined with dominantly convex enamel. In *Aplodontia* only the leading edge of the lingual enamel is convex. In the arvicolines convex enamel is not common, but may occur.

The lack of contact may be due to occlusal pressures lower than the force of resistance of the compressed food or simultaneous contact occurring elsewhere.

Polish. The surface characteristic in which there is little observable texture under magnifications as great at 10 000 diameters is called polish because it seems to result from abrasion by very fine or soft food material, and/or direct contact between enamel. It apparently is not produced by solution, for the internal structure of the enamel is not revealed, and because in many instances it does not extend into shallow recesses but is always present where enamel or food contact would normally occur. The most conspicuous instance in which polish does extend into pits and striae is explainable by other mechanisms (see *Peromyscus* in the section 'Systems of Wear').

Striations. Striated surfaces are defined as those containing randomly spaced grooves of varying diameter and length. These structures most likely result from small inorganic particles (e.g. detrital rock in the soil), which have been drawn across the surface of the enamel (or dentine) under pressure sufficient to cause gouging. For grooves to be produced, the particles must be harder than the enamel (or dentinal) surface, and the pressure not so great as to caused them to be crushed. Occurrences of very short striae may be the result of crushing of the particle.

Striae are most often arranged in parallel sets, although the degree of parallelism varies. More than one set may be superimposed on a single surface, and where otherwise parallel there are frequently a few divergent grooves. The direction of each stria on enamel must normally reflect a direction of jaw motion, and strict parallelism of sets implies unidirectional motion.

Furrows. This term is perhaps descriptive of the parallel fabric-like grooves in which the diameters and spacing are uniform. These structures clearly differ in their regularity of size and spacing from those called striae. They do, however, resemble striae in their high degree of parallelism, straightness, and alignment with the direction of occlusal motion.

They may represent the alternating rod and interprismatic substance of enamel, which tend to be oriented perpendicular to the enamel–dentine surface (p. 47 in Sicher and Bhasker, 1972). The enamel structure is not visible on other surfaces worn by the polishing and striating mechanisms discussed above, but it is revealed when acid is applied to the surface. Figure 5(A and B) shows the etched surface of upstroke enamel on the right M^1 of the same individual of *Microtus* which bears the furrows shown in Fig. 3(B, C and D). The rods are of approximately the same average spacing as the occlusal furrows. However, the diameter of an individual rod is not uniform, and the stereoscopic views show that each rises in its course toward the dentine (upper right) from a sulcus at the centre of the enamel, and changes direction from that near the external surface (lower left). The direction of the rods on the dentine side alternates in vertical sets at 60–80° angles to one another. Near the dentine interface the rods dip to a lower elevation. Neither the central sulcus, the convexity nor the lack of parallelism are matched by the furrow system of Fig. 3(B, C and D). It does not therefore seem likely that the furrowed pattern represents simply chemically etched enamel structure. The observed differences do not preclude the possibility that the flatness and greater regularity of the occlusal furrows resulted from simultaneous chemical and physical abrasion in which physical abrasion removed weakened interprismatic material, but only in the direction of occlusal motion.

Figure 5C shows the results of etching the lingual enamel on the left M^1 of the same individual of *Aplodontia* which displayed the furrow pattern of Fig. 4B. This enamel, although it corroded as rapidly as that of *Microtus*, did not yield as clear an isolation of the rods as did the arvicoline enamel, and the morphology of the rod arrangement is different. The rods and interprismatic substance in *Aplodontia* seem to be more equally resistant to acid than those in *Microtus*. However, as in *Microtus*, the rods seem to be less constant in their direction and parallelism than the furrows on the worn surface, and the two patterns are not greatly similar. Here also it is possible that a combination of physically and chemically abrasive activities caused the differences.

Alternatively, the furrows might have been caused by mastication of plant tissue containing a supportive skeleton of fine siliceous fibres of approximately 3 μm in diameter. The specimens displaying the furrow pattern are

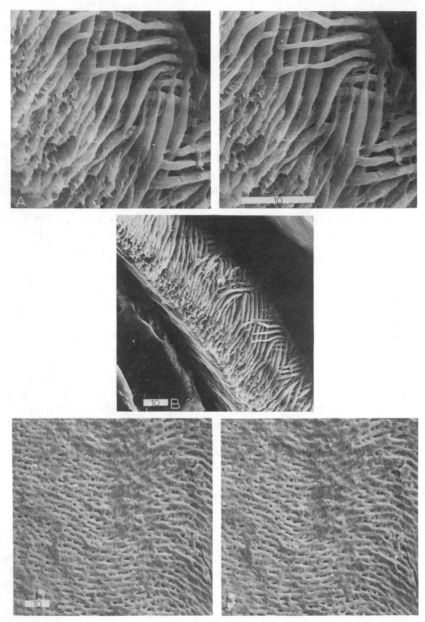

FIG. 5. SEM micrographs of etched enamel, showing rod morphologies. (A) *Microtus townsendi*, UWZ 26499, postero-lingual view, right M^1, upstroke enamel, stereo pair; dentinal platform off frame toward upper right. (B) Same, lower magnification. (C) *Aplodontia rufa*, UWZ 20502, antero-labial view, left M^1, lingual enamel, stereo pair. Scales: A, B and C—10 μm.

probably from the same geographic province and therefore may have had access to the same type of vegetation.

Several trapped individuals of the same species of *Microtus* held short segments of grass between the cheek teeth with the longitudinal axis and fibres oriented antero-posteriorly. In this position, uniformly spaced fibres sufficiently hard and of the proper size might produce a uniform pattern of furrows like those observed. However, acceptability of this explanation depends upon the yet undemonstrated existence of such siliceous spicules, and the hypothesis combining attributes of physical and chemical abrasion revealing selected rod outlines seems more likely.

Whatever the cause, the existence of the furrow pattern indicates that some individuals of the hypsodont taxa occasionally held an unusually abrasive substance in contact with the cheek teeth. The substance may have been a food with a strongly corrosive chemical action, a digestive fluid originating in the stomach, or perhaps food containing a siliceous skeletal fabric.

Fissures. Before they were polished, these structures were probably deep pits with vertical sides converging towards the centre of the crest. They are related to the direction of occlusal motion because they occur only on the upstroke side of the enamel crest, yet they are present on both the external as well as the dentinal edges. Their existence is evidently not dependent upon the precise structure of the enamel rod fabric, because the latter differs on the external and dentinal margins of the enamel (Fig. 5A and B). They are, on the other hand, dependent upon the existence of a relatively sharp edge. Where the enamel edge is well rounded, fissures are scarce. These structures therefore appear to be caused by stress concentrated on restricted areas of relatively weaker edges. Exceptionally resistant fibres and hard detrital particles caught between opposing edges of enamel would tend to provide high concentrations of stress and are probably necessary for the production of fissures.

Flaked Pits. The trailing edges of enamel usually bear relatively wide, shallow depressions as a result of loss of a flake-shaped chip. These structures are sometimes a short distance upstroke from the trailing edge (Fig. 2C, D and E), but are normally on the edge itself. The difference in shape compared to that of fissures is attributable to the different direction of stress with respect to the enamel corner. Where a trailing edge is supported by cementum (Fig. 3E) the enamel lacks flaked pits.

Pebbly Texture. This type of surface consists of relatively small, densely arranged pits of variable proportions. It is characteristic only of *Aplodontia* and *Hydrochoerus* among the forms examined, and probably results from some aspect of the diet or masticatory process peculiar to these forms. The enamel crests of *Aplodontia* and *Hydrochoerus* contain other types of wear in specific areas, so the pebbly texture is probably not the result of a different type of enamel structure, although some structural differences exist (Fig. 5B and C). The surfaces bearing the pebbly texture are facets, indicating that they contact or nearly contact the opposing enamel as they wear. If it were not for the association with facets, it might be inferred that this pattern was produced by a crushing motion normal to the surface, because of the poor development of striae. However, there is some directional elongation of the pits, more conspicuous in Fig. 4E of *Hydrochoerus* than in the other illustrations, and this, together with the disposition of direction-related fissures and flaked pits leaves no doubt about the prevalence of translatory motion.

If detritus or resistant particles are responsible, these did not remain intact after initial contact, otherwise striae would be present in place of pits. Assuming that hard particles caused the pits therefore leads to the implication that either the occlusal pressures were especially high, or the particles were not as hard as the presumed inorganic detrital grains producing striae elsewhere in these taxa and in the other forms. High occlusal pressures may be implied for *Hydrochoerus* by the arrangement of its masseter, which produces a class II lever system (p. 281 in Turnbull, 1970).

On the other hand, in the other hypsodont taxa examined, most of the food and detrital fragments were apparently excluded from compression between the interiors of the crests due to complete shearing between the leading edges. The lack of many detrital grooves on the pebbly-textured facets of *Aplodontia* and *Hydrochoerus* may be the result of similar action. If so, the pits may not be due to detritus but to the enamel facets being pressed against one another under pressure high enough to cause the surfaces to flake. Identical hardness of the opposing surfaces perhaps may, under sufficient pressure, cause frictional breakage of an irregular pattern. Prominences would produce local concentrations of stress and pitting on the opposing surface but, because they are no more resistant than the opposing surface, would not be capable of producing an elongate groove.

Systems of Wear

Seldom were any of the distinctive features of worn surfaces found to exist alone in either a taxon, a tooth or even a limited area of a tooth. Apparently the processes responsible for these features normally act in combinations as components in systems of wear. Total wear amounts to the sum of the wear produced by each of the components. The rate of wear of the system is the sum of the rates of the component processes. However, the characteristics of a given occlusal surface depend upon the ratios of the rates of wear of the component processes to one another. Evidence from the SEM enlargements provides information about only the last of these attributes, the ratio or relative contributions of the several component processes. The pattern in each of the genera examined seems to differ from that of the others in the relative contributions of the wear components, suggesting that each has a distinctive system if these specimens are representative.

Sciurus. The metaconid Phase I facet (Fig. 2C) is more completely dominated by detrital striations than any surface observed in the other taxa, excepting certain small areas in the microtines. As noted above, this does not indicate that detrital wear was more intense than in any other taxon, but that it was more intense than other sources of wear on this surface. The protoconid II facet (Fig. 2B) shows subequal contributions from the mechanisms of striation and polish, and the central region of the metaloph is dominated by polish.

The positional differences in the patterns of wear in this genus may be explained as consequences of differences in the intimacy of contact and availability of food. The Phase I contact would not receive as much food as

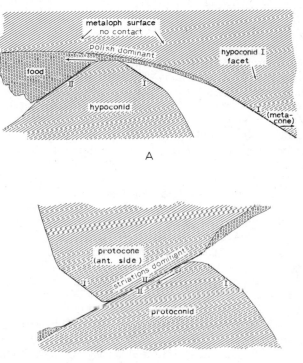

Fig. 6. Transverse sections through portions of M_1^2 in *Sciurus*, showing relationships of wear patterns to facet attitudes. Heavy lines mark facets; Roman numeral indicates phase when facet contacts opposing surface. (A) Occlusion stage intermediate between occurrence of Phase I and Phase II contacts. (B) Occlusion stage during occurrence of Phase II contacts.

the others because it is contacted by the opposing surface only at the commencement of the stroke, before much food can accumulate ahead of the metaconid. In contrast, both of the other surfaces receive the opposing cusps after the latter have moved some distance across the occlusal surface, pushing ahead an accumulating mass of food (Fig. 6A and B). The surface of the metaloph traversed by the hypoconid is not really a facet, because it is not entirely flat and the borders are indistinct. The hypoconid therefore doesn't normally attain close contact with it, and the dominating polish must result from food abrasion. The differences in wear on these three areas are therefore caused by differences in the relative amounts of food reaching each of the surfaces, as determined by the tooth morphology. The dominance of small striations is a two-fold consequence of the intimate contact of the surfaces:

(a) relatively small quantities of food being allowed between the contacts, and
(b) the likelihood that the occasional hard particle will be pressed into contact.

The relative rates of wear of the different surfaces are determinable only from indications of the thicknesses of tooth materials which have been removed. In *Sciurus* the Phase II facets of the four major cusps are the most heavily worn. The Phase I facets on the same cusps are less worn, but nevertheless significantly more so than other areas of the tooth. The "subfacets" of the protoloph and metaloph rank third, the basins or valleys between the cusps and lophs rank fourth, and the vertical labial and lingual surfaces of the teeth show no discernible wear in the earlier life of the individual. The dominant mode of wear in *Sciurus*, i.e. that dominating the surfaces with the highest rates, is detrital.

Peromyscus. The rounded occlusal surfaces of the enamel loops and the prevalence of polish in this taxon are products of food abrasion. However, the moderate frequency of striae indicates that detrital abrasion is also significant. Food abrasion is judged to be the dominant factor because the striae are typically polished; a relatively high rate of detrital abrasion would have significant numbers of unpolished striae and gouges, such as occur on the metaconid I and protoconid II facets in *Sciurus*. An alternative explanation is that the striae are highly polished because they occurred simultaneously during a short interval when the diet was different, followed by an interval of mastication of food lacking hard particles just prior to death. However, such an interpretation, if correct, does not alter the conclusion that the dominating factor of wear to the enamel was food abrasion, for the striae were undoubtedly inscribed upon a smoothly convex surface which was probably polished at the time. Furthermore, it isn't likely that all the striae were produced at the same time, because some, especially the fine ones of Fig. 1F, are more sharply edged than others.

Because the surfaces of Figs 1F and 2A are located on the side of the protocone, which in each case has been worn to its base, they are among the positions which must have experienced the higher rates of wear (the others are the positions of the other major cusps). The dominant process of wear in the specimens of *Peromyscus* was therefore apparently food polish, together with a major contribution from detrital abrasion.

The difference in wear exhibited by *Sciurus* and *Peromyscus* is less likely to be a result of difference in the diet, than of difference in the masticatory habits or mechanism. The diets are apparently quite similar. Nixon *et al.*

(1968) reported that the diet of the Eastern grey squirrel consisted mainly of nuts and seeds, but that arthropods comprised 15 % (by volume) and green vegetation (stems, roots and leaves, including 2 % grass leaves) 11 %. Animal matter (chiefly insects) amounted to as much as 87 % for short periods. In *Peromyscus maniculatus* (Flake, 1973) seeds and nuts (39 %) and arthropods (39 %) were eaten in equal abundance, and most of the remainder of the food consisted of green vegetation (13 %). These differences in the diet do not in themselves seem to account for the difference in wear.

The typical occlusal surface, on the other hand, is quite different in the two forms. That in *Peromyscus* is based upon a series of narrow enamel loops moving across opposing loops. The occlusal apparatus in *Sciurus* retains cusps through much of the individual's life. The cusps penetrate through the food and make contact with opposing cusps. For an individual of *Peromyscus* to attain the enamel loop condition it must undergo a relatively greater amount of wear than is typically evident in *Sciurus*. Because this more intensive wear is apparently not associated with a difference in texture of the food, it must have resulted from either a greater amount of chewing activity or a development of higher occlusal pressures (or both). Mastication in *Peromyscus* may involve greater chewing activity, during which, in the young individual, cusp–cusp contact and consequently relatively high pressures are attained. As the cusps become lowered, the areas of contact enlarge, reducing pressure until, in the mature stage, the force/area ratio is too low to cause constant enamel–enamel contact to be maintained. The insect cuticle may then be sufficiently tough to inhibit direct enamel contact after initial crushing. A fine subdivision of the chitinous material is probably unnecessary for digestion of the most nutritive portions of the insect.

Microtus and Lagurus. These taxa utilize an occlusal morphology which is highly modified from the primitive rodent occlusal configuration. As in *Peromyscus*, the cusps are rapidly worn away to produce a surface consisting of enamel loops and dentinal platforms. However, the inflexions of enamel are deeper, making the total length of enamel crest greater and increasing the rate of food subdivision (p. 520 in Rensberger, 1973). The enamel is thinner, which will produce a higher pressure/crest length ratio, the direction of occlusal motion is more nearly anterior and the occlusal surface is much flatter than that in *Peromyscus*.

The flatter overall occlusal surface and the faceted crests with relatively sharp edges imply intimate contact between the opposing surfaces. This explains the general lack of detrital abrasion on the crests of the upstroke sides of the dentinal platforms, yet its presence on the centres of the down-stroke crests. With opposing upstroke crests passing snugly, food is cleanly sheared at the leading edges, so that segments are pushed ahead of the two leading faces, but little passes between the contacting surfaces; detrital particles are similarly excluded and carried with the food. But the dentinal platforms, being partially recessed by differential wear, act as temporary reservoirs for food, which piles up in front of the downstroke crests. When enough food is compressed in front of a crest, some of it will wedge itself between the opposing crests and be carried over the enamel surface. When this happens, hard detrital particles embedded in the food will gouge the enamel as they pass.

The special concentration of detrital wear at the centres of the downstroke crests is a result of transverse movement of food along the crest when the latter is sloping gently in the direction of occlusal motion. The places of concentrated detrital abrasion are the points of convergence of such slopes. That detrital particles are directed by sloping crests is clearly demonstrated in *Hydrochoerus* (Fig. 4F). Here, coarse striae are parallel to the transverse downstroke crest where it bends slightly in the direction of occlusal motion, but are also parallel to the direction of motion where the crest is perpendicular to the latter.

Polish is the dominant feature of the worn enamel in the arvicolines. It is present on most surfaces, even those giving evidence of intensive detrital abrasion, and exists in the absence of much detrital wear over the greater length of occlusal enamel. Even where detritus has broken large segments of the poorly supported downstroke enamel down to the dentinal level, as in *Lagurus* (Fig. 2B), the rate of detrital abrasion must slow and await the advance of the polishing process on the upstroke enamel before much additional breakage can occur. Therefore, in these rapidly wearing ever-growing teeth, the rate of wear by polish is the determining factor in occlusal attrition.

The diet of *Microtus* is largely green vegetation, although in areas where this source is scarce in winter, bark may be important (p. 540 in Hall, 1946; p. 193 in Linsdale, 1938). Grass is a major component of the diet of *M. townsendi* in western Washington (personal observation). The diet of *L. curtatus*, the sagebrush vole, is foliage and cambium, especially that of *Artemisia* (p. 557 in Hall, 1946). The principal difference in the diets of *Peromyscus* and the arvicolines is the much greater percentage of fibrous vegetation in that of the latter. If the rate of wear in the arvicolines is dependent upon the rate of polishing abrasion, then the coarseness of the diet is not the direct cause of the high rate of crown reduction. Instead, the quantity of food consumed must have increased. This itself would be a correlate and consequence of the differences in diet, because the lower percentage of available nutrients in grasses and other vegetative parts compared to that of seeds and arthropods would increase the absolute volume of food required for maintenance.

Aplodontia. Although it is not the only type of wear in *Aplodontia*, pebbly texture is the dominant pattern of wear on the heavy lingual enamel crest. Some striae are present on this surface, but they are dominant only in restricted areas, as for example on the prominence separating the anterior and posterior facets. The striae on this prominence were not caused by cheek-tooth mastication, as discussed above. However, striae are dominant on the entire leading edge of the crest adjacent to the dentinal platform, where the enamel was reached only by food and abrasive detritus (and where also furrows of uncertain origin occur), but this is not the area of most intensive wear. The greater rate of wear to the enamel in this specimen occurred at the enamel–enamel contact, for this was the plane of loss of the larger volume of enamel (Fig. 7A). Had wear at the leading edge been more rapid, the shape of the surface would more closely resemble that of Fig. 7B. If the pebbly

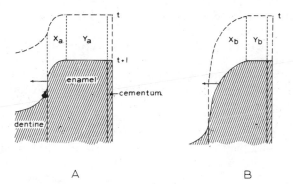

A   B

FIG. 7. The relationship of the rate of food abrasion and the degree of convexity of occlusal enamel. Transverse sections through lingual enamel of upper molar in *Aplodontia* as shown in Fig. 3E. (A) Faceted enamel crest. (B) Convex enamel. Direction of relative motion of surfaces shown by arrows. X and Y represent volumes of enamel removed during time *t* by, respectively, food abrasion and contact abrasion. The ratio of X to Y determines the shape of the occlusal surface.

texture is an effect of friction and high pressure at the enamel–enamel contact, then the wear in *Aplodontia* probably involves higher occlusal pressures than are attained by the other taxa (except *Hydrochoerus*, discussed below).

Although the greater rate of wear occurs on the occlusal facet, wear at the leading edge is relatively more intense than in any of the other taxa studied. This relationship may be a consequence of the diet of *Aplodontia*, which consists of coarser materials than are known in the diets of the other taxa. In the north-western United States, *Aplodontia* apparently has few limitations on the type of vegetation it can masticate, and consumes entire herbaceous plants, bark, foliage and young shoots of such woody plants as Douglas fir, western hemlock and cedar (Scheffer, 1929). Although experimental data on the failure thresholds of different plant materials is lacking, it seems likely that an especially high occlusal pressure is required for the diet of *Aplodontia*, and that this breaks down the leading edge more rapidly than in the arvicolines. The absence of wedge-shaped fissures along the leading edge may be due to the structural difference in the enamel rod fabric of these forms (Fig. 5B and C). Large flaked pits characteristic of the trailing edge of enamel in the arvicolines and *Hydrochoerus* are in part, at least, prevented in *Aplodontia* by the lingual lamina of cementum, which is absent in the other forms.

Hydrochoerus. Wear in this form shares attributes characteristic of both *Aplodontia* and the arvicolines. Pebbly texture is the dominant mode of wear, although in positions comparable to those where detrital wear is concentrated in the arvicolines, striae and the pebbly pattern are equally developed. As in the arvicolines, leading edges bear wedge-shaped fissures and trailing edges bear flaked pits, which correlate with the similarity of the gross enamel configurations in these groups. Both have numerous narrow enamel crests aligned transversely on the tooth-row. It is possible that the enamel structure is also similar, but I did not etch the enamel in *Hydrochoerus* because only one specimen was available.

Although the diet of this zoo specimen is uncertain, the probability that it was fed in captivity the same materials eaten by wild *Aplodontia* is low. The presence in both *Aplodontia* and *Hydrochoerus* of the pebbly texture therefore lends support to the theory that some aspect of the masticatory system, perhaps pressure, is responsible.

Hypsodonty

One apparent and somewhat unexpected implication of this study is that the dental surfaces in the brachyodont forms, whose diets consist of the more delicate kinds of foods, were dominated by detrital abrasion, whereas those of the more hypsodont taxa were not. Furthermore, wear in the hypsodont cricetids was dominantly polish, whereas that in the brachyodont cricetid, *Peromyscus*, exhibited a combination of both polish and detrital abrasion. These data are inconsistent with the common assumption that hypsodonty equates with excessively abrasive diets or ones containing large amounts of inorganic grit. Nor is the rough pebbly texture of the wear surfaces in *Aplodontia* and *Hydrochoerus* suggestive of simply abrasive foods or detritus, either of which would cause linear markings in forms chewing with a translatory motion.

The data, however, do not disallow increased chewing activity, or chewing under higher pressure, or both, as causes of higher rates of wear in the hypsodont taxa. In fact, the data suggest that both are involved. The lesser accessibility of nutrients in the diets of the hypsodont forms points toward increased consumption as a cause, and the nature of the pitted surfaces in *Aplodontia* and *Hydrochoerus* are suggestive of pressure as a major factor in these taxa.

SUMMARY

The occlusal surfaces of enamel in some herbivorous and partially insectivorous rodents were examined under SEM magnifications of up to 15 000 diameters. A number of distinctive features of wear were observed. Polish appears to have been caused by food abrasion and striations by hard detrital fragments. Wedge-shaped fissures were confined to relatively sharp leading edges of thin, vertical enamel and probably resulted from stress concentrated by resistant particles in the food. Shallow, flaked pits occurred typically on the trailing edges of vertical enamel where it was not supported by cementum. Facets probably resulted from intimate enamel–enamel contact, and convex enamel from absence of close contact. A pebbly texture of randomly arranged concentrations of small, shallow pits may have resulted from high occlusal pressure. A fabric-like pattern of furrows were of the average size and spacing of enamel rods, but where observed they appeared to be more uniform than the latter. The furrows suggested at least that some individuals had held an abrasive substance of unusual chemical or physical characteristics in contact with the occlusal surface.

Wear in *Sciurus* was dominated by detrital striations, whereas that in *Peromyscus* involved a subequal share of polishing abrasion. In the hypsodont arvicoline rodents the dominant mode of wear was polish. Wear in *Aplodontia* had produced extensive amounts of the pebbly texture, suggesting that mastication of the extremely fibrous diet of this genus perhaps involved high occlusal pressures. The occlusal surface of *Hydrochoerus* was dominantly pebbly, but also contained features characteristic of the arvicolines, which correlated with similarities in the thickness and arrangement of the enamel plates in the two groups.

The dominance of detrital wear in *Sciurus*, the most brachyodont form, and of polish or pebbly texture in the hypsodont forms, indicated that in the latter groups the selective advantage of high crowns was that they permitted larger volume mastication (especially in arvicolines) and higher occlusal pressures (especially in *Aplodontia* and *Hydrochoerus*) necessary for diets of lower nutrient concentrations and tougher materials.

ACKNOWLEDGEMENTS

Drs Mary R. Dawson (Carnegie Museum, Pittsburgh), William Turnbull (Field Museum, Chicago), and Albert Van der Meulen (Geological Institute, Utrecht) kindly read the manuscript and provided important suggestions. I am grateful for discussions with Dr Karen Hiiemae (Guy's Hospital Medical School, London), Dr Richard Kay, (Department of Anatomy, Duke University Medical Center), Dr William Turnbull (Field Museum of Natural History, Chicago) and Dr Donald Morris (Department of Anthropology, Arizona State University) on various aspects of this problem. Discussions with Dr O. J. Whittemore, Jr. and Dr William D. Scott (Department of Mining, Metallurgical and Ceramic Engineering, University of Washington) on the mechanical aspects of wear, and with Dr Alan Boyde (Department of Anatomy and Embryology, University College, London) on rodent enamel structure were very helpful. The SEM micrographs were made by Mrs Yorko Tsukada (Quaternary Research Center, University of Washington) and supported by NSF Grant number GB 35959.

REFERENCES

BUTLER, P. M. (1952a). The milk-molars of Perissodactyla, with remarks on molar occlusion. *Proc. zool. Soc. Lond.* **121**, 777–817.

BUTLER, P. M. (1952b). Molarization of the premolars in the Perissodactyla. *Proc. zool. Soc. Lond.* **121**, 819–843.

BUTLER, P. M. (1973). Molar wear facets of early Tertiary North American primates. *Symp. 4th Int. Cong. Primat.* (Montagna, Z. W. and Zingeser, M. R. eds), **3**, 1–27. Karger, Basel.

CROMPTON, A. W. and HIIEMAE, K. (1970). Molar occlusion and mandibular movements during occlusion in the American opossum, *Didelphis marsupialis J. Linn. Soc.* (*Zool*) **49**, 21–47.

EVERY, R. G. and KÜHNE, W. G. (1971). Bimodal wear of mammalian teeth. *J. Linn. Soc.* (*Zool*) **50**, Suppl. 1, 23–27.

FLAKE L. D. (1973). Food habits of four species of rodents on a short-grass prairie in Colorado. *J. Mammal.* **54**, 636–647.

GINGERICH, P. D. (1973). Molar occlusion and function in the Jurassic mammal *Docodon. J. Mammal.* **54**, 1008–1013.

HALL, E. R. (1946). "Mammals of Nevada". University of California Press, Berkeley.

HIIEMAE, K. M. and CROMPTON, A. W. (1971). A cinefluorographic study of feeding in the American opossum, *Didelphis marsupialis. In* "Dental Morphology and Evolution" (Dahlberg, A. A. ed.), pp. 299–334. University of Chicago Press, Chicago.

KAY, R. F. and HIIEMAE, K. M. (1974). Jaw movement and tooth use in Recent and fossil primates. *Am. J. phys. Anthrop.* **40**, 227–256.

LINSDALE, J. M. (1938). Environmental responses of vertebrates in the Great Basin. *Am. Midl. Nat.* **19**, 1–206.

MILLS, J. R. E. (1955). Ideal dental occlusion in the primates. *Dent. Practnr, Bristol* **6**, 47–61.

MILLS, J. R. E. (1963) Occlusion and malocclusion of the teeth of primates. *In* "Dental Anthropology" (Brothwell, D. R., ed.), pp. 29–52. Pergamon Press, Oxford.

MILLS, J. R. E. (1966). The functional occlusion of the teeth of the Insectivora. *J. Linn. Soc.* (*Zool*) **47**, 1–25.

MILLS, J. R. E. (1967). A comparison of lateral jaw movements in some mammals from wear facts on the teeth. *Archs oral Biol.* **12**, 645–661.

NIXON, C. M., WORLEY, D. M. and McCLAIN, M. W. (1968). Food habits of squirrels in southeast Ohio. *J. Wildl. Mgmt* **32**, 294–305.

RENSBERGER, J. M. (1973). An occlusion model for mastication and dental wear in herbivorous mammals. *J. Paleont.* **47**, 515–528.

RENSBERGER, J. M. (in press). Function in the cheek tooth evolution of some hypsodont geomyoid rodents. *J. Paleontol.*

SCHEFFER, T. H. (1929). Mountain beavers in the Pacific Northwest: their habits, economic status, and control. *U.S. Dept Agric. Farm. Bull.* **1598**, 1–18.

SICHER, H. and BHASKER, S. N. (1972). "Orban's Oral Histology and Embryology" 7th edition, 293 pp. C. V. Mosby, St. Louis, U.S.A.

TURNBULL, W. D. (1970). Mammalian masticatory apparatus. *Fieldiana, Geol.* **18**, 149–356.

26. Molar Cusp Nomenclature and Homology

P. M. BUTLER

Royal Holloway College, Englefield Green, Surrey, England

INTRODUCTION

Every student of comparative tooth morphology has first to overcome the rather considerable obstacle of a complicated nomenclature. This gives the impression that the subject is much more abstruse than it really is, with the result that many students are deterred from getting to grips with its more interesting problems. The Osborn system (1888, 1907) was based on a theory of molar evolution in the Mesozoic that has turned out to be wrong, and so the names given to the cusps no longer have a logical basis. The protocone of tribosphenic molars, thought by Osborn to be the oldest cusp, is now believed to be the youngest cusp of the trigon, dating only from the Cretaceous (Fig 1). In addition, there is no relationship between upper and lower cusps with similar names: paracone and paraconid, protocone and protoconid etc. Consequently, proposals have been made, most recently by Vandebroek (1961) and Hershkovitz (1971), to replace the Osborn system by new ones, believed by the authors to be more logical. However, the Osbornian names have been used so widely and for so long that a familiarity with them is essential to anyone who wishes to understand the literature, and the introduction of new terms only adds to the load on the memory. Furthermore, as will be argued below, the theoretical basis of the new systems is far from firmly established.

THE OSBORN SYSTEM
Pre-tribosphenic Molars

Osborn named the cusps in the order in which he believed they had appeared in phylogeny: first the protocone, then the paracone and the metacone, and finally the hypocone. It is now, I think, generally agreed that the cusp in triconodonts, symmetrodonts and pantotheres which Osborn called the protocone is homologous with the paracone of the tribosphenic molar. Therefore, if we use Osborn's names for the tribosphenic cusps, as I think we must, we cannot apply them to the pre-tribosphenic mammals in the way that he did. The original cusp cannot be called protocone, and another name must be found for it. Paracone, used by Butler (1939) and Patterson (1956), might

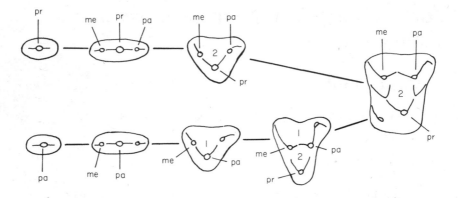

FIG. 1. The origin of the tribosphenic upper molar according to Osborn (upper sequence) and according to current opinion (lower sequence). Osborn confused the primary trigon (1) with the secondary trigon (2). me = metacone; pa = paracone; pr = protocone.

be considered etymologically objectionable. Bohlin (1945) proposed eocone, a term used by Simpson (1961) as well as by Vandebroek (1961). Crompton and Jenkins (1968) called it cusp A. My own preference is for eocone.

Osborn was correct in believing that mammalian molars had passed through a three-cusped stage (if minor cingulum cusps are ignored). Today we recognize this as a cynodont inheritance. He was also correct in believing that the originally straight row of cusps became converted into a V, though he mentioned (Osborn, 1907) the possibility that the accessory cusps (his paracone and metacone) might have arisen *in situ* already out of line with the protocone. Cusp rotation, about which much controversy raged in the early days, seems much more plausible today. As Crompton and Jenkins (1968) have pointed out, the angle of the V shows a wide range of variation within the order Symmetrodonta, and even differs from tooth to tooth along the jaw. What is called rotation is a change in the shape of the crown base, combined with a change in the distribution of growth in the epithelial sheet that folds to form the cusps. As a result, the eocone became the lingual cusp of a primary trigon, so called by Gregory (1916) to distinguish it from the secondary trigon of tribosphenic molars.

Anterior to the eocone in *Thrinaxodon*, *Eozostrodon* (*Morganucodon*) and *Kuehneotherium*, there is a cusp which Osborn would no doubt have homologized with the first of the three cusps of *Triconodon* and called the paracone. It is probably homologous with the anterior buccal cusp of the Upper Jurassic symmetrodont *Peralestes*, previously called parastyle but identified as a stylocone by Patterson (1956). Patterson gave the name stylocone to a cusp on the Forestburg molars (i.e. *Pappotherium* and *Holoclemensia*) which stands near the buccal edge of the tooth posterior to the parastyle. It is the equivalent of style *b* of opossums (Bensley, 1903), and Patterson homologized it with the main buccal cusp of *Melanodon* and other dryolestid pantotheres. His reason for regarding the cusp in *Peralestes* as a stylocone and not a parastyle was the existence in the Forestburg symmetrodont, *Spalacotheroides*, of an additional small cusp in the anterior side of the supposed stylocone. This additional cusp is represented in *Peralestes* by a ridge. Patterson believed that the parastyle was a new development, primitively absent. This would make the anterior cusp of *Kuehneotherium* a stylocone (Fig. 2).

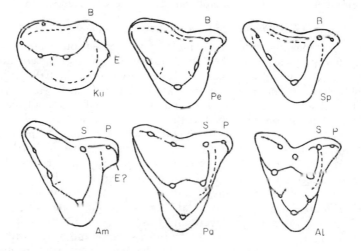

FIG. 2. Right upper molars of Mesozoic mammals to illustrate the possible homology of cusp *B* of *Keuhneotherium*. Teeth figured are those of: *Keuhneotherium, Peralestes, Spalacotheroides, Amblotherium* (a dryolestid), *Pappotherium* and *Alphadon* (Cretaceous didelphid). Not to scale. S = stylocone; P = parastyle.

I am not convinced by this argument, and believe that cusp B is the parastyle and not the stylocone. It is worn on its lingual surface by the tip of the protoconid, both in *Kuehneotherium* and in *Eozostrodon*, a function that characterizes the parastyle of pantotherian and tribosphenic molars. The stylocone of dryolestids and *Pappotherium* stands more posteriorly and is worn from the front; it extends the anterior wear facet of the paracone buccally. In *Kuehneotherium* there is a smaller cusp (E) at the anterior end of the lingual cingulum, involved in the same wear facet as cusp B. It occurs also in *Eozostrodon* and even in *Thrinaxodon*, always in a lingual position. It seems to be represented in tribosphenic molars by a slight elevation of the cingulum, lingual to the parastyle and rapidly removed by wear against the tip of the protoconid.

Posterior to the eocone in the Triassic mammals there is a cusp which I believe to be the metacone on the basis of its occlusal relations in *Kuehneotherium* (see p. 479 in Butler, 1972); if it is, it would be the only upper cusp for which Osborn's name can be retained. Behind it is a small posterior cusp (D of Crompton and Jenkins) which apparently has the function of locking the tooth to the next by fitting between B and E. It is absent in *Thrinaxodon*. This cusp seems to be the equivalent of the metastyle of tribosphenic molars, which fits against the lingual side of the parastyle of the following tooth.

Thus the oldest part of the mammalian upper molar appears to be the ectoloph of Osborn, consisting of parastyle, paracone (or eocone), metacone and metastyle. The lingual cusps, including the protocone, were added with the development of the tribosphenic pattern in the Cretaceous.

Lower molars and Upper–Lower Homologies

Osborn's nomenclature for lower molars was based on their supposed homology with upper molars, the buccal side of the lower molar corresponding to the lingual side of the upper. As lower molars bite lingually to uppers we would expect to find a mutual adaptation of the surfaces which occlude, i.e. the buccal surface of the lower teeth and the lingual surface of the upper teeth. When opposition developed at the tribosphenic stage a new relationship arose: the secondary trigon functions with the talonid and enlarges correlatively with it (Butler, 1961). But over and above such functional requirements, which make the patterns complementary and therefore different in the two jaws, there are factors which make them alike. The similarity is most striking in the earliest stages, and it is reflected in the nomenclature used by Crompton and Jenkins, who label corresponding cusps with the same letters, using capitals for upper teeth and lower case for lower teeth.

The three larger cusps of Triassic mammals are homologous with those of the trigonid of tribosphenic molars, and the names paraconid, protoconid and metaconid are unambiguous and should I think be retained. An alternative—parastylid, eoconid and metaconid—would emphasize the equivalence of upper and lower cusps, but this seems to me less important than the homology with the cusps of later mammals.

Some small cusps at the anterior and posterior ends of the tooth need mention. In *Kuehneotherium* there is a cusp *e* at cingulum level immediately anterior to the paraconid, and also cusp *f* of similar size standing more buccally. At the posterior end there is a cusp *d* which forms the rudimentary talonid and fits between *e* and *f* of the following tooth (lettering from Crompton and Jenkins 1968). Tribosphenic molars are locked together by the hypoconulid fitting between a ridge on the anterior surface of the paraconid and a cingulum which stands more buccally (Fig. 3). I believe the

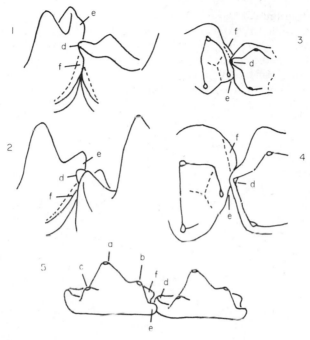

FIG. 3. To illustrate how the hypoconid (d) fits against the following tooth. 1. *Eodelphis* (Cretaceous didelphid), buccal view of right teeth. 2. *Centetodon* (*Geolabis*) (Oligocene insectivore), the same. 3. *Cimolestes* (Cretaceous palaeoryctid), crown view of left teeth. 4. *Propalaeosinopa* (Palaeocene pantolestid), the same. 5. *Kuehneotherium*, lingual view of two left teeth, cusps labelled according to Crompton and Jenkins (1968).

structures concerned with this function to be homologous throughout the mammals, and cusp *d* of *Kuehneotherium* to be the hypoconulid.

THE VANDEBROEK SYSTEM

Interpretation of Antemolar Patterns

Vandebroek (1961) begins by assuming that premolars and milk molars can be used to interpret the morphology of the molars. This is of course essentially the basis of the premolar analogy theory of Wortman (1902). By tracing the molar pattern forward from tooth to tooth it is seen to become simplified until eventually only a single cusp is left. The fact that this cusp is the paracone of Osborn, and not the protocone, led Wortman and his followers to reject the tritubercular theory. Wortman believed that the anterior cheek teeth, being farther removed from the jaw muscles, were less specialized than the molars and so retained a more primitive condition.

According to Vandebroek, the simplest antemolars in a wide variety of mammals have a common morphology that is independent of the molar pattern. There is an eocone, standing on a longitudinal crest, the eocrista, with buccal and lingual ridges (anticrista and epicrista). All forms of therian molar are derivable from this pattern, the mode of derivation being found by tracing the pattern through the more posterior premolars and milk molars. Thus Osborn's metacone arises on the eocrista posterior to the eocone, and is called the distocone, while Osborn's protocone arises on the epicrista and is called the epicone. The eocone is of course Osborn's paracone (Fig. 4).

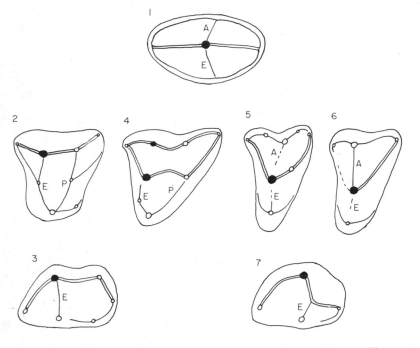

FIG. 4. Diagrams to illustrate Vandebroek's interpretation of molar patterns. The eocone is marked in black; eocrista is indicated by a double line; A—anticrista; E—epicrista.
1. The basic plan of simple antemolars.
2 and 3. Upper and lower molars of "euthemorphic" type, in which the eocrista remains more or less straight.
4. Upper molar of a marsupial, in which the eocrista divides. The lower molars resemble 3.
5, 6 and 7. Molars of "zalambdomorphic" type, in which the eocrista is markedly folded.
   (5. *Potamogale*; 6. A tenrecid, in which the anterior part of the eocrista has disappeared; 7. Lower zalambdomorphic molar.)

From an ontogenetic point of view, the non-molariform antemolars are probably best regarded as teeth whose development has been diverted from the molar path to various degrees, perhaps because they are situated near the margin of a molarization field, or because the cells from which they arise have lost their capacity to react (see Chapter 14). Products of the same gene system, antemolars evolve in many respects in parallel with the molars, although their simpler structure does not permit the expression of all the genes that influence the molar pattern. They could be regarded either as

potential molars or as degenerate molars, but in any case they should be
interpreted by comparison with the molars. Vandebroek on the other hand
interprets molars by comparison with antemolars. He ignores the fact that
even apparently simple antemolars may reflect some of the features of the
molar pattern with which they are associated.

Interpretation of Ridges: Buccal Stylar Cusps

Vandebroek's identification of molar cusps depends in very large measure
on the interpretation of ridges on the slopes of the antemolar eocones and
eoconids. Unfortunately, ridges vary considerably in their distinctness, from
sharp crests to mere rounded convexities. In Vandebroek's diagrams many

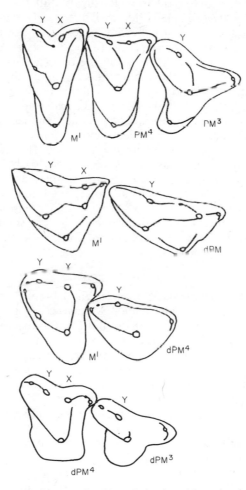

FIG. 5. Right upper teeth of mammals with well-developed buccal stylar cusps: *Potamogale*,
Didelphis, an unnamed Kimmeridgian dryolestid and *Tenrec*.

of them are indicated by dotted lines. Ridges are also, in my experience, less constant from tooth to tooth within a series than Vandebroek supposes.

As an example, consider his treatment of the buccal stylar cusps, which have a rather similar arrangement in dryolestid pantotheres, in didelphids and in zalambdodont insectivores (Fig. 5). Between the parastyle and the metastyle there are two cusps, or groups of cusps. Anterior to the bay in the buccal margin (ectoflexus of Van Valen, 1966) is the anterior buccal cusp, or stylocone (X), and more posteriorly are one or more posterior buccal cusps (Y). At intermediate stages of molarization the stylocone disappears (when the pattern is traced forward), the paracone approaches the buccal margin of the tooth, but the posterior buccal cusp remains. Teeth at this stage are dPM⁴ of an unnamed dryolestid from Portugal (Butler and Krebs, 1973), the milk molar of *Didelphis*, and PM³ and dPM³ of *Potamogale*. In such teeth the paracone (eocone) is usually connected by a ridge to the posterior buccal cusp, and also by an anterior ridge to the parastyle. As the stylocone develops with more complete molarization, the ridge to the posterior buccal cusp tends to disappear, and the anterior ridge is often diverted to join the stylocone. Vandebroek, when dealing with *Potamogale*, regards the postero-buccal ridge as an anticrista and the posterior buccal cusp as an anticone. He thinks that the stylocone is a specialized new development and calls it the mesio-anticone. But in other Tenrecidae such as *Setifer*, as well as in dryo-lestids, he identifies the stylocone with the anticone. The reason is that the anterior ridge of the eocone joins the stylocone in *Setifer* but not in *Potamogale*. On such a basis he puts *Potamogale* into a different superfamily from the other Tenrecidae. The marsupials are interpreted differently again: here the posterior buccal cusp is supposed to have split off from the metacone (distocone) and is called the exo-distocone, while the stylocone is named exo-eocone. Thus marsupials are considered to have a markedly different molar construction from the placentals.

The Eocrista of Lower Molars

A more fundamental disagreement between Vandebroek and the trituberculists is his interpretation of the metaconid. He believes that this cusp developed from the lingual crest of the eoconid, and not from the eocrista, and accordingly he names it epiconid. If he is correct, the third large cusp of triconodonts and symmetrodonts, which stands on the eocrista, cannot be a metaconid, and he regards it as a distoconid that disappears at the tribosphenic stage. Vandebroek is in fact in agreement with the view I held in 1939 when I distinguished between a "posterior accessory cusp", which develops on the posterior side of the protoconid, and a metaconid which arises more lingually.

It is a fact that in tribosphenic mammals the metaconid arises during molarization on the postero-lingual side of the protoconid, usually from a ridge in that position (Fig. 8). This is so in PM₃ of *Gypsonictops*, PM₃ of *Protungulatum* and PM₄ of *Purgatorius*, among Cretaceous mammals, as well as in numerous Tertiary mammals. I know of no case, except obviously specialized forms like Carpolestidae, where the metaconid arises directly posterior to the protoconid. The situation is complicated by the presence in a number of mammals of a posterior or postero-buccal ridge on which a cusp may develop: Miacidae and other Carnivora, Leptictidae, *Rhynchocyon*, Soricidae, Tenrecidae and *Didelphodus* among others. This cusp, the proto-stylid of Van Valen (1966), has been confused with the metaconid or with the hypoconid by various authors, but it is distinct from both. Its function is to shear against the antero-lingual surface of the paracone of the corresponding upper tooth, where the parastyle is anteriorly placed (Fig. 6). The metaconid

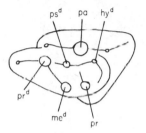

FIG. 6. To illustrate the occlusal relations of the "protostylid" (ps^d) of submolariform lower teeth.

(or the ridge from which it arises) shears against the anterior face of the upper protocone, and the hypoconid occludes posteriorly to the tip of the paracone.

The problem is to identify the eocrista on lower cheek teeth. In *Kuehneo-therium* and *Tinodon*, as one passes back along the series, the metaconid is seen to become progressively displaced lingually. Deviation of the eocrista is still more marked in pantotheres: between protoconid and metaconid it runs transversely to the tooth, and this part of the eocrista is represented on dryolestid premolars by a strong postero-lingual crest. The posterior part of the eocrista is the talonid crest, which in *Amphitherium* and *Peramus* can be traced up the posterior trigonid wall to the tip of the metaconid (Fig. 7). It is the "distal metacristid" of Fox (1975).

In tribosphenic molars a hypoconid differentiates on the talonid crest which then deviates towards the buccal side. Anterior to the hypoconid the eocrista is represented by the so-called oblique crest, and in *Kermackia* this connects to the tip of the metaconid as in pantotheres. However, in *Holoclemensia* the crest ends buccally to the tip of the metaconid, below the metaconid–protoconid notch (see Fig. 4 in Turnbull, 1971); in Late Creta-ceous mammals it fades out near the mid-point of the posterior trigonid wall, and in many Tertiary mammals it is still more buccal, merging into the base of the protoconid. This trend to displace the oblique crest buccally is associ-ated with the loss of the V-shape of the paracone, which occludes in the groove between the oblique crest and the trigonid, and with widening of the talonid basin. A parallel change takes place in less molariform teeth, where the talonid crest is no longer continuous with the postero-lingual crest that will form the

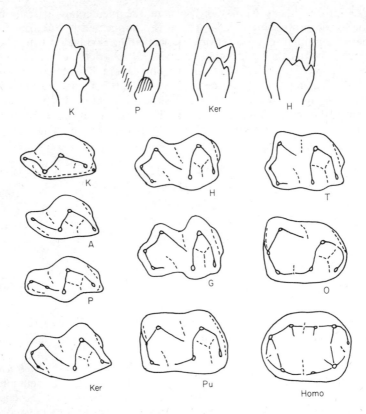

FIG. 7. To illustrate the different relations to the trigonid of the posterior part of the eocrista (oblique crest, anterior hypoconid crest) in lower molars. Above, posterior views of left lower molars of *Kuehneotherium, Peramus, Kermackia* and *Holoclemensia*. Below. crown views of left lower molars: *Kuehneotherium, Amphitherium, Peramus, Kermackia, Holoclemensia, Gypsonictops, Protungulatum, Talpavus, Omomys* and *Homo* foetus (dPM₄).

metaconid (Fig. 8). Usually it fades at the base of the protoconid, but sometimes it extends to the tip of that cusp, and an accessory cusp may develop on it, as in Leptictidae and often in man. A third ridge may develop on the protoconid in a more buccal position, and on this again a cusp may form, as in Soricidae.

Vandebroek's assumption that a crest running directly from protoconid to hypoconid is part of the eocrista (see Fig. 4 and his Plate 2) is erroneous, being based upon a secondary rearrangement of crests. Hence his thesis that the metaconid (epiconid) is equivalent to the protocone (epicone) is unacceptable, and the basis of his nomenclature breaks down. The same applies to the scheme of Hershkovitz (1971), which is founded on that of Vandebroek. Hershkovitz goes even farther in equating upper and lower cusps: for

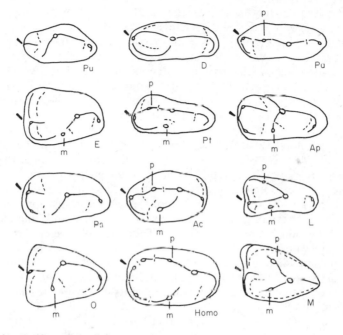

FIG. 8. Submolariform lower left antemolars.
Protungulatum PM$_3$, *Diacodexis* (artiodactyl) PM$_4$, *Palaeictops* (leptictid) PM$_3$, *Entomo-lestes* (erinaceoid) PM$_4$, *Protictis* (miacid) PM$_4$, *Aphronorus* (pentacodontid) PM$_4$, *Protoselene* (condylarth) PM$_4$, *Acmeodon* (palaeoryctid) PM$_4$, *Litomylus* (condylarth) PM$_4$, *Omomys* (primate) PM$_4$, *Homo* foetus dPM$_3$ and *Myosorex* (soricid) PM$_4$. m = metaconid; p = "protostylid". The pointer indicates the posterior end of the eocrista.

instance, he equates the metacone, present in the Triassic, with the hypo-conid, which did not arise until the Cretaceous.

MODIFICATIONS OF THE OSBORN SYSTEM

If we have to continue to use the Osborn system of nomenclature, at least for tribosphenic molars, let us keep it as simple as possible. Dental nomen-clature serves two purposes: it is an aid to description and an expression of homologies. To give a name to a feature, even if only a letter or number, individualizes it and fixes it in the mind as something worthy of special consideration. To give the same name to features on different teeth enables the reader to see how one tooth resembles or differs from another. As tooth patterns have been studied in much greater detail, names have been given to many features additional to those originally referred to by Osborn. Van Valen (1966) and Szalay (1969) have largely contributed to this development, and their system has been widely adopted by American authors, as may be seen in several chapters in this volume. It seems to me that, while some of the innovations are useful, others are unnecessary and merely increase the number of terms that the student has to learn.

Osborn's names for the cusps are retained, except that protoconule has been replaced by paraconule, a change which seems to me to have some advantage. The crests are given names mostly derived from cusps; thus we have in Szalay's system a postparacrista and a premetacrista, together making up the centrocrista which joins the paracone and metacone. While agreeing that crests should be defined from cusps and not the other way round as in Vandebroek's scheme, it seems unnecessary to give them Latin names. Either they lie on the slopes of cusps or they join two cusps, and can be named accordingly: thus posterior paracone crest, paracone–metacone crest etc. (cf. MacIntyre, 1966). Likewise, parts of the cingulum named paracingulum, precingulum etc could be named form the cusps to which they relate, thus paraconule cingulum, preprotocone cingulum etc., or where they are more extensive, to the topography of the tooth, as buccal cingulum (instead of ectocingulum). This takes up a little more space but in my opinion it makes for easier understanding. Moreover, the use of cristid and cingulid for the lower teeth would be made superfluous if for example the cristid obliqua of Szalay were called the anterior hypoconid crest, and the postcingulid the posthypoconid cingulum. I also see no reason why the well-established expressions trigon basin, trigonid basin and talonid basin should be given up in favour of Van Valen's protofossa, protofossid and postfossid, and I am glad to see that Szalay rejects these.

Hershkovitz (1971) lists 300 terms that have been applied to details of the tooth crown, and proposes a new system containing 92 terms. Under the heading of conules and styles, he gives names to 16 upper cusps and 18 lower cusps. As most of them are limited to single taxa there seems to be little point in trying to fit them into a common scheme for all mammals, especially as it would not be difficult by further search to add to the list. Special terms have come into use for features of the teeth or rodents, horses and other groups; Osborn (1898) himself introduced a nomenclature for rhinoceros teeth. This is inevitable, but if authors expect their papers to be read by more than a very narrow circle of specialists they should go to the trouble of explaining their terminology. Unfortunately they do not always do this.

All this adds up to a plea to keep the number of technical terms as small as possible. The aim should be to enable a student to understand a description once he has learnt the Osbornian names of the cusps.

Nomenclature in Relation to Homology

Teeth are comparatively simple structures, and the number of ways in which they can vary and evolve is limited. As a result, they are particularly subject to parallel evolution: most phylogenetic changes in the dentition have been repeated, in some cases many times. This has long been recognized in Tertiary mammals, where additional cusps like the hypocone, the mesostyle and the metastylid have been developed in group after group. When Early Cretaceous mammals are better known it will probably be found that other cusps have evolved more than once: the conules, the entoconid and perhaps

even the protocone and the hypoconid. It is clearly impracticable to give
different names to similar cusps because they originated independently,
especially as in many cases the exact origin is unknown. A name implies a
type of cusp, with characteristic topographical relations to other cusps and
characteristic functional relations to cusps of the opposing tooth. For
example, in many lines of ungulates and primates a metastylid differentiates
from the posterior surface of the metaconid. It takes over from the metaconid the function of shearing against the anterior face of the protocone,
preserving the contact as the protocone is displaced posteriorly away from
the metaconid.

There are of course difficult cases, arising from the fact that the cusps may
not be exactly alike, and one has to decide how different they should be
before the need arises to give them different names. The so-called pseudo-
hypocone of *Notharctus* and *Pelycodus* differs in its functions, as well as its
mode of origin, from the hypocone of other early primates, but the hypocone
of higher primates is more like that of *Notharctus* in function, although its
origin is unknown (Butler, 1973). Similarly, is a mesostyle which takes part
in the paracone–metacone notch, extending the shear against the hypoconid,
different from a mesostyle on the buccal cingulum which is independent of
the paracone–metacone crest?

It is now general practice to name the cusps of premolars and milk molars
from the molar cusps with which they are serially homologous. This is in
accordance with current ontogenetic views, mentioned earlier in this chapter.
The proposal of Scott (1892) to name the cusps according to the order of
their appearance in evolution (protocone, deuterocone, tritocone and tetar-
tocone) implied that antemolars evolved independently of the molars and
came to resemble them only through convergence: the premolar protocone
resembles the molar paracone. It is interesting to note that Scott, commenting
on the work of Taeker (1892), says that if it were proved that the order of
cusp development was the same in the molars as in the premolars and milk
molars, the special cusp nomenclature for premolars would be superfluous.
It is now well established that the paracone is the first cusp to develop in the
ontogeny of all upper teeth, and Scott's scheme has fortunately been
abandoned. Still more confusing was the application by Roth (1927) of
Scott's names to molar cusps.

Perhaps it is too much to hope that we have come to the end of the inven-
tion of schemes of cusp nomenclature. The Osborn system, as a method of
describing tribosphenic molars and their derivatives, i.e. the cheek teeth of
marsupials and placentals, has stood the test of time, and cannot now be
abandoned. Let those who are contemplating the introduction of new names
pause to consider whether in so doing they are advancing the subject or
making it more difficult to understand. Language is for communication.

SUMMARY

(a) Despite its faulty theoretical basis, the Osborn system of nomenclature
should continue to be applied to tribosphenic molars and their derivatives.

(b) Osborn's names for the upper cusps of triconodonts, symmetrodonts and pantotheres should be rejected, and it is suggested that the three main cusps should be called parastyle, eocone (or paracone) and metacone.

(c) The system of Vandebroek is unsatisfactory because (i) it ignores the effect of changes of molar pattern on antemolar structure, (ii) it depends too much on the identification of ridges, and (iii) it misinterprets the evolution of the metaconid.

(d) Introduction of new terms, additional to those used by Osborn, should be avoided as far as possible. Descriptions should be written so as to be understood by those with a knowledge only of the basic cusp nomenclature.

(e) Cusp names refer to species of cusp as defined by topographical and functional relations, and do not necessarily imply strict homology. Antemolar cusps are named from the molar cusps with which they are serially homologous.

REFERENCES

BENSLEY, B. A. (1903). On the evolution of the Australian Marsupialia, with remarks on the relationships of the Marsupialia in general. *Trans. Linn. Soc. Lond.* (*Zool.*) **9**, 83–217.

BOHLIN, B. (1945). The Jurassic mammals and the origin of the mammalian molar teeth. *Bull. Geol. Inst. Upsala* **31**, 363–388.

BUTLER, P. M. (1939). The teeth of the Jurassic mammals. *Proc. zool. Soc. Lond.* (B) **109**, 329–356.

BUTLER, P. M. (1961). Relationships between upper and lower molar patterns. Int. Colloq. on the Evolution of lower and non-specialised mammals. *Kon. Vl. Acad. Wetens. Lett. Sch. Kunst. België* **1**, 117–126.

BUTLER, P. M. (1972). Some functional aspects of molar pattern. *Evolution* **26**, 474–483.

BUTLER, P. M. (1973). Molar wear facets of Early Tertiary North American primates. *Symp. IV Int. Cong. Primat.* **3**, 1–27.

BUTLER, P. M. and KREBS, B. (1973). A pantotherian milk dentition. *Paläeont. Z.* **47**, 256–258.

CROMPTON, A. W. and JENKINS, F. A., JR. (1968). Molar occlusion in Late Triassic mammals. *Biol. Rev.* **34**, 427–458.

FOX, R. C. (1975). Molar structure and function in the Early Cretaceous mammal *Pappotherium*: evolutionary implications for Mesozoic Theria. *Can. J. Earth Sci.* **12**, 412–442.

GREGORY, W. K. (1916). Studies in the evolution of the Primates. *Bull. Am. Mus. nat. Hist.* **35**, 239–355.

HERSHKOVITZ, P. (1971). Basic crown patterns and cusp homologies of mammalian teeth. *In* "Dental Morphology and Evolution" (Dahleberg, A. A., ed.), pp. 95–150. University of Chicago Press, Chicago, U.S.A.

MACINTYRE, G. T. (1966). The Miacidae (Mammalia, Carnivora). Part I. The systematics of *Ictidopappus* and *Protictis*. *Bull. Am. Mus. nat. Hist.* **131**, 115–210.

OSBORN, H. F. (1888). The nomenclature of the mammalian molar cusps. *Am. Nat.* **22**, 926–928.

OSBORN, H. F. (1898). The extinct rhinoceroses. *Mem. Am. Mus. nat. Hist.* **1**, 75–164.

OSBORN, H. F. (1907). "Evolution of Mammalian Molar Teeth to and from the Triangular Type" (Gregory, W. K. ed.). Macmillan, New York and London.

PATTERSON, B. (1956). Early Cretaceous mammals and the evolution of mammalian molar teeth. *Fieldiana, Geol.* **13**, 1–105.

ROTH, S. (1927). La differenciacion del sistema dentario en los ungulados, notoungulados, y primates. *Rev. Mus. La Plata* **30**, 172–255.

SCOTT, W. B. (1892). The evolution of the premolar teeth in the mammals. *Proc. phil. Acad. nat. Sci.* **1892**, 405–444.

SIMPSON, G. G. (1961). Evolution of Mesozoic mammals. International Colloquium on the Evolution of lower and non-specialised Mammals. *Kon. Vl. Acad. Wetens. Lett. sch. Kunst. België* **1**, 57–95.

SZALAY, F. S. (1969). Mixodectidae, Microsyopidae and the insectivore-primate transition. *Bull. Am. Mus. nat. Hist.* **140**, 193–330.

TAEKER, J. (1892). "Zur Kenntnis der Odontogenese bei Ungulaten." Inaug. Diss., Dorpat.

TURNBULL, W. D. (1971). The Trinity therians: their bearing on evolution in marsupials and other therians. *In* "Dental Morphology and Evolution", (Dahlberg, A. A., ed.), pp. 151–179. University of Chicago Press, Chicago, Illinois.

VANDEBROEK, G. (1961). The comparative anatomy of the teeth of lower and non-specialised mammals. International Colloquium on the Evolution of lower and non-specialised mammals. *Kon. Vl. Acad. Wetens. Lett. sch. Kunst. België* **1**, 215–313 and **2**, 1–181.

VAN VALEN, L. (1966). Deltatheridia: a new order of mammals. *Bull. Am. Mus. nat. Hist.* **132**, 1–126.

WORTMAN, J. L. (1902). Studies of Eocene Mammalia in the Marsh Collection, Peabody Museum. *Am. J. Sci.* **13**, 39–46.

27. Teeth as an Indicator of Age in Man

A. E. W. MILES

Department of Anatomy, London Hospital Medical College, London

Because man has a special interest in his own species and because, for various reasons, including forensic ones, the assessment of age in *Homo sapiens* has practical value, there has been more intensive study of the human dentition as an indicator of age than that of other species.

Eruption of teeth, or to use a better term, tooth emergence, is very easy to observe and, as it occurs in accord with a well recorded time-table, it provides a simple method of assessing age. For example, if a child has a completely erupted deciduous dentition, it can be assessed to be not younger than 2 years; if the first or second permanent molars are emerging, the child can be assumed to be respectively about 6 or 12 years of age. Tooth emergence, consisting as it does of a series of episodes of short duration, is, however, of limited value and, after the age of 12 years, is of little use in most peoples of European origin because the third molars so frequently fail to emerge properly, if at all, because jaw growth does not provide enough space for them to emerge.

Girls tend to erupt their permanent teeth a few months earlier than boys even before puberty (Friedlaender and Bailit, 1969), but sex differences in emergence of the deciduous dentition are much less and more doubtful (Infante, 1974). Deciduous tooth emergence is significantly more advanced in babies of high birth weight (Billewicz *et al.*, 1973). Differences between various racial groups have been recorded and can therefore be taken into account (Eveleth, 1966; Eveleth and de Souza Frietas, 1969; Friedlaender and Bailit, 1969). For instance, the permanent teeth emerge several months earlier in both sexes in Chinese (Lee *et al.*, 1965) and in negroids both in North America (Garn *et al.*, 1973b) and in Africa (Houpt *et al.*, 1967) than in caucasoids. However, account must also be taken of socio-economic differences; poverty level existence appears to delay tooth emergence slightly (Garn *et al.*, 1973a; Kaul *et al.*, 1974) although there are studies which appear to contradict this (Bambach *et al.*, 1973).

Longitudinal and cross-sectional radiographic studies of the state of development of the dentition (Israel and Lewis, 1971), including the stages of growth of the roots at various ages, provide a similar body of records on which age can be assessed. Sex differences in these aspects of tooth development are much less than for tooth emergence, and study of the immature dentition either radiographically or in skeletalized material by direct observation, using charts such as that prepared by Schour and Massler (1941) and reproduced in many textbooks (Fig. 1) for comparison, enables age to be

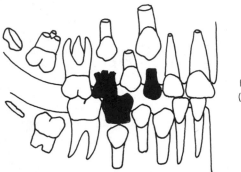

10 years
(±9 months)

FIG. 1. A typical re-drawn part of the Schour and Massler (1941) chart.

assessed up to 12 years with an error of only a few months (Miles, 1958 1963a). Thereafter, the error increases so that, by 14–15 years of age, the error can be as large as 2 years; it can be even larger in late adolescence when the state of growth of the third molar is the sole criterion, the root of the second molar being usually complete by 15 years. The root of the third molar is complete at about 20 years so that tooth development as an age indicator using radiography is virtually limited to the first two decades of life.

The origins of this chart (Fig. 1) and its limitations have been discussed in an earlier review (Miles, 1963b) in which details of the chronology of tooth development are discussed more fully than is possible here. The principal defect of the chart is that its value is virtually limited to ages below 15 years because no stages of growth of the third molars are recorded for the ages between 15 and 21 years. This is a deficiency made good by Moorrees et al. (1963), who present in a graphic form (part of which is depicted in Fig. 2) data for all the permanent teeth, including both the third molar and sex differences, based upon a longitudinal radiographic study of 134 children.

A similar but more diagrammatic chart based upon a variety of literature sources, but not including any of the data of Moorrees et al. (1963) nor any data for the third molar, is available in Johanson (1971, see his p. 24) and Gustafson and Koch (1974).

As there is close correlation between tooth development in the four jaw quadrants, it is common practice to use the radiographs of one quadrant

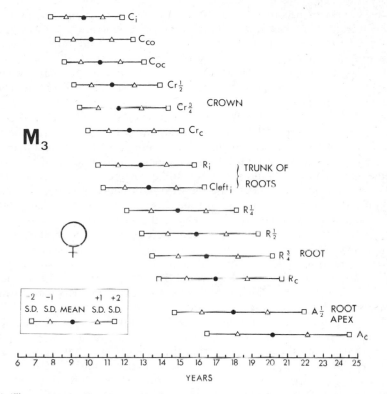

FIG. 2. The norms for development of the human third molar. A typical portion of the chart provided by Moorrees et al. (1963).

only in determining age. Usually a mandibular quadrant is chosen because mandibular radiographs tend to be less distorted.

Demirjian et al. (1973) have proposed a system, which unfortunately does not take account of the third molars, in which each tooth is given a numerical score according to which of eight stages of development it has reached. The score is based upon a total of 100 achieved by females at 16 years of age when the roots of second molars are complete.

After emergence, teeth undergo changes with advancing age which provide a basis for the estimation of age, but they are less reliable than the changes which take place during tooth development. If the dentition is put to good use, as it must be for survival in any relatively primitive population, then the crowns of teeth begin to show signs of wear; the tips of the cusps wear away and, because teeth are capable of slight individual movements and rub against one another, there is wear at the approximal surfaces of contact between adjacent teeth in the arch which tends to be regularly proportional to the amount of occlusal wear.

Occlusal cusps are gradually reduced in height and in due course the occlusal surfaces become flat, or rather cupped out because dentine wears more quickly than enamel. Eventually, in advanced age, the crowns become destroyed and the teeth are lost through abscesses and other *sequelae* of excessive wear. However, the nature of the diet of most of us is such that wear of the teeth is not nearly as great as this. In archaic populations, on the other hand, tooth wear probably provides the best indicator of age if it can be used systematically.

An example can be drawn from the remains of about 200 Anglo-Saxon of about 200 A.D. (Miles, 1962). The material ranged from complete skulls to fragments only of the jaws. About 30 were young enough for their ages to be assessed from the stage of tooth development. Tooth wear in this young group showed an orderly progression with advancing age, and second molars could be matched for wear against first molars which had been functional for more or less the same period of time. From this it seemed that it takes a little longer for a second molar to wear to the same extent as a first molar; in fact there is a gradient of rate of wear between the three molars. This has been commented on by other workers (Murphy, 1959; Pal, 1971). I estimated that this gradient could be expressed as $6 : 6 \cdot 5 : 7$; in other words, it takes 7 years for the third molar to show the same amount of wear as the first molar does in 6 years. This formula was applied in the calculations of age from tooth wear about to be described.

On the group of 30 dentitions of ages up to about 20 years, which could be regarded as of "known age", it was possible to base a system of gradual extrapolation with the assumption that the rate of wear, having been shown to be regular or constant during youth, would remain more or less so during later life. First, the ages of those dentitions which showed only slightly greater wear than those of the "known age" group were assessed by a careful comparison of the wear of their second and third molars with first and second molar wear of those of "known age". Groups of dentitions were then selected which showed still greater degrees of wear and their wear compared with that of those already estimated, making appropriate adjustments with the gradient formula, until eventually those of the 20 to 30-year group, and in due course even later ages, were being used for comparison in the same way that those of the "known age" had been.

Figure 3 illustrates the principle. The 18-year-old specimen was estimated to be so because M_3 was emerging and its root was not completely formed. The M_1, having begun to function at 6 years, shows 12 years of wear and M_2, having begun to function at 12 years, shows 6 years of wear. The other dentitions depicted have been selected as examples of extrapolation derived from the molar-tooth wear of the 18-year-old one.

It is evident that, with the further extension of the system, its reliability would tend to decrease. When those dentitions with really advanced wear and associated tooth loss were reached, subjective adjustments for this were made on the basis that it would tend to increase the rate of wear of those teeth that remained.

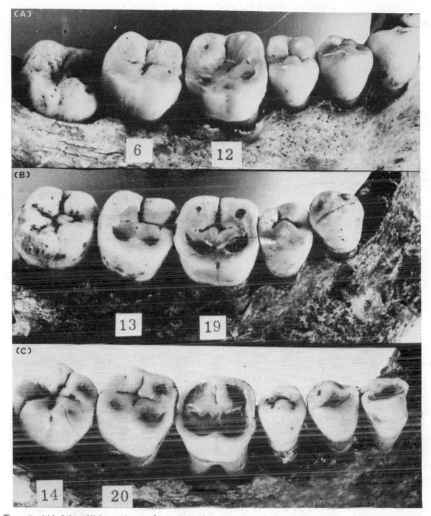

Fig. 3. (A) Mandible estimated, mainly from state of eruption of M_3, to be aged about 18 years. (B) Mandible of which M_2 shows degree of wear similar to M_1 in 18-year-old specimen. Hence assessed to be that of 25-year-old individual. (C) Mandible of which M_3 shows degree of wear comparable to M_2 at 25 years and M_1 at 18 years. Hence estimated to be aged about 32 years. (Reproduced by permission from Miles, 1962).

The system can only be applied, and it has been by others (Woo and Bai, 1965; J. A. Hopson, personal communication), to groups of skulls in which there is a considerable amount of tooth wear and which contain a large enough young group of which the ages can be estimated from their growing dentitions.

Changes other than wear occur in teeth with advancing age. Gustafson (1966) has described six such changes (Fig. 4) and uses them as the basis of a system for assessing age. The gum margin tends to recede with age, the basis of the saying "getting long in the tooth". Whether this recession is a physiological ageing process or the product of the chronic gum inflammation that is practically universal is not important in the present context. The pulp gets

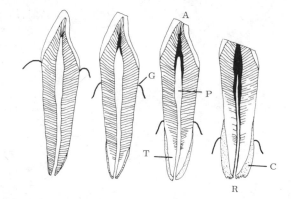

Fig. 4. Diagrammatic representation of sections of teeth of increasing age from left to right, derived from Johanson (1971). A = attrition; P = pulp, the size of which is dimished by continued deposition of dentine (in black); G = gum margin; T = translucency; C = cementum; R = resorption.

smaller with age as a result of deposition of dentine, partly in response to tooth wear. Cementum on the root surface gets thicker, and areas of resorption, either of the original root surface or of later-formed cementum, tend to accumulate with age.

Of special importance is a process of mineralization of the contents of the dentinal tubules which leads to translucency of the dentine and seems to begin at the root apex, at about 30 years of age. This translucency extends gradually towards the crown of the tooth and, in really advanced age, may involve the greater part of the root (Fig. 5).

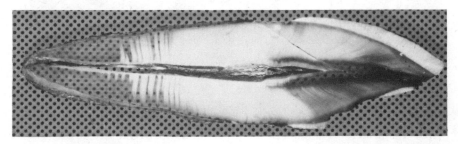

Fig. 5. Longitudinal ground section of an incisor of a man aged 52 years. × 4. (Reproduced by permission from Miles, 1963b).

In a Gustafson system, each of these six features is scored subjectively on a 0–3 scale and the total score is read off on a regression line prepared from the total scores for teeth of known age. The disadvantage of the system is that it assumes that all the six factors are equally correlated with age, whereas they are not. Figure 6 shows the correlation coefficients for the various features and the intercorrelations between them for 200 incisors of known

	AGE	T_{mm}	T	A	G	P	C	R
AGE	I							
TRANSLUCENCY in mm	+0·69	I						
TRANSLUCENCY VALUES	+0·70	+0·87	I					
ATTRITION VALUES	+0·58	+0·47	+0·52	I				
GINGIVAL VALUES	+0·64	+0·55	+0·62	+0·54	I			
PULP VALUES	+0·58	+0·54	+0·57	+0·47	+0·46	I		
CEMENTUM VALUES	+0·59	+0·63	+0·67	+0·40	+0·39	+0·55	I	
RESORPTION VALUES	+0·28	+0·29	+0·29	+0·21	+0·29	+0·31	+0·18	I

FIG. 6. The correlation coefficients between known age for 200 incisors and the scores for the six Gustafson criteria and for the measured amount of translucency are given in the left-hand column. The intercorrelations between the various criteria are given in the other columns.

age. Only root translucency with a correlation coefficient of about 0·7 and 0·87 is reassuringly high. The values for root resorption, by contrast, are so low that it can contribute little in value to the system.

Johanson (1971) has produced figures very similar to these and has gone much further, improving the Gustafson system in two ways: by enlarging the scale of points from 0–3 to 0–6 and by using a multiple regression line which, in effect, is a formula which gives greater weight to those criteria which are highly correlated with age and less to those which are less well correlated.

It is inappropriate here to discuss these matters in a forensic context but it will be evident that those who use these methods, involving as they do, subjective judgements, need to keep in constant practice, which is rarely possible. There could be large advances if some form of measurement could be substituted for a ranking system. Unfortunately a measuring method only appears to be practicable for root translucency and cementum thickness.

Figure 5 depicts a moderately typical example of root translucency and, although obviously measurement on a millimetre scale with eye-piece graticule or measuring microscope, or even with an ordinary micrometer (Bang and Ramm, 1970), could only be approximate and would involve making additions for the more or less isolated zones of translucency, it is possible to obtain worthwhile measurements on ground sections cut as far as possible in to the central long axis of the root. Plane of section appears to be more important than thinness of section or its standardization. Sections must, however, be mounted in water; if they are dehydrated and mounted in Canada balsam, the balsam enters the patent tubules of the dentine and renders all the dentine about equally translucent.

These relatively crude measurements of translucency show a quite close correlation with age (Fig. 7), though there are many measurements which

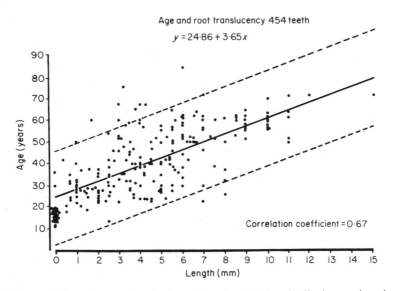

FIG. 7. The relation of age to length of translucent root in longitudinal ground sections of 454 human teeth.
——————— (solid line) calculated regression line.
— — — — (broken line) 95% confidence limits.

fall outside the 95% confidence limits. Not only is no great experience required to prepare and measure ground sections in this way, but it would seem not absolutely necessary for every worker to prepare his own regression line.

The thickness of cementum is measurable. Zander and Hürzeler (1958) used an optical projection method on transverse sections of teeth and it should be possible to use a similar method on longitudinal sections to obtain a measurement of the mean thickness of cementum in the selected plane or section.

Clearly there is room for further investigation into the use of teeth as indicators of age and for refinements of the methodology. A moderate amount is known about change in the chemical composition of the dental tissues with age; for example, the enamel surface takes up ions from the saliva and from food so that the surface layers of enamel after the passage of years become enriched in various elements such as fluorine, iron, lead and zinc (Brudevold and Söremark, 1967). There would seem to be possibilities in this of some sort of age indicator, but much more data would need to be collected, very laboriously, before this became a practical piece of methodology.

REFERENCES

BAMBACH, M., SARACCI, R. and YOUNG, H. B. (1973). Emergence of deciduous teeth in Tunisian children in relation to sex and social class. *Hum. Biol.* **45**, 435–444.

BANG, G. and RAMM, E. (1970). Determination of age in humans from root dentin transparency. *Acta odont. scand.* **1**, 3–35.

BILLEWICZ, W. Z., THOMSON, A. M., BABER, F. M. and FIELD, C. E. (1973). The development of primary teeth in Chinese (Hong Kong) children. *Hum. Biol.* **45**, 229–241.

BRUDEVOLD, F. and SÖREMARK, R. (1967). Chemistry of the mineral phase of enamel. *In* "Structural and Chemical Organization of Teeth" (Miles, A. E. W. ed.), Vol. II, pp. 247–277. Academic Press, London and New York.

DEMIRJIAN, A., GOLDSTEIN, H. and TANNER, J. M. (1973). A new system of dental age assessment. *Hum. Biol.* **45**, 211–227.

EVELETH, P. B. (1966). Eruption of permanent dentition and menarche of American children living in the tropics. *Hum. Biol.* **38**, 60–70.

EVELETH, P. B. and DE SOUZA FREITAS, J. A. (1969). Tooth eruption and menarch of Brazilian-born children of Japanese ancestry. *Hum. Biol.* **41**, 176–184.

FRIEDLAENDER, J. S. and BAILIT, H. L. (1969). Eruption times of the deciduous and permanent teeth of natives on Bougainville Island, territory of New Guinea: A study of racial variation. *Hum. Biol.* **41**, 51–65.

GARN, S. M., NAGY, J. M., SANDUSKY, S. T. and TROWBRIDGE, F. (1973a). Economic impact on tooth emergence. *Am. J. phys. Anthrop.* **39**, 233–238.

GARN, S. M., SANDUSKY, S. T., NAGY, J. M. and TROWBRIDGE, F. L. (1973b). Negro-Caucasoid differences in permanent tooth emergence at a constant income level. *Archs oral Biol.* **18**, 609–615.

GUSTAFSON, G. (1966). "Forensic Odontology". Staples Press, London.

GUSTAFSON, G. and KOCH, G. (1974). Age estimation up to 16 years of age based on dental development. *Odont. Revy.* **3**, 1–10.

HOUPT, M. I. ADU-AYEE, S. and GRAINGER, R. M. (1967). Eruption times of permanent teeth in the Brong Ahafo Region of Ghana. *Am. J. Orthod.* **53**, 95–99.

INFANTE, P. F. (1974). Sex differences in the chronology of deciduous tooth emergence in white and black children. *J. dent. Res.* **53**, 418–421.

ISRAEL, H. and LEWIS, A. B. (1971). Radiographically determined linear permanent tooth growth from age 6 years. *J. dent. Res.* **40**, 334–342.

JOHANSON, G. (1971). Age determinations from human teeth. *Odont. Revy.* **22**, supplement, 21.

KAUL, S., SAINI, S. and SAXENA, B. (1975). Emergence of permanent teeth in school-children in Chandigarh, India. *Archs oral Biol.* **20**, 587–593.

LEE, M. M. C., LOW, W. D. and CHANG, K. S. F. (1965). Eruption of the permanent dentition of Southern Chinese children in Hong Kong. *Archs oral Biol.* **10**, 849–861.

MILES, A. E. W. (1958). The assessment of age from the dentition. *Proc. R. Soc. Med.* **51**, 1057–1060.

MILES, A. E. W. (1962). Assessment of the ages of a population of Anglo-Saxons from their dentitions. *Proc. R. Soc. Med.* **55**, 881–886.

MILES, A. E. W. (1963a). Dentition in the estimation of age. *J. Dent. Res.* **42**, 255–263.

MILES, A. E. W. (1963b). The dentition in the assessment of individual age in skeletal material. *In* "Dental Anthropology" (Brothwell, D. R., ed.), pp. 191–209 Pergamon Press, Oxford.

MOORREES, C. F. A., FANNING, E. A. and HUNT, E. E. JR. (1963). Age variation of formation stages for ten permanent teeth. *J. dent. Res.* **42**, 1490–1502.

MURPHY, T. (1959). Gradients of dentine exposure in human tooth attrition. *Am. J. phys. Anthrop.* **17**, 179–186.

PAL, A. (1971). Gradients of dentine exposure in human molars. *J. Ind. anthrop. Soc.* **6**, 67–73.

SCHOUR, I. and MASSLER, M. (1941). The development of the human dentition. *J. Am. dent. Ass.* **28**, 1153–1160.

WOO, J.-K. and BAI, H.-Y. (1965). Attrition of molar teeth in relation to age in Northern Chinese skulls. *Vertebrata palasiatica, Peking* **9**, 217–222. In Chinese, with English summary.

ZANDER, H. A. and HÜRZELER, B. (1958). Continuous cementum apposition. *J. dent. Res.* **37**, 1035–1044.

28. Molar Attrition in Medieval Danes

DOROTHY A. LUNT

University of Glasgow Dental School, Glasgow, Scotland

INTRODUCTION

An aspect of dental attrition which has not yet been fully investigated is the extent to which the rate of attrition varies from one population to another. If the teeth of a modern population consuming a soft and highly refined diet are compared with those of a people living under so-called "primitive" or natural conditions, the difference in rate of attrition is obvious. Studies of American Indians from the southwestern United States and Mexico (Molnar, 1971) and of Natufians (Smith, 1972) suggest that there are also significant differences in attrition rates between closely related population subgroups, all subsisting on an unrefined diet, and that these differences may be related to variations in the diet.

What remains to be established is whether such differences can be demonstrated in other parts of the world, particularly in Europe; whether populations living in different areas but consuming a similar type of unrefined diet will show a similar rate of attrition; and what degree of variation exists in the attrition rates of populations subsisting on different types of diet.

In order to study European populations whose diet was unrefined, it is necessary to turn to skeletal material of prehistoric and medieval periods. This has the disadvantage that usually neither the sex nor the age of an individual skull is known. In many cases the sex may be assessed with moderate accuracy from various features of the skeleton. Age assessment is much more difficult: cranial suture closure, which has often been used, is unreliable. At present the exact age of a person at death cannot be deduced by examination of the skeleton.

Since attrition is related to the age of an individual, comparison between the absolute amounts of attrition observed in two populations is meaningless unless the age-distribution of the two populations is similar, and this cannot be established in most skeletal collections. Other methods have therefore been devised in order to compare rates of attrition in different populations. Gradients of attrition have been used for this purpose, with the differences in attrition between pairs of teeth forming the basis of comparison, instead of absolute amounts of attrition.

A major difficulty in the anthropological study of attrition has been the establishment of a suitable scale on which it may be graded. Broca had published the first scale of attrition by 1879, and since then there have been several variants of his system (e.g. Davies and Pedersen, 1955; McCombie, 1957; Devoto *et al.*, 1971). All of these methods employ a four, five or six point scale, whose steps are so large that they do not permit detailed assessment of the progress of attrition. In addition, in some cases one or more of the criteria used are highly subjective. In other studies the scale has been applied in a different manner (Smith, 1972), or additional aspects of attrition have been included (Molnar, 1971).

In 1959, Murphy introduced a more elaborate scale for the assessment of molar attrition. This scale is based on the exposure of dentine in individual molar cusps and has a greater number of steps, which allows much finer grading of attrition over part of the total attrition range. The method has the further advantage of being entirely objective.

METHODS
Grades of Attrition

The method of recording attrition used in the present study was that of Murphy (1959a, b). The grades of attrition are illustrated diagrammatically in Fig. 1. Each molar was considered to consist of four major cusps and the

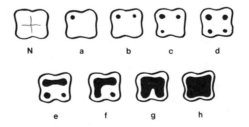

FIG. 1. Diagrammatic representation of the nine grades of attrition. N = enamel facets, no dentine exposure. *a–d* = dentine exposure in isolated areas on cusps. *e–h* = coalescence of exposed dentine areas.

small distal cusp which may be present on first and third mandibular molars was ignored. The letter N represented the stage of attrition with enamel facets only, and no exposure of dentine. Dentine exposure appeared first as isolated patches at the tips of the cusps, and the successive stages were indicated by the letters *a–d*. This was followed by progressive coalescence of the exposed areas of dentine, indicated by the letters *e–h*. At stage *g* all the dentine areas had coalesced but there was still an island or peninsula of enamel, while at stage *h* the entire occlusal surface was formed by dentine, surrounded by a rim of enamel.

Once stage *h* had been reached, further attrition could not be graded by this method. It should be realized that some stages on this attrition scale may occupy quite a long period, and that obvious differences in degree of attrition may be observed between teeth which have to be classified under the same letter (Fig. 2). Further, the amount of attrition between one grade and the

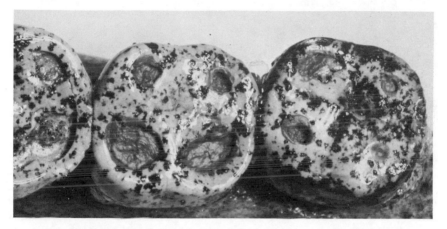

Fig. 2. Left side of mandible. Both second and third molars must be assigned to attrition grade *d* though there is an obvious difference in the amounts of wear they have undergone. (The teeth in this specimen were affected by a mottled black post-mortem deposit, and the exposed areas of dentine have been painted in order to distinguish them.)

next is not necessarily the same throughout. However, any further subdivision of the steps on this scale would have been purely subjective and therefore was not attempted.

Gradients of Attrition

When the grades of attrition had been assessed, gradients of attrition were calculated, either between pairs of molars in the same quadrant (intermolar gradients) or between pairs of molars in opposing jaws (interjaw gradients), according to the method of Murphy (1959b). The gradient was recorded as the number of stages on the attrition scale between the two teeth. The gradient was negative if the first tooth showed a greater degree of attrition than the second tooth, and positive if the attrition of the second tooth was greater than that of the first. In the case of interjaw gradients, the maxillary tooth was considered as the first member of the pair. An example is shown in Fig. 3.

Statistics

In making comparisons between population groups, it is necessary to use

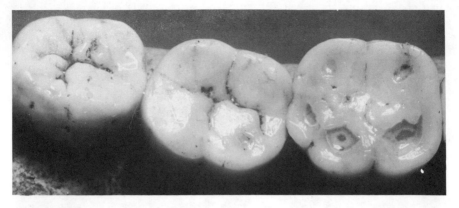

FIG. 3. Right side of mandible. The first molar is in grade d and the second molar in grade a: the gradient M_1–M_2 is therefore -3. With the third molar in grade N, the gradient M_2–M_3 is -1, and the overall gradient M_1–M_3 is -4.

some form of statistical preparation of the data, and in this type of study care must be exercised in the selection of statistical methods. Neither grades nor gradients of attrition are measured on an interval scale and therefore the use of parametric statistical methods is not appropriate. The data is at best measured on an ordinal scale, and non-parametric tests in the form of ranking tests should be employed. The methods used in the present study were the Wilcoxon matched-pairs signed-ranks test and the Mann–Whitney U test.

MATERIAL

The study was carried out on two collections of medieval skeletons from Denmark, one from the monastery graveyard at Aebelholt, the other from the cemetery of the leper hospital in Naestved. Both burial places were in use between the mid thirteenth and mid sixteenth centuries, but individual skeletons could not be more closely dated.

Almost equal numbers of male and female skeletons were recovered during the excavations at Aebelholt. This shows that not only the monks but also members of the local lay population were buried there. The leper hospital at Naestved also served a relatively restricted area, and the skeletons from the two sites may be considered to be reasonably representative of the local Danish population in the late Middle Ages. It is not known whether the sites differed with respect to the socio-economic class of the persons buried there. (For further details of the material, see Møller-Christensen, 1953, 1958; Lunt, 1969.)

The criteria initially adopted in selecting skulls for study were as follows. Firstly, the skull must have all six permanent molars present and in normal function and occlusion on at least one side. Secondly, if a skull had a normal complement of molars on one side, but data for the other side were lacking as the result of *in vivo* loss of teeth, or as the result of severe caries, then this skull was excluded since these conditions might cause abnormal masticatory patterns and perhaps abnormal attrition on the intact side.

Differences in Attrition on Right and Left Sides

The first observation was that a considerable degree of asymmetry often occurred in attrition, between right and left sides of the jaw. This contrasted with the statement by Murphy (1959b) that in his Australian Aborigine dentitions, right and left sides were "largely mirror images of one another" in respect of the degree of attrition.

The observed right–left differences were tested for statistical significance, using the Wilcoxon matched-pairs signed-ranks test. As expected, no significant difference was observed, i.e. attrition was not consistently greater on one side than on the other.

Because of the considerable degree of asymmetry observed in some individuals, however, it was decided to use data from the left side only in further comparisons, and not to substitute data from the right side in cases where the left side was incomplete.

Sex Distribution of Skulls in Study

Using the selection criteria outlined above, some 15% of the total adult skeletal material proved suitable for further study. The skeletons had already been sexed as far as possible, and the sex distribution of the skulls used in the present study is shown in Table I. There were more males than females in the Aebelholt group, while the balance was slightly in favour of the females in the Naestved group.

TABLE I. Sex distribution of skulls.

	Males	Females	Sex unknown	Total
Aebelholt	38	24	16	78
Naestved	21	26	8	55
Total	59	50	24	133

DISTRIBUTION OF ATTRITION IN MEDIEVAL DANES

Further study of attrition in the medieval Danes was carried out by comparing frequency distributions of the data, using ranking tests.

Comparison of Grades of Attrition in Maxilla and Mandible

Examination of the data for the medieval Danes showed that in both population groups and both sexes there was a distinct trend towards more advanced attrition in the mandibular teeth than in the maxillary teeth of the same individual.

The Wilcoxon matched-pairs signed-ranks test was applied to the data, and showed that the difference was statistically significant in most instances (Table II). The most highly significant differences were to be found in the second molars throughout.

Murphy (1959b) also found that, in the Australian Aborigines, attrition of mandibular molars was usually more advanced than that of maxillary molars.

TABLE II. Comparison of grades of attrition
in mandibular and maxillary teeth.

	n	M^1 vs. M_1	M^2 vs. M_2	M^3 vs. M_3
Aebelholt males	38	N.S.	$P < 0·02$	$P < 0·05$
Aebelholt females	24	N.S.	$P < 0·01$	N.S.
Naestved males	21	$P < 0·05$	$P < 0·01$	$P < 0·05$
Naestved females	26	$P < 0·05$	$P < 0·01$	$P < 0·02$

N.S. = no significant difference.

Sex Comparison of Grades and Gradients of Attrition

The data were next tested for possible differences in attrition between the sexes, using the Mann–Whitney U test. First, the distribution of grades of attrition was examined. No significant differences in the distribution of grades of attrition were observed between males and females of the Aebelholt group, nor between males and females of the Naestved group, nor when the population subgroups were combined (Table III).

The process was repeated using gradients of attrition, since slight variations in attrition of adjacent teeth, if occurring in opposite directions in the sexes, might produce a significant difference in the gradients. No significant sex differences were observed in the intermolar gradients of attrition when the Aebelholt and Naestved material was treated separately. But when the two groups were combined, the gradients between M_1 and M_2 were significantly smaller in the females than in the males (Table III).

Interjaw gradients showed no significant differences between males and females (Table III).

One significant difference in the mandibular intermolar gradients does not indicate any general tendency towards differences in attrition between the sexes. Caution must be exercised in interpreting these data because of the

TABLE. III. Comparison of grades and gradients
of attrition in males and in females.

	Aebelholt	Naestved	Aebelholt + Naestved
Grades of attrition			
M^1	N.S.	N.S.	N.S.
M^2	N.S.	N.S.	N.S.
M^3	N.S.	N.S.	N.S.
M_1	N.S.	N.S.	N.S.
M_2	N.S.	N.S.	N.S.
M_3	N.S.	N.S.	N.S.
Intermolar gradients			
M^1–M^2	N.S.	N.S.	N.S.
M^2–M^3	N.S.	N.S.	N.S.
M^1–M^3	N.S.	N.S.	N.S.
M_1–M_2	N.S.	N.S.	$P < 0.01$
M_2–M_3	N.S.	N.S.	N.S.
M_1–M_3	N.S.	N.S.	N.S.
Interjaw gradients			
M^1 M_1	N.S.	N.S.	N.S.
M^2–M_2	N.S.	N.S.	N.S.
M^3–M_3	N.S.	N.S.	N.S.

N.S. = no significant difference.

age-related nature of attrition, and the lack of information concerning individual age in the Danish skulls. Had there been consistently significant differences in the same direction between the sexes, it would have been impossible to say whether these were due to differences in the age distribution of males and females, or whether they were due to differences in the rates of attrition in the sexes. Lack of statistical significance in the results indicates either that there are real differences between the sexes in both age distribution and rate of attrition and that these differences are opposite and equal, or that there are no real differences either in age distribution or in rate of attrition. The latter seems the more probable explanation.

Group Comparison of Grades and Gradients of Attrition

Differences in grades and gradients of attrition between the population subgroups from Aebelholt and Naestved were next evaluated. The Mann–Whitney U tests showed that there were no significant differences between these groups in the distribution of grades of attrition, either when males and

TABLE IV. Comparison of grades and gradients of attrition
in Aebelholt and in Naestved subgroups.

	Males	Females	Males + Females
Grades of attrition			
M^1	N.S.	N.S.	N.S.
M^2	N.S.	N.S.	N.S.
M^3	N.S.	N.S.	N.S.
M_1	N.S.	N.S.	N.S.
M_2	N.S.	N.S.	N.S.
M_3	N.S.	N.S.	N.S.
Intermolar gradients			
M^1–M^2	N.S.	N.S.	N.S.
M^2–M^3	N.S.	N.S.	N.S.
M^1–M^3	N.S.	N.S.	N.S.
M_1–M_2	N.S.	N.S.	N.S.
M_2–M_3	N.S.	N.S.	N.S.
M_1–M_3	N.S.	N.S.	N.S.
Interjaw gradients			
M^1–M_1	N.S.	N.S.	N.S.
M^2–M_2	N.S.	$P < 0.05$	N.S.
M^3–M_3	N.S.	N.S.	N.S.

N.S. = no significant difference.

females were compared separately, or when all the material in each group
was pooled; this of course allowed inclusion of the unsexed skulls (Table IV).

Nor were there significant differences between the groups as far as the
intermolar gradients were concerned (Table IV).

The females of the two groups showed one significant difference, i.e. in
the interjaw gradient between the second molars. There was no significant
difference in this gradient between the males of the two groups, and when
the skulls of both sexes were pooled, the difference between the females was
masked (Table IV).

One significant difference in interjaw gradients in the females does not
allow of any general hypothesis of differences in attrition between the Aebelholt and Naestved subgroups, and it may be suggested that the age distribution of the skulls and the rate of attrition are similar in the two groups.

Frequency Distribution of Attrition Data in Danes

Since there were no major differences between the sexes and none between
the population subgroups, all the data could be combined to provide overall

frequency distributions of grades and gradients of attrition in the medieval Danes (Tables V, VI and VII; Figs 4, 5 and 6).

The frequency distributions of grades of attrition in the first molars showed peaks at grade d (Fig. 4). Unless this stage was generally reached at an age which had an unusually high mortality rate, this suggests that the time taken for a tooth to pass from grade d to grade e may have been greater than the time taken for the phase c to d.

Some 30–40% of second molars were still in grade N, and roughly 70% of third molars were at this stage (Fig. 4).

Of the intermolar gradients, those between the second and third molars in both jaws showed peaks at zero gradient (Fig. 5). The gradients between first and second molars, and between first and third molars were largely negative, with peaks at -3 and -4. Very few positive gradients were observed, i.e. it was very seldom that a molar showed a more advanced degree of attrition than those anterior to it in the arch.

The interjaw gradients showed peaks at zero gradient, but also displayed a relatively high proportion of positive gradients and few negative gradients (Fig. 6). This bore out the finding, already shown to be statistically significant by the Wilcoxon test, that mandibular teeth often showed a greater degree of attrition than their maxillary counterparts.

COMPARISON OF MEDIEVAL DANES WITH OTHER POPULATIONS

It would have been interesting to compare the findings on attrition in the medieval Danes with the results published for Anglo-Saxon and nineteenth century English skulls by Lavelle (1970) who also used the Murphy system of grading dentine exposure. However, grade N of attrition was not used by Lavelle, and this implies that an additional criterion was employed in the selection of skulls: that all molars including third molars must have reached the stage of dentine exposure. Thus only the more advanced stages of attrition have been studied by Lavelle, and his results are not comparable with those obtained for the medieval Danes. Furthermore, some of the figures given by Lavelle in his table of gradients do not appear to be consistent with the data provided for grades of attrition.

Only the results published by Murphy (1959b) for Australian Aborigines appear to be comparable with the data from the present study. Some of the findings for the Australian Aborigines are similar to those for the medieval Danes: a very high proportion of intermolar gradients are negative, and a high proportion of interjaw gradients are positive in both groups.

More detailed comparisons pose certain problems. Murphy (1959b) and Lavelle (1970) compared gradients of attrition by calculation and analysis of mean gradients, a procedure which is statistically unsound since it involves parametric statistical methods.

The frequency distributions of the gradients of attrition in different populations could be compared using the Mann–Whitney U test, but this procedure also may be unsound, particularly when the distribution of grades of attri-

TABLE V. Frequency distribution of grades of attrition in medieval Danes.

Grade	Maxilla						Mandible					
	M^1		M^2		M^3		M_1		M_2		M_3	
	n	%	n	%	n	%	n	%	n	%	n	%
N	3	2·3	52	39·1	104	78·1	0	0	41	30·8	86	64·6
a	6	4·5	38	28·6	16	12·0	2	1·5	17	12·8	17	12·8
b	13	9·8	21	15·7	3	2·3	7	5·3	18	13·5	8	6·0
c	16	12·0	8	6·0	2	1·5	12	9·0	17	12·8	7	5·3
d	43	32·3	2	1·5	0	0	54	40·6	20	15·0	6	4·5
e	15	11·3	5	3·8	6	4·5	18	13·5	5	3·8	4	3·0
f	13	9·8	4	3·0	1	0·8	12	9·0	8	6·0	2	1·5
g	9	6·7	1	0·8	0	0	15	11·3	3	2·3	1	0·8
h	15	11·3	2	1·5	1	0·8	13	9·8	4	3·0	2	1·5

TABLE VI. Frequency distribution of intermolar gradients in medieval Danes.

Gradient	Maxilla						Mandible					
	M^1–M^2		M^2–M^3		M^1–M^3		M_1–M_2		M_2–M_3		M_1–M_3	
	n	%	n	%	n	%	n	%	n	%	n	%
−8	0	0	0	0	5	3·8	0	0	0	0	1	0·8
−7	3	2·3	0	0	8	6·0	0	0	0	0	5	3·8
−6	4	3·0	2	1·5	8	6·0	1	0·8	2	1·5	9	6·7
−5	11	8·3	1	0·8	22	16·5	3	2·3	2	1·5	15	11·3
−4	32	24·0	2	1·5	38	28·6	33	24·8	12	9·0	59	44·3
−3	37	27·8	5	3·8	24	18·0	30	22·5	12	9·0	22	16·5
−2	26	19·5	18	13·5	16	12·0	34	25·5	23	17·3	14	10·5
−1	13	9·8	40	30·0	7	5·3	19	14·3	30	22·5	6	4·5
0	7	5·3	64	48·1	4	3·0	12	9·0	48	36·1	1	0·8
+1	0	0	0	0	1	0·8	1	0·8	3	2·3	0	0
+2	0	0	0	0	0	0	0	0	1	0·8	1	0·8
+3	0	0	0	0	0	0	0	0	0	0	0	0
+4	0	0	1	0·8	0	0	0	0	0	0	0	0

TABLE VII. Frequency distribution of interjaw gradients
in medieval Danes.

Gradient	M^1–M_1		M^2–M_2		M^3–M_3	
	n	%	n	%	n	%
−3	4	3·0	0	0	0	0
−2	5	3·8	2	1·5	2	1·5
−1	8	6·0	8	6·0	3	2·3
0	62	46·6	56	42·1	92	69·1
+1	32	24·0	27	20·3	18	13·5
+2	17	12·8	20	15·0	9	6·7
+3	5	3·8	15	11·3	5	3·8
+4	0	0	3	2·3	3	2·3
+5	0	0	0	0	1	0·8
+6	0	0	2	1·5	0	0

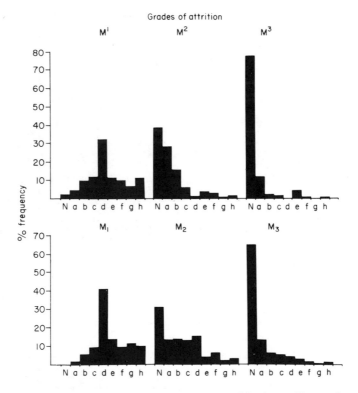

FIG. 4. Percentage frequency distributions of grades of attrition in maxillary and mandibular molars of medieval Danes.

Intermolar gradients of attrition

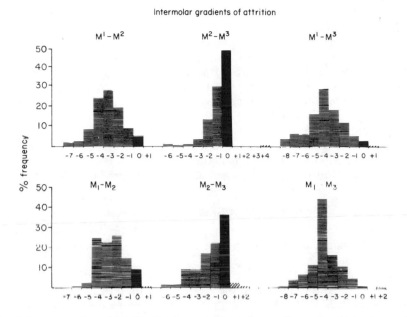

FIG. 5. Percentage frequency distributions of intermolar gradients of attrition in maxilla and mandible of medieval Danes.

Interjaw gradients of attrition

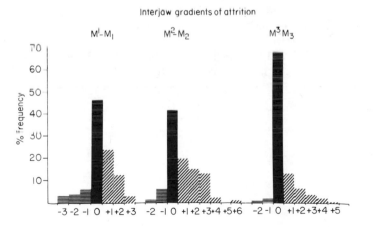

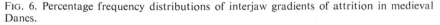

FIG. 6. Percentage frequency distributions of interjaw gradients of attrition in medieval Danes.

tion in one or other population is unknown. When comparison of frequency distributions is carried out using ranking tests, it is assumed that a gradient of, say, 3 always represents a greater difference in attrition between two molars than does a gradient of 2. But so little is known about the amount of attrition involved in passing from one grade to the next, that this simple assumption about gradients may not be correct: e.g. a gradient of 2 between grades *e* and *g* might represent a greater difference in attrition than a gradient of 3 between grades *a* and *d*.

If comparisons are made between two populations in which the proportion of high and low grades of attrition varies markedly as the result of differences in the age-distribution of the populations, then the use of simple frequency distributions of attrition gradients could lead to errors in the assessment of attrition rates.

Grade-related Gradients of Attrition

I should therefore like to suggest that a more realistic comparison between populations might be achieved by the use of gradients related to the grade of attrition of one of the teeth, preferably the first molar.

For the medieval Danes, the frequency distributions of the intermolar gradients of attrition, related to the grade of attrition of the first molar, are shown in Tables VIII–XI. It should perhaps be pointed out here that it is not strictly necessary to calculate attrition gradients in order to set out the data in this way: the same tables would result if the grades of attrition for the first molar were plotted against the grades of attrition for the second molar or for the third molar. However, if gradients have already been calculated, it is less confusing if grades are used on one coordinate and gradients on the other.

The gradients between first and third molars (M^1–M^3 and M_1–M_3) were naturally the largest and showed the widest distribution (Tables VIII and IX). The diagonal line of figures within each table represents the maximum

TABLE VIII. Distribution of gradients M^1–M^3 related to the grade of attrition of M^1.

Stage of M^1	Gradient M^1–M^3											
	-8	-7	-6	-5	-4	-3	-2	-1	0	$+1$	$+2$	Total
N									3			3
a							6					6
b						13						13
c					16							16
d				37	4	1				1		43
e			14	1								15
f		5	6		1		1					13
g	5	2	1			1						9
h	5	3	1	1		3	1		1			15
Total	5	8	8	22	38	24	16	7	4	1		133

TABLE IX. Distribution of gradients M_1–M_3 related to the grade of attrition of M_1.

Stage of M_1	Gradient M_1–M_3											
	-8	-7	-6	-5	-4	-3	-2	-1	0	$+1$	$+2$	Total
N												
a								2				2
b							7					7
c						12						12
d					48	3	2	1				54
e				11	3	1	2	1				18
f			3	2	3	2		1			1	12
g		2	6	2	2	2	1					15
h	1	3			3	2	2	1	1			13
Total	1	5	9	15	59	22	14	6	1		1	133

TABLE X. Distribution of gradients M^1 M^2 related to the grade of attrition of M^1.

Stage of M^1	Gradient M^1–M^2											
	-8	-7	-6	-5	-4	-3	-2	-1	0	$+1$	$+2$	Total
N									3			3
a								6				6
b							12	1				13
c						10	5	1				16
d					19	17	4	1	2			43
e				1	6	7	1					15
f				5	5	1		2				13
g		1	2	2	2		1	1				9
h		2	2	3		2	3	1	2			15
Total		3	4	11	32	37	26	13	7			133

possible gradient at any given stage, i.e. when the third molar is still at grade *N*. In the maxilla (Table VIII), maximum gradients were observed up to grade *c* of the first molar, and it was only when the first molar reached grade *d* that some gradients fell below the maximum, i.e. dentine was now being exposed in some third molars. With advancing attrition of the first molar, there was a tendency for attrition gradients to drop further below the maximum as wear of the third molar increased, but at grades *f*, *g* and *h* of the first molar there were still fairly high proportions of maximum gradients. Attrition thus exhibits a considerable degree of variability especially in the more advanced stages and cannot be a reliable indication of the age of an individual.

TABLE XI. Distribution of gradients M_1–M_2 related to the grade of attrition of M_1.

Stage of M_1	Gradient M_1–M_2											Total
	−8	−7	−6	−5	−4	−3	−2	−1	0	+1	+2	
N												
a								2				2
b							6			1		7
c						8	4					12
d					25	11	7	8	3			54
e					1	3	6	8				18
f					5	2	2	1	2			12
g			1	3		5	3		3			15
h					2	1	6		4			13
Total			1	3	33	30	34	19	12	1		133

In the mandible the situation was similar (Table IX) with gradients below the maximum appearing at grade d of the first molar. At grades f, g and h of the first molar, a slightly smaller proportion of gradients reached the maximum, i.e. wear of the mandibular third molars was more rapid than that of the maxillary third molars.

A similar pattern was seen in the distribution of the gradients between first and second molars (Tables X and XI). By grade b of the first maxillary molar, dentine exposure could occasionally be observed in the second molar (Table X), and by grade d of the first molar a large proportion of second molars showed dentine exposure. With the more advanced grades of attrition of the first molar, few maximum gradients were observed.

This was even more marked in the mandible (Table XI), showing that the rate of attrition of mandibular second molars was more rapid than that of maxillary second molars.

One disadvantage of this method is that it requires a fairly large quantity of data. The Danish material was not sufficient to allow comparisons between males and females or between the Aebelholt and Naestved subgroups to be carried out by means of grade-related gradients. But if data for other sufficiently large population groups were presented in the same way, it would be possible to make comparisons between the frequency distributions of gradients of attrition at specific grades of first molar attrition, and it should then be possible to establish whether different populations show variations in the progress of attrition. This could be particularly valuable where the distribution of the grades of attrition is known to be different in two populations.

SUMMARY

Molar attrition has been studied in two skeletal collections of the medieval period from Denmark. Exposure of dentine has been the basic criterion used in the assessment of the degree or grade of attrition. Gradients of attrition have been employed to indicate the relationship between the grades of attrition of different teeth in an individual.

While marked differences in grades of attrition may exist between right and left sides in an individual, the population groups do not show a significantly greater degree of attrition on one side than on the other. However, there is a statistically significant tendency for grades of attrition to be more advanced in mandibular than in maxillary teeth.

There is no consistent difference in the distribution of grades and gradients of attrition, either between males and females, or between the population subgroups.

An attempt has been made to refine the use of attrition gradients by relating them to the grade of attrition of the first molar. When the data for the medieval Danes are displayed in this way, in the form of "grade-related gradients", it is observed that variability of attrition gradients increases with advancing attrition of the first molar. It is suggested that grade-related gradients may prove a more suitable means of investigating possible population differences in the rate of attrition than the methods used previously.

ACKNOWLEDGEMENTS

I wish to thank Rigsantikvar Professor Dr P. V. Glob of the National Museum, Copenhagen and Professor Dr V. Møller-Christensen, Københavns Universitets Medicinsk Historisk Museum, for permission to study the skeletal collections from Aebelholt and Naestved.

I am indebted to Mr A. D. McLaren of the University of Glasgow for advice on statistical problems.

I should also like to thank Mr J. B. Davies and the staff of the Photography Department, University of Glasgow Dental School, for their assistance with the illustrations.

REFERENCES

BROCA, P. (1879). Instructions relatives à l'étude anthropologique du système dentaire. *Bull. Soc. Anthrop. Paris* **2**, 128–152.

DAVIES, T. G. H. and PEDERSEN, P. O. (1955). The degree of attrition of the deciduous teeth and first permanent molars of primitive and urbanised Greenland natives. *Br. dent. J.* **99**, 35–43.

DEVOTO, F. C. H., PERROTTO, B. M. and BELLOTTA, A. R. (1971). Dental attrition in the pre-Columbian population of Tastil (Salta, Argentina). *J. dent. Res.* **50**, 1162–1163.

LAVELLE, C. L. B. (1970). Analysis of attrition in adult human molars. *J. dent. Res.* **49**, 822–828.

LUNT, D. A. (1969). An odontometric study of mediaeval Danes. *Acta. odont. scand.* **27**, suppl. 55.

McCOMBIE, F. (1957). Dental epidemiology in Malaya. I. The problem and a programme of research. *J. Can. dent. Ass.* **23**, 623–632.

MØLLER-CHRISTENSEN, V. (1953). "Ten lepers from Naestved in Denmark". Danish Science Press, Copenhagen.

MØLLER-CHRISTENSEN, V. (1958). "Bogen om Aebelholt kloster" Dansk Videnskabs Forlag, Copenhagen.

MOLNAR, S. (1971). Human tooth wear, tooth function and cultural variability. *Am. J. phys. Anthrop.* **34**, 175–189.

MURPHY, T. (1959a). The changing pattern of dentine exposure in human tooth attrition. *Am. J. phys. Anthrop.* N.S. **17**, 167–178.

MURPHY, T. (1959b). Gradients of dentine exposure in human molar tooth attrition. *Am. J. phys. Anthrop.* N.S. **17**, 179–186.

SMITH, P. (1972). Diet and attrition in the Natufians. *Am. J. phys. Anthrop.* **37**, 233–238.

29. The Use of Teeth for Estimating the Age of Wild Mammals

P. MORRIS

Zoology Department, Royal Holloway College, Egham, Surrey

INTRODUCTION

Age-related changes in an organism may affect growth, maturation, behaviour and taxonomic criteria. They are a vital factor in the analysis of population structures, survival rates and other parameters essential to the formulation of wildlife management programmes. A method of assessing the age of individual animals may provide a valuable insight into many aspects of a species' biology. Studies which disregard the age factor contain a built-in flaw which may well invalidate the whole investigation.

Most age-determination methods originate in studies of man, and were only later applied to wild mammals as the need arose for population analysis and management. Techniques used by the wildlife biologist often seem to lack finesse, but the standards of accuracy to which his laboratory-based, often anthropocentric, colleagues are accustomed are inappropriate yardsticks by which to judge work carried out under difficult conditions in the field.

The student of human-age criteria has the invaluable advantage that his subjects usually know how old they are and have birth certificates to prove it. The wildlife biologist can rarely check his estimates of age, important though these may be. Despite the difficulties, the commercially valuable mammals (especially whales, seals and deer) have been intensively investigated and many of the techniques developed have now been applied to other species. In an earlier paper (Morris, 1972), the major methods of assessing age in mammals were reviewed with particular reference to methodological details, and Spinage (1973) has provided an excellent analysis of the use of teeth for age determination, particularly in African mammals. The present review attempts to incorporate some of the more recent work and wasteful repetition of references cited in these earlier papers has been avoided.

Using teeth to estimate age is not a new idea. The saying "Never look a gift horse in the mouth" (to check its age!) is attributed to St. Jerome of the fifth century, and 300 years earlier still, Pliny the Elder wrote in his second book on natural history a remarkably detailed account of how to age a horse from its teeth. The particular value of teeth for age determination stems partly from their durability, which ensures their availability, even after decomposition or major trauma. In addition, since all age-determination techniques rely upon some persistent sign of the passage of time remaining discernible in the body, teeth are especially helpful since they change constantly and progressively with increasing age. It is useful to consider the various changes that take place in the teeth, as their nature and extent provide the clues we seek in order to assess the age of their owner.

Tooth Eruption and Replacement

A diphyodont dentition is one of the definitive characteristics of mammals. The teeth erupt in an orderly sequence, and in most species (though not all), two or more deciduous teeth may be lost and replaced by elements of the permanent dentition. The sequential loss and replacement of teeth may take place over an extended period and the stage attained is a guide to the age of an animal. An individual's dentition may be checked against known minimum and maximum ages for the replacement or eruption of particular teeth—a simple technique employed by veterinarians, wildlife biologists and anthropologists to make a rough estimate of age.

Even this simple procedure is not universally applicable. In the hedgehog (*Erinaceus europaeus*) for example, tooth replacement is complete within 3 or 4 months—less than 5% of the animal's potential lifespan—and in certain seals, tooth replacement is complete before birth. The eruption sequence is also not constant for all members of the same order (Slaughter *et al.*, 1974).

Some mammals have unusual patterns of tooth replacement which can be very helpful. In the elephants (*Elephas* and *Loxodonta*) each half of each jaw contains only six teeth, at most only two of which are in wear at any one time. As each tooth is worn away it moves forward in the jaw until its posterior remnant is finally lost. Meanwhile the next tooth in the set moves in behind it to assume the role of the main functional molar. This procession of teeth through the jaw continues for most of the 60–80-year lifespan of the elephant and identifying which of its six teeth are actually in wear provides a rough guide to age. Laws (1966) and Sikes (1966, 1968) have refined the technique using the transverse lamellae of which the teeth are comprised as the basis for a more precise description of the dentition, permitting definition of fairly narrow age classes.

Certain of the Sirenia have a similar aberrant pattern of tooth replacement and could perhaps be aged by a comparable method. In macropod marsupials the molars erupt and move forwards in the jaw. Both the eruption stages and the forward progression have been used to assess age in these animals (Maynes, 1972).

Many herbivores (notably rodents and certain perissodactyls) have teeth which erupt continuously to compensate for the attrition of their occlusal surfaces caused by mastication of vegetation contaminated by grit, and as an adaptation to permit consumption of plants (especially grasses) with a high silica content. Continuously growing teeth, by their very nature, tend to retain a similar appearance throughout life and are therefore not generally very useful as guides to age. In the special case of continuously growing rodent (and lagomorph) incisors, a change does take place with age. As the animal gets older, its skull enlarges and the curvature of its incisors also increases to maintain a fairly constant relationship with the size of the growing skull. The radius of curvature might be equated with age, or perhaps (knowing that rodent incisors conform to a logarithmic spiral and the rate at which they grow) a predictive formula might be devised to relate shape to age. Logical though these approaches may appear, study of incisor teeth in known-age brown rats (*Rattus norvegicus*) yielded equivocal results which suggested only that incisor growth did not follow a simple geometrical course and was unlikely to form the basis for a valid method of age determination (S. Fargher, unpublished).

The canines of foxes appear to erupt continuously, but no new enamel is added to the crown once it has first pierced the gum. Continued eruption therefore increases the distance between the proximal margin of the enamel and the alveolus. Allen (1974) found this method provided a simple and swift field method for identifying juveniles of *Vulpes fulva*, though there was some overlap of age classes in older animals.

In the bank vole (*Clethrionomys glareolus*) and other congeneric species, the molars continue to grow after weaning, but the open roots begin to close at the age of about 3 months (Southern, 1964). As each tooth erupts further, its root becomes divided into two parts, whose increasing length has been frequently used as a criterion for age determination. However, root division has been reported to commence at 2 months by some authors and at up to 6 months by others. Moreover, Lowe (1971) has demonstrated that the chronology of development varies as between captive and free living animals and it seems likely that environmental factors may influence the validity of this technique.

Tooth Wear

Since mastication usually results in tooth wear, the age of an animal has frequently been assessed based upon the degree of attrition exhibited by its teeth. The usual practice is to use a set of drawings or photographs illustrating progressive stages of tooth wear and match animals of unknown age against this standard series. The simplest assessments are purely subjective and very liable to be influenced by proficiency and past experience of the investigator.

Gilbert and Stolt (1970) found that ten biologists, using tooth wear to assess age in a sample of deer, averaged only 58 % correct. Nevertheless, subjective estimates of tooth wear are a familiar and easily used criterion for the assessment of age.

Methods of quantifying tooth wear vary according to the types of teeth under investigation. In insectivores and carnivores, for example, pointed cusps become blunted, even obliterated, and measurements record the diminishing height of the tooth crown. This pattern of wear is particularly evident in the soricine shrews which have a red pigment in the enamel. This disappears with increasing age as the cusps are worn away, and in older animals the normally deep-red teeth appear predominantly white. Actual measurements of wear on the first lower molar were used by Crowcroft (1957) in his study of shrew populations. The method was further refined by Dapson (1968), working on the short-tailed shrew (*Blarina brevicauda*): in an effort to reduce the detrimental effect of anomalous wear patterns in individual teeth, he devised a wear index based upon the summed heights of seven different cusps on three molars.

In herbivorous mammals (particularly ungulates and rodents), where the teeth tend to be broader and flatter, diminishing height of the tooth crown tends to be less evident than changes in the patterns of dentine and enamel on the occlusal surfaces. In young animals, the teeth are capped with enamel and its subsequent attrition progressively reveals more of the underlying dentine. The total area of exposed dentine may be determined directly using a measuring grid. Alternatively, areas of dentine may be drawn on paper (using a camera lucida), cut out and weighed to provide an index of relative size.

Usually, accurate studies of tooth wear in wild species have been confined to dead specimens where the skull is available for careful laboratory examination. However, objective studies are possible in living animals and may be very useful in validating results obtained from skulls. In his study of the Defassa water buck, Spinage (1967) used "Plasticine" to take impressions of teeth in immobilized animals which were then released. When recaptured subsequently, fresh dental casts revealed the progress of tooth wear during a known time interval under natural conditions. A similar technique has also been applied to deer, but would be difficult to use on smaller animals. Substituting wax or resins for "Plasticine" would enhance this technique, but such materials are often not readily available to the field biologist.

Since all teeth are made of the same basic materials, they might be expected to have broadly similar physical properties. One is tempted to speculate that perhaps the rate of attrition may follow a reasonably close relationship with the passage of time in most mammals with basically similar dentitions. Spinage (1971) has proposed the use of a conceptual wear model which could be applied to groups (though not single individuals) of ungulates to estimate age when no known-age specimens were available for comparison. At least it might provide rough estimates as the basis for management policies whilst more reliable data are amassed.

The actual nature of such a wear model is open to speculation. One might imagine that as more soft dentine becomes exposed, the rate of attrition will increase. However, Spinage (1973) has made the contrary assertion, namely that tooth wear follows a negative exponential and the rate of attrition per unit time decreases with age. This suggestion is based upon the idea that a greater surface area is brought into wear, and as the tooth crowns become more polished, food slides over them more easily causing less abrasion. Although Spinage published his negative exponential curve without labelling the axes and without the data upon which it was based, the postulated curve agrees well with actual measurements taken from free-living deer in America and gazelles in Africa (Spinage, personal communication). A recent study (S. Fargher, unpublished) of molar wear in *Rattus norvegicus* confirms that in this species too, the rate of wear per unit time decreases with age, perhaps fitting the negative exponential curve of Spinage, even though rat teeth are quite different in size and structure from those of the ungulates upon which he has worked.

Whereas rodent and ungulate species may have a relatively standard diet, omnivores do not and are perhaps less likely to conform to a general pattern of tooth wear. Individuals eating gritty food will suffer accelerated attrition of the teeth compared with conspecifics which dine on carrion or table scraps. Seasonal variations occur in the amounts of grit ingested with the food of grazing animals. Even among insectivorous bats, where the diet is fairly uniform, tooth wear is an unreliable guide to age (Hall *et al.*, 1957). Hibernating mammals might also be expected not to conform to a standard pattern of tooth wear as their teeth are not used for several months each year. Tooth shape may also affect rates of wear. In sheep (*Ovis aries*), for example, the incisors are broader at their occlusal surfaces than at the gum so they may wear more rapidly in older animals as the same mechanical stress is applied to a smaller area.

These and many other factors which seem to invalidate any attempt to predict general patterns of tooth wear are largely based upon conjecture and call for critical investigation.

Combination of Tooth Eruption and Wear to Estimate Age

Many investigators have employed combined analysis of tooth-eruption stages with assessment of tooth wear for age determination. The two techniques complement each other well. Teeth do not usually show much sign of wear in juveniles, the age group in which eruption is still likely to be in progress; once the full dentition has erupted, this method ceases to be useful but by then measurable wear has taken place. The various weaknesses of the tooth-wear technique are thus avoided among the most numerous (juvenile) part of a population sample. Lowe (1967) found this combined technique to be the best available for determining age in red deer (*Cervus elaphus*), with a success rate of 88 %.

Growth of Teeth

Estimates of age may be based not only on material lost from a tooth but also in what is added to it. After eruption, secondary dentine is formed, lining the pulp cavity, and also cement is deposited around the roots. Both processes provide clues to age.

The young tooth has a relatively large pulp cavity; in an older tooth the cavity is largely occluded by thick layers of dentine around its walls. Decreasing pulp-cavity size is very evident in a series of radiographs of jaws of different ages (Kleymann, 1972). The same changes are demonstrable using sectioning techniques but these are less suitable for use on live animals. Dolgov and Rossolimo (1966) cut transverse sections of canine teeth and recorded the ratio between the pulp-cavity diameter and that of the tooth as a whole. The ratios permitted separation of age classes in the Arctic fox (*Alopex lagopus*), but male and female animals had to be considered separately.

The demonstration by Schour and Hoffman (1939) that the rate of apposition of dentine in ten species of vertebrates averaged 16 μm day^{-1}, offers the tempting prospect that the thickness of dentine might be used as a direct indication of true age. One millimetre of dentine would represent approximately 2 months' growth. For the hedgehog, this rate would approximately fit the observed rapid development of secondary dentine within the first few months of life; but in this species (and probably many others), once maturity is reached further changes in the pulp cavity are minimal. The naivety of translating Schour and Hoffman's findings to a direct measure of age is illustrated by reference to "Ahmed", the famous African elephant who died recently. His tusks were 2·9 m long. Growing these at 16 μm day^{-1} would have taken him over 500 years! In fact, Schour and Hoffman's observations do not provide a simple key to age in teeth because the actual mass of dentine present is not simply due to 16 μm increments being added to the dentine tubules, but also the number of tubules present.

Incremental Lines in Cement and Dentine

A far more satisfactory method of using the growth of dentine and cement as a guide to age is based upon the fact that the growth of both these tissues is susceptible to variations which cause these tissues to assume a layered rather than homogeneous structure. The fluctuations are apparently the result of environmental influences and the layers can usually be correlated with regular events in the animal's life, thus providing a guide to true age.

The causal origins of incremental lines have been the subject of considerable debate in the literature. Enough evidence has now accumulated from many studies of the teeth of wild mammals of known age to make it fairly conclusive that the lines are the result of fluctuations in the rate and nature of the deposition of these calcified tissues and that these fluctuations closely reflect major events in the animal's life. In temperate-zone mammals it appears that a narrow, denser band corresponds to winter growth, contrasting with a wider, less dense zone deposited during the summer months. Incremental lines tend to be less distinct in areas where winter conditions do not impose a significant check on growth. For example, roe deer (*Capreolus capreolus*) from Northumberland had clear laminations in the cementum pads of their molars, whereas those from Cranbourne Chase did not (White, 1974). Outside the temperate zone, incremental lines are often either undetectable or correlated with seasonal changes in rainfall or breeding cycles, but relatively little investigatory work has been done, such as, for example, where two distinct wet or dry seasons occur annually.

Incremental lines in human teeth have been known for a long time and their occurrence in wild mammals is not a new discovery. However, it was not until 1952 that Laws suggested they might be used to estimate age in marine mammals. A flurry of investigation, mainly of seals and whales, followed (reviewed by Jonsgard, 1969), but it was still another 7 years before Sergeant and Pimlott (1959) applied the technique to a land animal (the moose, *Alces alces*), and paved the way for literally hundreds of studies on wild mammals.

Incremental lines in dentine are particularly obvious in stained sections of teeth, but opinions differ as to their value for age determination. Secondary dentine seems to be particularly liable to include multiple accessory "growth lines", in addition to the annual ones. These bear no consistent relationship to an animal's age and cause confusion when counts are made. Moreover, deposition of secondary dentine slows after maturity is reached, and is anyway limited in extent by the space available within the pulp cavity. An exception is provided by the canines of pinnipedes and also the simple conical teeth of odontocete whales. In these animals, orientation of the dentine is such that growth can continue unimpeded, and over 20 annual incremental lines may be present (Laws, 1952).

Incremental lines are usually studied in tooth sections. These are prepared either by cutting and grinding or by decalcification, followed by sectioning with a cryostat or by conventional wax-block embedding techniques. A variety of staining techniques has been employed and the use of polarized light has sometimes proved advantageous. In some studies, particularly on deer and whales, thin sections have not been prepared; instead teeth have been bisected and polished, the incremental lines being viewed by reflected rather than transmitted light. In the literature there has been considerable confusion caused by the use of differing techniques. Authors have used varying terminology to describe incremental lines, adjectives like "dense", "dark", "light", "opaque" and "translucent" being employed to characterize the zone of growth relating to a particular season. In fact the actual appearance of the laminations depends upon the manner in which the teeth are prepared and examined, and this should always be made clear.

Tooth sectioning requires more equipment and expertise than most techniques and usually must be carried out in the laboratory; matters of considerable concern to the field biologist. Tooth sectioning is also unsuitable for use on living animals, though an anaesthetized animal might be deprived

490 P. MORRIS

of one of its minor teeth without undue inconvenience, a practice which has been used on grizzly bears (*Ursus horribilis*) in the Yellowstone National Park (Craighead *et al.*, 1970). There are problems, however, even with dead animals. The proud slayer of a trophy animal is reluctant to permit the mutilation of his prize or may insist on a taxidermist making costly restorations of missing teeth when the specimen is mounted. This problem is particularly serious because game animals are the very species with which the biologist is most likely to be concerned and the trophy specimens are likely to be the older animals least well represented and most needed in population studies.

Other difficulties result from resorption or hypertrophy of cement, fractures and pathological disorders. Various investigators have failed to find a consistent relationship between age and cementum lines, or have obtained different counts among the teeth of the same animal (perhaps overlooking the fact that some teeth may have erupted a year or more before others even begin to form). In some species (e.g. the bobcat, *Lynx rufus* and the coyote, *Canis latrans*), the first darkly staining layer does not develop until an age of 20 months or more, i.e. during the second winter (Crowe, 1972), calling attention to the need for each species and each investigation conducted to be afforded individual consideration.

With small mammals, problems arise from cement layers being so thin as to be barely discernible. Even in large animals a substantial proportion may have cementum layers too poorly differentiated to permit reliable counting (18 % in a study of deer by Douglas, 1970). In practice, the use of cementum lines is often a matter of interpretation rather than simple counting (Jensen and Nielsen, 1968; Grue and Jensen, 1973), calling for experience and inviting the same criticisms of subjectivity so frequently levelled at tooth-wear studies.

Nevertheless, incremental lines in teeth (especially in cement) are of widespread occurrence among mammals (thoroughly reviewed by Klevezal and Kleinenberg, 1967, covering the extensive Russian as well as Western literature), and have been reliably linked with age in many diverse species from various habitats. Cementum lines are now one of the more popular and widely used age-determination criteria.

The greatest single advantage of incremental lines is that age is revealed directly in terms of units of time, usually years or seasons. Other criteria, such as tooth wear or eruption sequences merely sort animals into arbitrary groups which, although related to age, still do not directly indicate how old an animal is.

COMPARISON OF TECHNIQUES

Counting incremental lines creates a comforting impression of precision, bolstered by the knowledge that many biologists have by now demonstrated the basic validity of relating these annuli to chronological age. Satisfied that cementum lines indicate true age, students of age-determination methods are now using this technique to assess the relative accuracy of various others.

Such comparisons usually serve to discredit the tooth-wear method. Karnukova (1971) is one of the few recent authors to conclude that tooth-wear assessments are still preferable to cementum annuli as indicators of age in rats (as did Lowe, 1967, working on red deer).

A more typical study by Kerwin and Mitchell (1971) on pronghorn antelope (*Antilocapra americana*) revealed that ages estimated on the basis of tooth wear were up to 5 years in error when compared with counts of cementum lines. The age of younger animals was frequently underestimated using the tooth-wear technique, and overestimated in older individuals. A similar situation was reported in the White-tailed deer by Gilbert and Stolt (1970) who found that 37% of their age estimates were incorrect. They also noted that none of their animals of over 5·5 years-old was correctly assigned to its age group based upon tooth wear alone. Lockard (1972) found 26% of deer were wrongly aged by the user of tooth-wear characteristics, inaccuracies being more frequent among older animals. Even in yearlings there were discrepancies between estimates based upon tooth wear and cementum structure. Robinette *et al.* (1957) devised a numerical molar index, but when tested against counts of cementum annuli this has proved no more accurate than visual estimation (Erickson *et al.*, 1970).

DISCUSSION

Discussing the merits of various techniques and methodological refinements of them may distract from the most fundamental question of all: are any of them really valid? Recent contributions to the literature are often very forthright, giving the impression that a few simple procedures will provide an authoritative determination of age. Perhaps authors are reluctant to admit uncertainty, or editors wish to minimize discursive material; but the impression is easily gained that age determination in wild animals has become almost as straightforward as it is for modern man.

It should not be forgotten that each investigator reports only what is found for a particular population at a given place and time. The results may not be universally applicable, nor should they be considered so. In both wild and domestic mammals, the development and wear of the dentition are known to respond to mechanical and environmental stress. Quantities of minerals in the diet may affect tooth hardness, amounts of grit ingested will affect attrition. Pathological conditions or uneven wear may stimulate hypertrophy of the cement and dentine in individuals. Variability may arise as a result of genetic factors; for example, one strain of laboratory mice carrying a gene for syndactylous toes also suffers from very soft teeth. Evidence from agricultural stock also suggests that tooth and jaw defects may be inherited.

Spinage (1973) rejects criticisms relating to significant variability among wild animals, pointing out that most stem from observations of domestic species which are not selected for the quality of their dentition nor properly adapted to the diet upon which they are often forced to live. He suggests that in the long evolutionary history of mammals, when teeth have proved very adaptable, natural selection would have eliminated extremes of variability. The contrary assertion by Chaplin (1971) that wild species would be more variable than domestic ones because they experience a greater diversity of conditions, is debatable and ignores the fact that under domestication the full spectrum of genetic variants may actually be encouraged to survive (even the most grotesque ones like Pekinese and bulldogs).

It seems reasonable to assume that members of the same wild population, from a similar habitat, will exhibit relatively little variability; but studies on one group should not be applied directly to another just because both are of the same species. Certainly it is unwise to use animals raised in captivity as the basis for validating age criteria in wild mammals, a practice often employed where free-living animals of known age are not available.

Greater consistency might be expected among those age criteria which follow clearly defined stages rather than progressive change, such as, for example, the sequence of tooth eruption. However, even this process can be experimentally manipulated and does not always follow a fixed chronology, as seen in man at least. Incisor teeth appear in babies (eagerly anticipated by parents) at about the fifth month, but cases are known where they are already present at birth (Louis XIV being a famous example). Similar deviations occur in domestic mammals, sometimes as the result of genetic factors, and are not unknown in the wild. The presence of supernumary teeth is another potentially confusing feature shared by man and wild mammals.

The problem of reliability begs the question of just how accurate age assessment needs to be. To the wildlife biologist, concerned with whole populations rather than individuals, anything better than 50% accuracy is likely to be more useful than misleading in management programmes. In many cases there is probably no real need to know an animal's age to within less than about 10% of its probable lifespan, except for personal satisfaction and academic interest.

The quest for total accuracy is a futile one unless the effects of human expertise and error can be eliminated. Further, if accuracy is sought for the purpose of population analysis, it will likely be thwarted by the inevitable bias introduced in sampling wild populations.

Reliability of age estimates will be improved by the use of combined techniques. Gustafson's technique (1950) summing numerical scores for several different criteria and the more recent scoring method of Demirjian et al. (1973) demonstrate the principle applied to human teeth and point the way for wildlife biologists to follow. Combined techniques would be further improved if they took account not only of dental age criteria, but skeletal and other features also.

CONCLUSION

Teeth provide a variety of valuable clues to the age of an animal, and the wildlife biologist has a wide selection of age-determination techniques available to him. Broadly speaking, the simplest methods will give the quickest but least reliable results. Reliability will be increased (even up to the 100 % level according to some authors) if incremental lines can be counted, especially in cement, but this technique is expensive and time-consuming. The best compromise is to employ a simple method (e.g. based upon tooth eruption, pulp-cavity occlusion or some non-dental criterion) to sort out the numerous juveniles from a population sample, and subject only the remainder to more definitive laboratory examination.

The choice of methods will also be governed by the material available and the constraints of working in the field; but simplicity and low cost are likely to be prime considerations, often taking precedence over the need for accuracy. Meanwhile, the wildlife biologist should also watch his laboratory-based colleagues in case they come up with any new ideas.

REFERENCES

ALLEN, S. H. (1974). Modified techniques for ageing red fox using canine teeth. *J. Wildl. Mgmt* **38**, 152–154.

CHAPLIN, R. E. (1971). "The Study of Animal Bones from Archaeological Sites." Seminar Press, London and New York.

CRAIGHEAD, J. J., CRAIGHEAD, F. C. and McCUTCHEN, H. E. (1970). Age determination of grizzly bears from fourth premolar tooth sections. *J. Wildl. Mgmt* **34**, 353–363.

CROWCROFT, P. (1957). "The Life of the Shrew." Reinhardt, London.

CROWE, D. M. (1972). The presence of annuli in bobcat cementum layers. *J. Wildl. Mgmt* **36**, 1330–1332.

DAPSON, R. W. (1968). Reproduction and age structure in a population of short tailed shrews *Blarina brevicauda*. *J. Mammal.* **49**, 205–214.

DEMIRJIAN, A., GOLDSTEIN, H. and TANNER, J. M. (1973). A new system of dental age assessment. *Hum. Biol.* **45**, 211–227.

DOLGOV, V. A. and ROSSOLIMO, O. L. (1966). Changes with age of some structural features of the skull and baculum in carnivorous animals, and procedures for age determination in the Arctic fox (*Alopex lagopus*). (In Russian). *Zool. Zh.* **45**, 1074–1080.

DOUGLAS, M. J. W. (1970). Dental cement layers as criteria of age for deer in New Zealand with emphasis on red deer, *Cervus elaphus*. *N.Z. Jl Sci. Technol.*, **13**, 352–358.

ERICKSON, J. A., ANDERSON, A. E., MEDIN, D. E. and BOWDEN, D. C. (1970). Estimating ages of mule deer—an evaluation of technique accuracy. *J. Wildl. Mgmt* **34**, 523–531.

GILBERT, F. F. and STOLT, S. L. (1970). Variability in aging Maine White tailed deer by tooth wear characteristics. *J. Wildl. Mgmt* **34**, 532–535.

GRUE, H. and JENSEN, B. (1973). Annular structures in canine tooth cementum in red foxes (*Vulpes vulpes* L.) of known age. *Dan. Rev. Game Biol.* **8**, 1–12.

GUSTAFSON, G. (1950). Age determinations on teeth. *J. Am. dent. Ass.* **41**, 45–54.

HALL, J. S., CLOUTIER, R. J. and GRIFFIN, D. R. (1957). Longevity records and notes on tooth wear of bats. *J. Mammal* **38**, 407–409.

JENSEN, B. and NIELSEN, L. B. (1968). Age determination in the red fox (*Vulpes vulpes* L.) from canine tooth sections. *Dan. Rev. Game Biol.* **5**, 1–15.

JONSGARD. A. (1969). Age determination of marine mammals. *In* "The Biology of Marine Mammals" (Anderson, H. T., ed.), pp. 1–30 Academic Press, London and New York.

KARNUKOVA, N. G. (1971). Age determination of brown and black rats. (In Russian.) *Ekologiya* **2**, 71–76.

KERWIN, M. L. and MITCHELL, G. J. (1971). The validity of the wear-age technique for Alberta pronghorns. *J. Wildl. Mgmt* **35**, 743–747.

KLEVEZAL, G. A. and KLEINENBERG, S. E. (1967). Age determination of mammals from annual layers in teeth and bones. Translation by Israel Program for Scientific Translations, Jerusalem, 1969.

KLEYMANN, M. (1972). Age caused changes of the pulp cavity in the roe deer. (In German.) *Z. Jagdwiss* **18**, 36–39.

LAWS, R. M. (1952). A new method of age determination in mammals. *Nature, Lond.* **169**, 972–973.

LAWS, R. M. (1966). Age criteria of the African elephant *Loxodonta a. africana*. *E. Afr. Wildl. J.* **4**, 1–37.

LOCKARD, G. R. (1972). Further studies of dental annuli for aging White tailed deer. *J. Wildl. Mgmt* **36**, 46–55.

LOWE, V. P. W. (1967). Teeth as indicators of age with special reference to red deer (*Cervus elaphus*) of known age from Rhum. *J. Zool., Lond.* **152**, 137–153.

LOWE, V. P. W. (1971). Root development of molar teeth in the bank vole (*Clethrionomys glareolus*) *J. Anim. Ecol.* **40**, 49–61.

MAYNES, G. M. (1972). Age estimation in the Parma Wallaby, *Macropus parma* Waterhouse. *Aust. J. Zool.* **20**, 107–118.

MORRIS, P. (1972). A review of mammalian age determination methods. *Mamm. Rev.* **2**, 69–104.

ROBINETTE, W. L., JONES, D. A., ROGERS, G. and GASHWILER, J. S. (1957). Notes on tooth development and wear for Rocky Mountain mule deer. *J. Wildl. Mgmt* **21**, 134–153.

SCHOUR, I. and HOFFMAN, M. M. (1939). Studies in tooth development. 1. The 16 microns calcification rhythm in the enamel and dentin from fish to Man. *J. dent. Res.* **18**, 91–102.

SERGEANT, P. E. and PIMLOTT, D. H. (1959). Age determination in moose from sectioned incisor teeth. *J. Wildl. Mgmt* **23**, 315–321.

SIKES, S. K. (1966). The African elephant, *Loxodonta africana*: a field method for the estimation of age. *J. Zool., Lond.* **150**, 279–295.

SIKES, S. K. (1968). The African elephant, *Loxodonta africana*: a field method for the estimation of age. *J. Zool., Lond.* **154**, 235–248.

SLAUGHTER, B. H., PINE, R. H. and PINE, N. E. (1974). Eruption of cheek teeth in Insectivora and Carnivora. *J. Mammal.* **55**, 115–125.

SOUTHERN, H. N. (ed.) (1964). "The Handbook of British Mammals." Blackwell Scientific Publications, Oxford.

SPINAGE, C. A. (1967). Ageing the Uganda Defassa Waterbuck *Kobus defassa ugandae* Neumann. *E. Afr. Wildl. J.* **5**, 1–17.

SPINAGE, C. A. (1971). Geratodontology and horn growth of the impala (*Aepyceros melampus*) *J. Zool., Lond.* **164**, 209–225.

SPINAGE, C. A. (1973). A review of the age determination of mammals by means of teeth, with especial reference to Africa. *E. Afr. Wildl. J.* **11**, 165–187.

WHITE, G. (1974). Age determination of roe deer (*Capreolus capreolus*) from annual growth layers in the dental cementum. *J. Zool., Lond.* **174**, 511–516.

30. Age Structure of a Sample of Subfossil Beavers (*Castor fiber* L.)

D. F. MAYHEW

University Museum of Zoology, Cambridge

INTRODUCTION

The development in recent years of techniques for assessment of absolute age from skeletal structures represents a major advance in mammalogy. Laws (1953) demonstrated annual layering in the dentine of teeth of the Southern elephant seal (*Mirounga leonina* L.). Many species of mammal have since been investigated and it has been possible in most cases to relate known age to periodic layering in the bones or in the teeth. This work has been reviewed by Klevezal' and Kleinenberg (1969), Morris (1972) and Spinage (1973).

In Recent mammals knowledge of age enables estimation of the ontogenetic component of intraspecific variation and provides the basis for studies of population biology. Methods of age determination based on the presence of periodic layers in skeletal structures are also applicable in principle to fossil material, particularly when the details have been tested on recent populations of the same species. This chapter describes age assessment of subfossil beaver material and discusses population characteristics based on this sample in the light of information from Recent animals.

The annual layers in the cheek-tooth cement of Recent beavers of known age were described independently by van Nostrand and Stephenson (1964) and Klevezal' and Kleinenberg (1969). The Russian workers also found annual periosteal adhesion layers in the mandible. Conventional methods of age determination were compared with results from dental characters and basal cement-layer counts by Larson and van Nostrand (1968) who concluded that previous techniques such as weight, pelt size, skull and external morphological measurements were not adequate indicators of age after the first year.

Larson (1967) discussed the age structure of trapped samples of Maryland

(U.S.A.) beavers using ages determined by dental characters including basal cement-layer counts. This study appears to provide the only accurate information on Recent beavers suitable for comparison with the results from the subfossil sample. Methods of age determination of subfossil beaver remains from Denmark were discussed by Hatting (1969a) in a paper which was seen after the present study was completed. Hatting demonstrated that periodic layering was visible in the basal cement of subfossil beaver cheek teeth. However, technical difficulties (which are avoided here) compelled her to reject age determination by basal cement-layer counts in favour of radiography which provided less precise results.

MATERIAL

This study is based on a sample of subfossil beaver remains representing 58 animals from the Cambridgeshire fen region. The specimens are kept in the University Museum of Zoology (UMZC) and the Sedgwick Museum of Geology, Cambridge, and they were collected during peat digging and drainage operations mainly during the last century. Many of the remains appear to represent complete skeletons, but as only the larger bones were collected, determination of sex according to the presence or absence of a baculum (Osborn, 1953) was not possible. Radiocarbon dating (J. Jewell, personal communication) and palynological evidence (P. Gibbard, personal communication) support the conclusion that the remains are derived from a population living in the fen region during Bronze Age times c. 3000 years B.P.

METHODS

Little protein matrix remains in the otherwise excellently preserved bone of the subfossil remains and investigation of mandible periosteal layers in decalcified section (Klevezal' and Kleinenberg, 1969) was not pursued. Basal cement layers were visible in longitudinal polished sections of each cheek tooth in a single individual and there seemed to be little difference between teeth in the ease of counting these layers. Van Nostrand and Stephenson (1964) suggested that the lower first or second molars were most suitable for age determination of Recent beavers although extraction of these teeth involved breaking the mandible. This procedure was apparently followed by Hatting (1969a) who noted that subfossil material was irreplaceable and that unnecessary damage should be avoided. The lower third molar is held in place by the bone at the top of the alveolus and is consequently present in most subfossil mandibles. Removal of a small piece of bone at the rear of the tooth allowed extraction and on the grounds of availability and ease of removal the third molar was chosen for age determination even though van Nostrand and Stephenson (1964) suggested that it was the least suitable of the mandibular teeth. Other mandibular and maxillary teeth were examined in specimens lacking the lower third molar.

Van Nostrand and Stephenson (1964) recommended grinding longitudinal sections using a fine textured circular grindstone, a method which optimizes visualization of the cement layers but sacrifices half of the tooth. While such a procedure is acceptable in studies of Recent mammals, it may be considered to reduce the research or display value of subfossil specimens. A solution adopted here was to grind the base of the tooth obliquely so that the emergent crown of the tooth was undamaged while the cement layers were visible at the base. Grinding was performed with a mechanical wheel using three grades of carborundum and the ground surface was finished with a buffing wheel.

Ontogenetic changes in the dentition of beavers have been discussed by Klevezal' and Kleinenberg (1969), van Nostrand and Stephenson (1964) and Larson and van Nostrand (1968). Information from these sources is summarized here. The teeth erupt in the following order: deciduous molar, first molar, second molar, third molar, premolar. The eruption of the deciduous molar occurs at the age of about one month (Hatting, 1969a) and the three molars are erupted by 6 months. The premolar comes into wear between 10 months (Hatting, 1969a) and 1 year (van Nostrand and Stephenson, 1964). At eruption the four cheek teeth of the permanent dentition consist of hypsodont crowns of enamel, dentine and cement with the enamel folded in the characteristic 3 + 1 pattern of castorids. Enamel formation continues at the base until the second year when the open bases of the teeth become filled with dentine and cement. The first conspicuous cement layer is formed in the third year. By the end of the fourth year the openings at the bases of the teeth are closed by cement which is deposited in annual layers of similar thickness for the rest of the life of the animal. Cement accretion does not entirely compensate for the reduction of crown height by wear and so the alveolar depth decreases with age. The assessment technique proposed by van Nostrand and Stephenson (1964), based on the state of eruption, the degree of closure of the basal openings and the amount of basal cement deposition, was used here.

Because of differential staining by brown humic substances from the peat in which they were buried, the annual layers in the cement of subfossil specimens were more readily visible than those of Recent teeth. Seen in reflected light, each annual unit consisted of a broad light line and a thin dark line (Fig. 1) and this agrees with the findings of Klevezal' and Kleinenberg (1969). The age of adult beavers was assessed by adding 2 to the number of annual units counted. The age class of juveniles (1 or 2) was decided by reference to the presence of the deciduous molar and the degree of closure of the cheek-tooth bases. Although the pattern of annual layers in the cement was sometimes complicated by the presence of accessory lines, the interpretation of these was aided by experience and the similarity in thickness of the annual units after the third year. Specimens which could not be aged consistently, including those in which layers were indistinct or absent, were excluded from the present study.

It is uncertain whether the apparent absence of cement layering observed in some subfossil specimens is due to physiological or *post mortem* reasons.

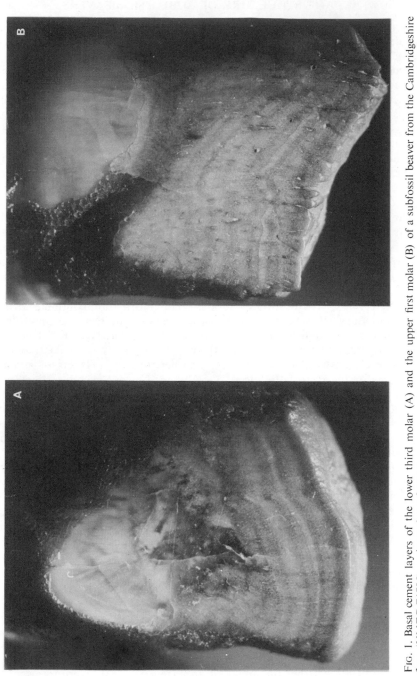

Fig. 1. Basal cement layers of the lower third molar (A) and the upper first molar (B) of a subfossil beaver from the Cambridgeshire fens (UMZC E1795), estimated age 9 years.

No layers were found in the basal cement of a Recent beaver from a zoo-logical garden. That the variation in optical density of the cement is depend-ent on general rather than local metabolism is shown by the presence of a similar complex of layers in upper and lower teeth of the same animal (Fig. 1).

It is believed that the ages determined for the sample by basal cement-layer counts are accurate in general to ± 1 year although an error of ± 2 years is possible in the case of old animals.

AGE STRUCTURE

Application of this method of age determination to 58 subfossil specimens led to the age-group distribution given in the second column of Table I. The oldest animal was in its twelfth year. Hatting (1969a) mentions an animal of 14 years in her study of Danish subfossil remains. Beavers may live much longer than this in the wild and an animal 20 years of age was noted by Larson (1967). The maximum age attained in captivity appears to be 23 years and 6 months (a Russian animal, L. S. Lavrov, personal communication). However, these ages may be regarded as exceptional because the crowns of the lower second and third molars may be completely worn away by the age of 17 years (L. S. Lavrov, personal communication). Of 143 specimens examined by Larson (1967), only the old animal of 20 years noted above was over 13 years. Investigations on large samples bring out the difference between the mean and the potential lifespans of wild animals. The mean longevity of the subfossil sample, obtained by dividing the total number of animal years

TABLE I. Life table for *C. fiber* based on a subfossil sample of 58 individuals.

age group (x)	a	d_x	l_x	q_x	e_x
0–1	5	86	1000	86	5·26
1–2	6	103	914	113	4·71
2–3	3	52	811	64	4·24
3–4	7	121	759	159	3·50
4–5	5	86	638	135	3·07
5–6	8	138	552	250	2·47
6–7	4	69	414	167	2·12
7–8	7	121	345	351	1·45
8–9	9	155	224	692	0·96
9–10	3	52	69	754	0·99
10–11	0	0	17	(0)	(1·5)
11–12	1	17	17	1000	0·5

a = sample number in each age group.
d_x = mortality (animals dying in age group x).
l_x = survivorship (animals surviving at beginning of x).
q_x = mortality rate (per thousand during x).
e_x = life expectancy of animals aged x.
(Based conventionally on a cohort size of 1000).

lived by the sample number, was between 5 and 6 years. According to a current handbook on "Growth" (Altman and Dittmer, eds, 1962) the "average lifespan" of beavers is 20–25 years. However, the source references do not support this conclusion and the information given here indicates that such an estimate refers rather to the maximum age achieved in captivity.

POPULATION CHARACTERISTICS

Investigations of number, density, age structure and reproductive rates form a central part of ecological studies of Recent populations. Deevey (1947) reviewed work on population dynamics of Recent species and Kurten (1953) estimated population characteristics of certain extinct animals. Work on mammalian life tables was critically reviewed by Caughley (1966) and investigation of human population biology from the Palaeolithic to the present has been attempted by Acsadi and Nemeskeri (1970). Reference should be made to these sources for the methods of calculating population characteristics as well as for discussion of the assumptions made in the calculations and conditions necessary for their application.

Although the difficulties of calculating population characteristics of fossil mammals have been pointed out, the possibility of obtaining all relevant information is limited even in studies of Recent wild populations. Population size is rarely known, not all animals dying will be noticed and age determinations of living and dead animals may be difficult. In practice, the information obtained concerns the age of specimens in living or dead samples. There are two approaches to the investigation of population characteristics of Recent animals. One method follows the time course of natural mortality in a cohort of the population as might be done in bird-ringing studies. This leads to knowledge of the age structure of a dead sample and these ages form a mortality (d_x) series. A life table calculated on this basis is known as "horizontal" or "dynamic". The other method takes a census or random sample which enables estimation of the age structure of the living population, and these ages form a survivorship (l_x) series. With knowledge of age-specific mortality rates, a "time-specific" or "vertical" life table may be constructed. Thus a population can be summarized by two different forms of life table, the characteristics of which will be the same only if the population remains stationary (in size and age structure) for a period exceeding the potential longevity of the species.

Palaeontological information for population investigations consists of more or less accurately aged samples from death assemblages. Mortality rates are not known (although they may be estimated); it is exceedingly unlikely that all members of the sample started life together; and the age structure of available samples is prevented by preservation and collection bias from representing that of the original graveyard population. Because mortality rates are not known, the construction of life tables for fossil populations requires the assumption that the population was stationary (in age structure and size) for the period in which the sample accumulated. Death assemblages consist of the results of disease, old age, predation and accidents; the proportion which each has contributed cannot be known. Such composite data (Kurten, 1953) may be analysed as a mortality (d_x) series if believed to result from natural mortality or as a survivorship (l_x) series if believed to reflect the age structure of a living population which perished in a catastrophe. These considerations are now discussed with reference to the subfossil sample.

Observations on the ecology of Recent beavers support the view that in the absence of human interference the numbers of beavers in a population change little with time. This stability appears to be at least partly due to their territorial nature and to the insulation from short-term climatic effects afforded by their winter food store. The isolation of family groups within territories also has the important effect of preventing the spread of epidemic disease which is unknown in beavers according to Elton (1966). The dating evidence suggests that the subfossil remains accumulated in a geologically short space of time—perhaps 1000 years. In view of the probable stability of wild beaver populations, the assumption of a stationary population essential for the construction of a life table does not seem unreasonable. Hunting activities by Bronze Age man are, however, a possible complicating factor.

The causes of mortality of most of the subfossil sample cannot be deter-

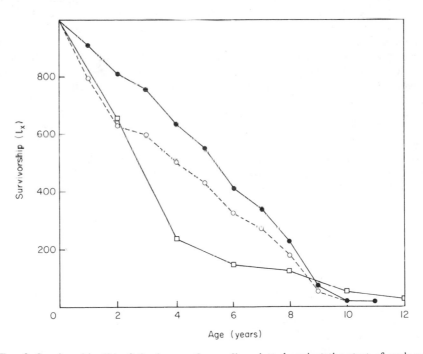

FIG. 2. Survivorship (l_x) of the beaver *Castor fiber* plotted against the start of each age interval. ●, subfossil, Cambridgeshire fens, from Table I; ○, subfossil, Cambridgeshire fens, adjusted data (see text); □, Recent, North America, recalculated from Larson (1967).

mined. Two specimens appear to have died as a result of abscesses at the base of the cheek teeth and a third showed signs of periodontal disease. None of the animals had worn-out or deficient dentitions. Although Hatting (1969b) described Danish subfossil beaver mandibles which had apparently been used by man as scrapers, there is no evidence of human use or damage in the sample from the Cambridgeshire fens. Finally, these deposits provide no evidence that death resulted from a catastrophe. This suggests that the sample represents the results of natural mortality and that it should be treated as a mortality (d_x) series in life-table calculations (Table I).

The survivorship curve from Table I is given in Fig. 2. On linear axes the plot is a diagonal line indicating low juvenile mortality and approaching the shape of that of man and other protected populations (Lack, 1954). However, another source of bias needs to be considered before accepting this result. The subfossil sample consists of museum specimens and isolated teeth were not included in this study. Juvenile specimens in which the bone was more fragile were less attractive to collectors and were less likely to be preserved. Sampling, collection and preservation bias have all tended to reduce the number of juveniles (age groups 1 and 2) in the sample. The bone of the mandible becomes more solid from the third year on and it is unlikely that bias exists between age groups later than 2 years. Although the extent of the bias against juveniles is unknown it is possible to test the effect of adjustments of a certain order on the life table. In Fig. 2 an adjusted survivorship plot is given which is based on the assumption that the numbers in the first and second age classes represent one-third and one-half respectively of the true values (a reasonable estimate of possible bias). Apart from the increased juvenile mortality in the adjusted plot the difference between the curves is not great.

DISCUSSION

Information on the age structure of Recent beaver populations is limited. Larson (1967) gave the age structure of a trapped sample of beavers from Maryland (U.S.A.), with ages determined by basal cement-layer counts. This information, which is the best available to date, was reworked to provide a survivorship curve (Fig. 2) suitable for comparison with the results of the present study. The shape of this curve for a Recent population differs considerably from the original plot of the subfossil sample and implies a much greater mortality in the first 5 years of life of Recent animals. It seems probable, however, that the differences between the results are more likely to be due to factors biasing the samples. It has been noted above that the number of juvenile animals in the subfossil sample does not represent that resulting from the original mortality. The effect of an adjustment to allow for this is to depress the first part of the survivorship plot. The data given by Larson (1967) for Recent animals are also subject to sample errors, but in this case these result in overestimation of the number of juveniles. The population sampled was increasing throughout the 5-year study period and this implies a higher proportion of juveniles than in a stationary population. The proportion of young to old beavers decreased consistently and significantly through the study period. If the population size and structure were changing, a survivorship curve fitted to lumped data covering 5 years must be treated with some reservation. The sampling method (trapping) must undoubtedly have led to bias in favour of younger less experienced individuals and the procedure also resulted in removal of samples from the living population, affecting subsequent samples, and creating conditions for population growth. Larson (1967) noted that:

> The data . . . are probably indicative of conditions found in an increasing beaver population as it is first subjected to trapping.

On the basis of Larson's data, a survivorship curve for a Recent stationary population would be expected to lie above the Recent plot in Fig. 2.

The available information from subfossil and Recent samples could therefore be considered to define the limits of a survivorship curve of a stationary beaver population. While it should not be assumed that a particular curve is species-specific and still less that survivorship curves are classifiable into types, plots within the limits of those discussed above have also been found for Middle Pleistocene samples of *Castor fiber* (Mayhew, 1975). Caution is necessary in interpreting population information based on such small samples. Subfossil and fossil material is, however, capable of providing information on absolute age, and the age determinations on which the calculations here are based are of the same order of accuracy as those of Recent animals. The information given here substantially modifies previous estimates of average age and survivorship of beavers.

Investigation of the ontogenetic age of the subfossil beaver remains has also provided a firm basis for interpreting variation within and between populations through the calibration of age related changes such as growth and tooth wear. The timing and pattern of epiphyseal fusion appear to vary between populations and the epiphyses of the limb bones are not all fused at 2 years of age (cf. Hatting, 1969a). Consideration of ontogenetic changes in tooth wear leads to the conclusion that the Pleistocene species *Castor plicidens* Major is a junior synonym of *C. fiber*, based on specimens of advanced age.

It is perhaps self evident that whereas museum collections of Recent material reflect the relative abundance of the living with a preponderance of juveniles, fossil samples reflect a graveyard population in age structure and are further biased by destruction and non-recovery of juveniles. In these circumstances accurate methods of age determination are essential for sound comparisons of fossil and Recent material.

SUMMARY

The ages of a sample of 58 subfossil beavers (*Castor fiber* L.) were determined by counts of annual cement layers at the bases of the cheek teeth and by reference to other dental characters. The oldest animal in the sample was in its twelfth year and the average lifespan was between 5 and 6 years. A life table constructed from the data yielded a diagonal survivorship curve which undoubtedly underestimated juvenile mortality, and this contrasted with a survivorship curve from a Recent population biased in favour of juveniles. It was suggested that values for a stationary beaver population would lie in between these two extremes. The practical and theoretical importance of applying accurate methods of age determination to fossil and Recent skeletal material has been briefly indicated.

Acknowledgements

I would like to thank Dr K. A. Joysey for critical discussion and advice, and Drs J. Jewell, P. Gibbard and L. S. Lavrov who generously provided information. This study was carried out during the tenure of a S.R.C. research studentship.

References

Acsadi, G. and Nemeskeri, J. (1970). "History of Human Life Span and Mortality." Akad. Kiado, Budapest.

Altman, P. L. and Dittmer, D. S. (eds) (1962). "Growth." Federation of American Societies for Experimental Biology, Washington.

Caughley, G. (1966). Mortality patterns in mammals. *Ecology* **47**, 906–918.

Deevey, E. S. (1947). Life tables for natural populations of animals. *Q. Rev. Biol.* **22**, 283–314.

Elton, C. (1966). "Animal Ecology". Methuen, London.

Hatting, T. (1969a). Age determination for subfossil beavers (*Castor fiber* L.) (Mammalia) on the basis of radiographs of the teeth. *Vidensk. Meddr dansk naturh. Foren.* **132**, 115–128.

Hatting, T. (1969b). Er baeverens taender benyttet som redskaber i Stenalderen i Danmark? *Aarbøger for nordisk Oldkyndighed og Historie* (1969) 116–126.

Klevezal', G. A. and Kleinenberg, S. E. (1969). Age determination of mammals from annual layers in teeth and bones (translated from Russian). Israel Program for Scientific Translations, Jerusalem.

Kurten, B. (1953). On the variation and population dynamics of fossil and recent mammal populations. *Acta zool. fenn.* **76**, 5–122.

Lack, D. (1954). "The Natural Regulation of Animal Numbers". Clarendon Press, Oxford.

Larson, J. S. (1967). Age structure and sexual maturity within a western Maryland beaver (*Castor canadensis*) population. *J. Mammal.* **48**, 408–413.

Larson, J. S. and van Nostrand, F. C. (1968). An evaluation of beaver aging techniques. *J. Wildl. Mgmt* **32**, 99–103.

Laws, R. M. (1953). A new method of age determination in mammals with special reference to the Elephant seal (*Mirounga leonina*). *Scient. Rep. Falk. Isl. Dep. Surv.* **2**, 1–11.

Mayhew, D. F. (1975). The Quaternary history of some British rodents and lagomorphs. Ph.D. Thesis, University of Cambridge.

MORRIS, P. A., (1972). A review of mammalian age determination methods. *Mammal Review*, **2**, 69–104.

OSBORN, D. J. (1953). Age classes, reproduction and sex ratios of Wyoming beaver. *J. Mammal.* **34**, 27–44.

SPINAGE, C. A. (1973). A review of age determination of mammals by means of teeth with especial reference to Africa. *E. Afr. Wildl. J.* **11**, 165–188.

VAN NOSTRAND, F. C. and STEPHENSON, A. B. (1964). Age determination for beavers by tooth development. *J. Wildl. Mgmt* **28**, 430–434.

31. Fluorescent Bone Histology in Incident Ultraviolet Light

F. L. D. STEEL and J. A. FINDLAY

Department of Anatomy, University College, Cardiff, Wales

The use of tetracyclines as a fluorescent marker for studying the growth of bone has long been recognized (e.g. Milch *et al.*, 1958; R. W. Fearnhead, personal communication). Most of the observations have been made by passing ultraviolet radiation through thin, ground, undecalcified sections. We believe, however, that there are certain advantages in the incident illumination of thick sections of bone. These are quickly and easily prepared, easily preserved and, in particular, make possible the production of close serial fluorescence photomicrographs of sufficient quality to allow three dimensional reconstruction of the growing surface. It is with this last hope in mind that we have taken some preliminary photomicrographs, which we believe to be histologically acceptable, and it is these which are shown here.

The method used has been previously described (Findlay *et al.*, 1974; but see also figure legend). All the specimens shown were taken from two oxen previously injected with 12 mg/kg body weight oxytetracycline hydrochloride and made available to us by our collaborators Mr T. M. Leach and Dr R. W. Pomeroy of the Meat Research Institute, Langford. Of these oxen, one, No. 3, was given a single injection and the other, No. 128, four injections.

The fluorescent lines corresponding to the inner surface of the periosteum immediately following the times of four tetracycline injections in ox 128 may be clearly seen in Fig. 1A; so can the endosteal line representing a single injection in ox 3 in (B). The bright profiles in (C) indicate osteons forming at the time of injection in ox 3. Figure 1D shows that osteogenesis in ox 128 at the time of the first injection, though not the second, appears to occur in multiple planes. This might be due either to the existence of simultaneous layers of ossification or to the folding of a single layer. Although this appearance has been observed before (A. Boyd, 1974, personal communication),

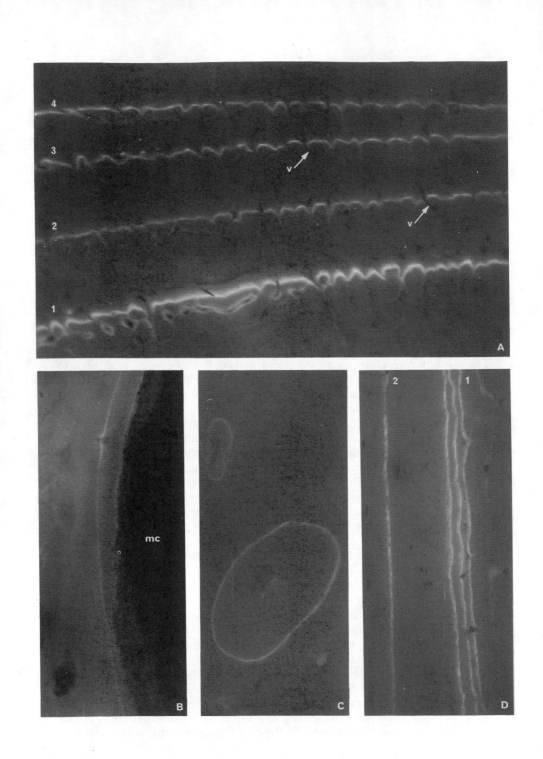

it has not, so far as we are aware, been reported in the literature. A further interesting formation is shown by all four lines in Fig. 1A. The layers of osteogenesis are either corrugated or consist of discrete stud-like elevations. These elevations are rounded on their outer aspect but are separated from their neighbours by acutely angled clefts through which vascular channels frequently run. All of these phenomena could be much better understood were they to be studied in serial sections.

Although serial sections of bone may be taken with a saw, the saw cut is necessarily too wide to allow truly adjacent regions to be examined and is therefore unlikely to assist in the interpretation of the appearances described above. We are awaiting the completion of a machine (at present being built) which will allow wet carborundum powder to grind away the surfaces of pieces of bone by a measured amount in a given time. By this means strictly adjacent serial sections should be obtainable by photographing the surfaces at intervals. It seems likely that this method, which as a *sine qua non* depends on pictures of the kind displayed here, may yield useful results.

REFERENCES

FINDLAY, J. A., LEACH, T. M., POMEROY, R. W. and STEEL, F. L. D. (1974). Growth changes in the mandible of the ox. *Acta anat.* **88**, 125–136.
MILCH, R. A., RALL, D. P. and TOBIE, J. E. (1958). Fluorescence of tetracycline antibiotics in bone. *J. Bone Jt Surg.* **40A**, 897–910.

FIG. 1. Incident fluorescence photomicrographs of thick sawn and polished coronal sections of ox mandibles. Source 200 W ultra-high-pressure mercury arc. Exciter filter 3 mm BG 3 + 4 mm BG 38 (for residual red absorption) and barrier filter K510. Incident illuminator adjusted to reflect at 455 nm.

(A) Ox No. 128, posterior premolar region of left half-mandible. Note characteristically irregular fluorescent lines, described in text, representing subperiosteal bone deposition following tetracycline injections numbered 1–4; vascular channels (v). × 36.

(B) Ox No. 3, posterior end of diastema of left half-mandible. Note: single endosteal line; mandibular canal (mc). × 43.

(C) Ox No. 3, from same section as (B). Note: large and small fluorescent profiles of osteons presumably at different stages of development at the time of tetracycline injection. × 108.

(D) Ox No. 128, from same section as (A) Note: fluorescent lines representing tetracycline injections 1 and 2—the first appears triple as speculated upon in the text. × 43.

32. A Comparison of Morphological and Gravimetric Methods of Estimating Human Foetal Age from the Dentition

D. A. LUKE

Dental School, Newcastle upon Tyne

M. V. STACK

MRC Dental Unit, Bristol

and

E. N. HEY

MRC Reproduction and Growth Unit, Newcastle upon Tyne

INTRODUCTION

Traditionally, the age of a human foetus is estimated from its crown–rump (CR) length using data relating length to age such as that provided by Streeter (1921). All foetuses, however, do not grow at the same rate and therefore size is an unsatisfactory indication of the age of an individual specimen. The dentition provides a suitable alternative to body size for estimating foetal age because dental development proceeds throughout intra-uterine life following a well established pattern of events. Furthermore, studies of post-natal dental development indicate that the dentition is relatively less affected than the rest of the body when nutritional conditions vary in man (Garn *et al.*, 1965), or are experimentally altered in the pig (Tonge and McCance, 1973) and in the rat (DiOrio *et al.*, 1973).

  Garn *et al.* (1970) have shown that during the first trimester of intra-uterine life, dental development can be used as a reference standard for embryological status. They defined eight stages of early tooth formation and found a high correlation between tooth stage and CR length. However, due to individual variation in foetal growth rate, the use of the dentition for the determination of age requires that dental development be related to age itself rather than to CR length. Two methods can be used for this purpose:

(a) Kraus and Jordan (1965) have related foetal age to the morphological stages of calcification of the occlusal surface of each deciduous molar, and

(b) Stack (1964) has demonstrated that, during the last trimester, foetal age is linearly related to the square root of the weight of mineralized tissue in the deciduous teeth.

In the present investigation a method of estimating foetal age based on the Kraus stages of molar calcification has been compared with Stack's gravimetric method using a group of human foetuses of known gestational age, some of which had experienced conditions *in utero* which restricted their growth.

MATERIALS

The dentitions examined were from 32 human foetuses, aged from 22 to 42 weeks, each of which had died from an acute condition during the perinatal period, the majority within 24 h of birth and none more than 5 days after birth. The gestational age of each foetus was known from reliable information of the date of the last menstrual period and was confirmed by a well documented history of the pregnancy itself. Nine foetuses were classified as growth-retarded or "light-for-dates" (LFD) since they were below the tenth

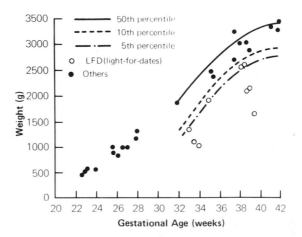

FIG. 1. Weight and gestational age of 32 human foetuses. Percentiles are from Thomson *et al.* (1968).

percentile of weight for gestational age given by Thomson *et al.* (1968). Figure 1 demonstrates that the LFD foetuses are considerably growth-retarded being, as a group, well below the tenth percentile. The other foetuses are regarded as normal in the sense that each is within one standard deviation of the mean weight for its age. Figure 2 shows that the LFD foetuses are also considerably shorter in CR length than those of normal weight.

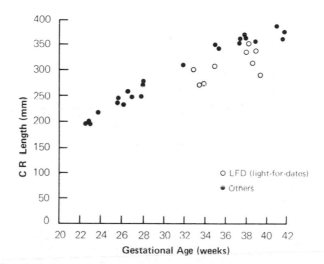

FIG. 2. CR length and gestational age of normal and LFD foetuses.

MORPHOLOGICAL METHOD OF ESTIMATING FOETAL AGE

Deciduous molar tooth germs were removed intact from one side of the dentition, fixed in 10% neutral formalin and stained with 1 : 1000 aqueous sodium alizarin sulphonate for 10 min. Kraus and Jordan (1965) have given a number to each stage of progressive calcification of the occlusal surface demonstrated by this technique. In Tables I–IV of their monograph these authors also give the foetal age, in weeks after fertilization, appropriate to each stage of molar development. This information was used to estimate the age of each foetus in the present study. Two weeks were added to the fertilization age given by Kraus and Jordan to make the estimated age comparable with the menstrual age derived from the clinical history. In the majority of cases, the age estimate was taken as the mean of the ages given for the four deciduous molars from one side of the dentition. Occasionally, if the age for a particular tooth stage was imprecise, e.g. 32+ weeks after fertilization at stage number 15 of the upper first deciduous molar, this was taken as 32 weeks if the age as assessed from the other three molars indicated 32 weeks or less. If the development of the other three molars indicated an age of more than 32 weeks, the age of the foetus was estimated from these three teeth

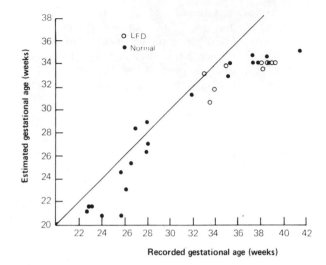

FIG. 3. Gestational age estimated from the data of Kraus and Jordan (1965) compared with clinically recorded age. The line is at $x = y$.

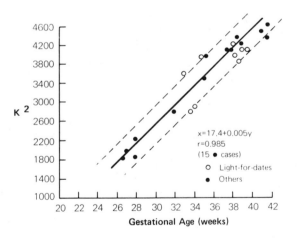

FIG. 4. Sum of Kraus stages of four deciduous molars from one side of the dentition (K) related to gestational age. Limits are at $2 \times$ s.d.

only. Cases in which two teeth were imprecisely aged from the Kraus and Jordan tables were omitted. Estimates of 30 cases made in this way were, on average, 2·5 weeks below the actual age (Fig. 3).

Because of the error in estimating foetal age by the direct use of the Kraus and Jordan data, an alternative method was devised. The sum (K) of the Kraus stage numbers of the four deciduous molars from one side of the dentition was related to clinically recorded gestational age using 15 normal-weight foetuses (Fig. 4). K was squared to improve the rectilinear relationship and a line fitted by the method of least squares. The equation to this line,

$$\text{Age (weeks)} = 17\cdot4 + 0\cdot005 \; K^2 \; (\text{s.d.} = 1)$$

can be used to estimate foetal age with a very good chance of the result being within 2 weeks of the actual age.

In order to compare the growth-retarded and normal-weight foetuses with respect to deciduous molar development, a group of nine normal foetuses was selected in such a way that the mean age of its members was similar to that of the LFD group (Table I). The mean sum of Kraus stages of the LFD

TABLE I. Developmental stages of molars in relation to gestational age.

LFD Foetuses		Normal Foetuses	
Foetal age (weeks)	Sum of Kraus stages	Foetal age (weeks)	Sum of Kraus stages
33·0	60	27·0	44
33·6	53	31·9	53
34·0	54	35·3	63
35 0	63	37·4	64
38·1	65	37·4	64
38·3	63	37·9	64
38·7	62	41·0	67
39·0	64	41·6	68
39·4	64	41·7	66
Mean 36·6	61	36·8	61

group was found to be the same as that of the normal-weight group, suggesting that growth-retarded foetuses are not retarded in this morphological aspect of their dental development. The accuracy of the K^2 regression equation given above, was tested by using it to estimate the age of each of the nine LFD and nine normal-weight foetuses shown in Table I.

GRAVIMETRIC METHOD OF ESTIMATING FOETAL AGE

Stack (1971) has given equations relating foetal age to dry weight of mineralized tooth tissue, based on the dentitions of 30 foetuses who failed to survive birth because of acute conditions. The equation in the case of the upper central deciduous incisor is: Age (weeks) = $2 \; (W^{\frac{1}{2}} + 19)$, where W is the weight (mg) of the tooth pair. For the upper lateral incisors, the appropriate terms are $2 \; (W^{\frac{1}{2}} + 23)$; for the lower centrals $2\cdot78 \; (W^{\frac{1}{2}} + 19)$; and for the lower laterals $2\cdot63 \; (W^{\frac{1}{2}} + 23)$. Using these equations, a mean estimate of foetal age was obtained from four (occasionally three) incisors from one

side of each dentition of the LFD and normal-weight foetuses shown in
Table I.

RESULTS

Clinically recorded ages were compared with estimates derived by using the
incisor-weight method and the K^2 regression equation (Fig. 5). Using the

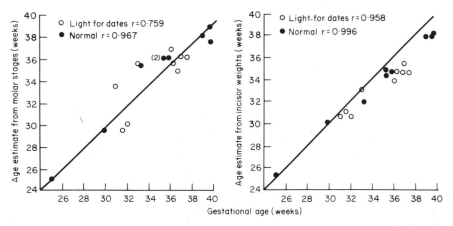

FIG. 5. Age estimated by the molar-stage method and by the incisor-weight method compared with clinically recorded gestational age. Lines are at $x = y$.

gravimetric method, the mean error was found to be 1·4 weeks for the LFD
foetuses and 1·0 week for the normal-weight group. When the molar-stage
method was used, mean errors for the two groups were, respectively, 1·7
weeks and 0·9 week. By means of the incisor-weight method, the ages of the
LFD group were underestimated to a greater extent than those of the normal
group, by an average of 0·5 week. This difference is only of marginal statistical
significance, suggesting that there is little retardation of this gravimetric
aspect of tooth development in growth-retarded foetuses.

Correlation coefficients were calculated between the two age estimates and
three other numerical observations: actual foetal age, CR length and body
weight (Table II). Ten correlations were thus produced for each of the two
groups of foetuses shown in Table I. All ten correlations for the LFD group
were below the corresponding correlations for the normal-weight group:
mean "r", using the z-transform, was 0·84 for the LFD group and 0·97 for
the normal group. The coefficient between actual foetal age and the age
estimated from incisor weight matches that for body weight and crown–
rump length in the LFD group and, in the normal group, is the highest of the
ten. Correlation coefficients between actual age and the age estimated by the
gravimetric method were higher than similar correlations for the molar-
stage method, especially for the LFD group. On the other hand, for both
LFD and normal-weight groups, correlation coefficients between actual

TABLE II. Correlations between recorded ages, estimated ages, body weights, and crown–rump lengths in light-for-dates foetuses (and normal foetuses, in brackets). Pearson product-moment coefficients "r".

	Body Weight	Crown–rump	Estimate (molars)	Estimate (incisors)
Foetal age	0·744 (0·973)	0·683 (0·945)	0·759 (0·967)	0·958 (0·996)
Body weight		0·960 (0·966)	0·830 (0·957)	0·813 (0·968)
Crown–rump			0·768 (0·964)	0·781 (0·943)
Estimate (molars)				0·812 (0·951)

foetal age and CR length were lower than those between foetal age and age estimated by either the molar-stage or incisor-weight method.

DISCUSSION

The tendency to underestimate foetal age by the direct use of the Kraus and Jordan data, may be explained as follows:

(a) The foetal specimens used by Kraus and Jordan and those used in the present study were derived from different populations and racial differences occur in the rate of foetal growth (Ounsted and Ounsted, 1973) and of dental development (Kraus and Jordan, 1965).

(b) Human foetal material, comprising infants who failed to survive birth, may contain a substantial proportion of specimens derived from pregnancies during which conditions of intra-uterine growth were less than optimal. If the Kraus and Jordan material included a relatively large proportion of such growth-retarded infants, age estimates based on CR length would tend to be less than the true age.

It is of interest that Gruenwald (1973), who used the data of Kraus and Jordan to estimate foetal age from mandibular molar development, also found that such estimates were less than the clinically recorded age by some 2–3 weeks.

The regression equation relating molar developmental stage to foetal age gives more satisfactory estimates of age between 24 and 42 weeks, than the Kraus and Jordan data. The line cannot, however, be extrapolated much below 24 weeks of gestational age. For example, the equation suggests that the earliest Kraus stage of molar development would occur at 17·4 weeks, whereas Kraus and Jordan give the age of this event as 14–14·5 weeks of gestation. The comparison of the molar-stage and incisor-weight methods of estimating foetal age demonstrates that although the mean error produced by each method is similar, correlation coefficients between actual and estimated age are higher in the case of the gravimetric method. The incisor-weight method is perhaps being more severely tested than the molar-stage method: the former was originally devised using a group of foetuses distinct from those of the present investigation, whereas the molar-stage method was partly based on the normal-weight foetuses which were later used to assess its accuracy.

Technically, it is probably easier to remove, at autopsy, the mineralized parts of deciduous incisors than to remove intact molar tooth germs, so that, from a practical viewpoint, the method of choice is that of Stack. In using this gravimetric method to estimate foetal age it is necessary to exclude cases which have suffered from those conditions which Stack (1963) has demonstrated may cause a reduction in the weight of mineralized tooth tissue. These include CNS defects, pre-eclamptic toxaemia and antepartum haemorrhage as well as other miscellaneous and multiple pathological conditions. A molar-stage method may be useful for estimating the age of an early foetus in which calcification has not begun or has not progressed very far, provided that data of Kraus and Jordan are first checked, using foetuses of known gestational age. Certainly, between 24–42 weeks of gestation, dental methods of estimating foetal age are more reliable than the use of CR length.

REFERENCES

DiORIO, L. P., MILLER, S. A. and NAVIA, J. M. (1973). The separate effects of protein and calorie malnutrition on the development and growth of rat bones and teeth. *J. Nutr.* **103**, 856–865.

GARN, S. M., LEWIS, A. B. and KEREWSKY, R. S. (1965). Genetic, nutritional and maturational correlates of dental development. *J. dent. Res.* **44**, 228–241.

GARN, S. M., BURDI, A. R., MILLER, R. L. and NAGY, J. M. (1970). Prenatal dental development as a reference standard for embryological status. *J. dent. Res.* **49**, 894.

GRUENWALD, P. (1973). Disturbed enamel formation in deciduous tooth germs. *Archs Path.* **95**, 165–171.

KRAUS, B. S. and JORDAN, R. E. (1965). "The Human Dentition Before Birth". Henry Kimpton, London.

OUNSTED, M. and OUNSTED, C. (1973). "On Fetal Growth Rate". Clinics in Developmental Medicine, No. 46, Heinemann, London.

STACK, M. V. (1963). Retardation of foetal dental growth in relation to pathology. *Archs Dis. Childh.* **38**, 443–446.

STACK, M. V. (1964). A gravimetric study of crown growth rate of the human deciduous dentition. *Biol. Neonat.* **6**, 197–224.

STACK, M. V. (1971). Relative rates of weight gain in human deciduous teeth. *In* "Dental Morphology and Evolution" (Dahlberg, A. A., ed.), pp. 59–62. University of Chicago Press, Illinois.

STREETER, G. L. (1921). Weight, sitting height, head size, foot length and menstrual age of the human embryo. *Contrib. Embryol.* **55**, 145–170.

THOMSON, A. M., BILLEWICZ, W. Z. and HYTTEN, F. E. (1968). The assessment of foetal growth. *J. Obstet. Gynaec. Br. Commonw.* **75**, 903–916.

TONGE, C. H. and McCANCE, R. A. (1973). Normal development of the jaws and teeth in pigs and the delay and malocclusion produced by calorie deficiencies. *J. Anat.* **115**, 1–22.

Index